Morphofunctional Nutritional Assessment in Clinical Practice

Morphofunctional Nutritional Assessment in Clinical Practice

Guest Editors

Daniel-Antonio de Luis Roman
Juan J. López-Gómez

MDPI • Basel • Beijing • Wuhan • Barcelona • Belgrade • Novi Sad • Cluj • Manchester

Guest Editors
Daniel-Antonio de Luis Roman
Center of Investigation of Endocrinology and Nutrition
Universidad de Valladolid
Valladolid
Spain

Juan J. López-Gómez
Center of Investigation of Endocrinology and Nutrition
Universidad de Valladolid
Valladolid
Spain

Editorial Office
MDPI AG
Grosspeteranlage 5
4052 Basel, Switzerland

This is a reprint of the Special Issue, published open access by the journal *Nutrients* (ISSN 2072-6643), freely accessible at: https://www.mdpi.com/journal/nutrients/special_issues/03JJMY36VN.

For citation purposes, cite each article independently as indicated on the article page online and as indicated below:

Lastname, A.A.; Lastname, B.B. Article Title. *Journal Name* **Year**, *Volume Number*, Page Range.

ISBN 978-3-7258-4595-8 (Hbk)
ISBN 978-3-7258-4596-5 (PDF)
https://doi.org/10.3390/books978-3-7258-4596-5

Contents

nutrients

MDPI

Editorial

Morphofunctional Nutritional Assessment in Clinical Practice: A New Approach to Assessing Nutritional Status

Daniel-Antonio de Luis Roman [1,2,*] and Juan José Lopez Gomez [1,2]

1 Servicio de Endocrinología y Nutrición, Hospital Clínico Universitario de Valladolid, 47003 Valladolid, Spain
2 Instituto de Endocrinología y Nutrición (IENVA), Universidad de Valladolid, 47003 Valladolid, Spain
* Correspondence: dluisro@saludcastillayleon.es

This Special Issue of *Nutrients* titled "Morphofunctional Nutritional Assessment in Clinical Practice" is oriented to the diagnosis of disease-related malnutrition (DRM). Disease-related malnutrition is a highly prevalent pathology which has become a great challenge to healthcare systems. This disease has a prevalence between 20 and 50% in hospitalized patients [1,2]. Malnutrition can be associated with other conditions such sarcopenia, defined as a loss of muscle mass and function. This disease was described as a primary condition associated with aging and frailty but the European Working Group on Sarcopenia in Older People (EWGSOP2) highlighted that secondary sarcopenia is associated with several diseases [3]. The adequate diagnosis of malnutrition and sarcopenia are based in tests to evaluate dietary intake, body composition, muscle strength and function, and biochemical parameters, which is called morphofunctional nutritional assessment [4]. However, the diagnosis of DRM is difficult because it does not depend only on body weight at a given time, but also on its evolution and the underlying pathological situations; thus, malnutrition is often underdiagnosed and undertreated [5], and is a serious health risk to patients. Therefore, the clinical use of body composition measurements is essential for the adequate assessment of this malnutrition, especially in the evaluation of muscle mass and function. In this context, nutritional assessment can no longer be based on classical anthropometric measurements. The concept of morphofunctional nutritional assessment postulates that the diagnosis and monitoring of nutritional status must be carried out using techniques and biomarkers that evaluate intake, anthropometry, body composition, muscle strength and function, which include techniques such as bioelectrical impedance analysis or nutritional ultrasound, and new biological parameters as well. This new diagnostic approach can help us to evaluate patients at risk of malnutrition and allow for the early diagnosis of DRM and personalized treatment for this condition.

Therefore, we are faced with a transition period in the area of nutritional assessment and there is no global consensus on the approach to DRM assessment. Many parameters have been used, such as body weight loss, body mass index, muscle mass, or dietary intake, which are included in most malnutrition screening tools [6], while other techniques, such as functional parameters, have gradually gained attention [7]. Nowadays, the criteria of DRM established by the Global Leadership Initiative on Malnutrition (GLIM) has enabled a more comprehensive nutritional assessment by including the evaluation of muscle mass, disease inflammation, and dietary intake [8]. The evaluation of body composition, especially muscle mass, is an important component of the diagnosis of malnutrition and sarcopenia, and it plays an essential role in monitoring the nutritional treatment of DRM. Nevertheless, the diagnosis of muscle quantity and quality is also difficult. Some techniques are not accurate such as anthropometric parameters or that use estimations based on bioimpedanciometry. Moreover, there are some tests like computerized tomography and magnetic resonance imaging that are considered gold standards but are more expensive, with potential side effects and are not feasible in routine clinical practice [9].

In this context, new easy and cheap techniques such as ultrasonography have demonstrated utility in morphofunctional evaluation. For example, parameters of the phase angle of BIA were correlated with muscle area through ultrasound, muscle echo intensity of the rectus femoris of the quadriceps, serum protein, quality of life SF-36, and strength physical performance [10]. Muscle ultrasound is a simple method to evaluate muscle mass in a consultation or at the bedside in hospitalized patients; it is an economic and non-invasive test and allows us to assess several muscular groups. These new approaches, including other techniques such as bioelectrical impedance analysis (BIA), dynamometry, or functional tests (for example, chair test, time up, and go test) to measure functionality could be included in usual clinical practice [7] in order to realize a holistic evaluation of the patient. It is also interesting to evaluate patients with structured nutritional tests that combine different parameters, such as the Mini Nutritional Assessment Short Form (MNA-SF) and the Subjective Global Assessment (SGA). The SGA and MNA-SF are considered adequate tools to diagnose malnutrition, with predictive value for mortality [11]. Finally, new biomarkers can help us in this morphofunctional assessment. For example, serum resistin levels [12] are associated with low skeletal muscle mass in obese women over 60 years of age and other potential molecules need attention in this area [13].

To summarize, it is necessary to implement this new concept of nutritional evaluation in the management of patients and in clinical research in nutrition. Thus, the implementation of these tools is recommended to improve diagnosis, treatments, and patient outcomes in the field of DRM [14].

Conflicts of Interest: The authors declare no conflict of interest.

References

1. Álvarez Hernández, J.M.P.V.; León-Sanz, M.; García de Lorenzo, A.; Celaya-Pérez, S.; García-Lorda, P.; Araujo, K.; Sarto Guerri, B.; on behalf of the PREDyCES®researches. Prevalencia y costed de la malnutrición en pacientes hospitalizados: Estudio PREDyCES®. *Nutr. Hosp.* **2012**, *16*, 1049–1059.
2. Merker, M.; Felder, M.; Gueissaz, L.; Bolliger, R.; Tribolet, P.; Kägi-Braun, N. Association of Baseline Inflammation with Effectiveness of Nutritional Support Among Patients with Disease-Related Malnutrition: A Secondary Analysis of a Randomized Clinical Trial. *JAMA Netw. Open* **2020**, *3*, e200663. [CrossRef] [PubMed]
3. Cruz-Jentoft, A.J.; Bahat, G.; Bauer, J.; Boirie, Y.; Bruyère, O.; Cederholm, T. Sarcopenia: Revised European consensus on definition and diagnosis. *Age Ageing* **2019**, *48*, 16–31. [CrossRef] [PubMed]
4. García-Almeida, J.M.; García-García, C.; Ballesteros-Pomar, M.D.; Olveira, G.; Lopez-Gomez, J.J.; Bellido, V. Expert Consensus on Morphofunctional Assessment in Disease-Related Malnutrition. *Grade Rev. Delphi. Study. Nutr.* **2023**, *15*, 612.
5. Fry, C.M.; Rame, S.; Hubbard, G.P.; Stratton, R.J. GP patient data bases show that malnutrition is under-reported and under-treated inpatients with chronic disease. *Clin. Nutr. ESPEN* **2017**, *22*, 120–121. [CrossRef]
6. Reber, E.; Gomes, F.; Vasiloglou, M.F.; Schuetz, P.; Stanga, Z. Nutritional Risk Screening and Assessment. *J. Clin. Med.* **2019**, *8*, 1065. [CrossRef] [PubMed]
7. García, C.G.; Almeida, J.M.G.; Aguilar, I.M.V.; Castañeda, V.B.; Guerrero, D.B. Morphofunctional assessment of patient nutritional status: A global approach. *Nutr. Hosp.* **2021**, *38*, 592–600. [CrossRef] [PubMed]
8. Cederholm, T.; Jensen, G.L.; Correia, M.I.T.D.; Gonzalez, M.C.; Fukushima, R.; Higashiguchi, T.; Baptista, G.; Barazzoni, R.; Blaauw, R.; Coats, A.J. GLIM criteria for the diagnosis of malnutrition—A consensus report from the global clinical nutrition community. *Clin. Nutr.* **2019**, *1*, 207–217.
9. Barazzoni, R.; Jensen, G.L.; Correia, M.I.; Gonzalez, M.C.; Higashiguchi, T.; Shi, H.P.; Bischoff, S.C.; Boirie, Y.; Carrasco, F.; Cruz-Jentoft, A.; et al. Guidance for assessment of the muscle mass phenotypic criterion for the Global Leadership Initiative on Malnutrition (GLIM) diagnosis of malnutrition. *Clin. Nutr.* **2022**, *41*, 1425–1433. [CrossRef] [PubMed]
10. Primo, D.; Izaola, O.; Gómez, J.J.L.; de Luis, D. Correlation of the Phase Angle with Muscle Ultrasound and Quality of Life in Obese Females. *Dis. Markers* **2022**, *9*, 7165126. [CrossRef] [PubMed]
11. Sánchez-Torralvo, F.J.; Pérez-Del-Río, V.; García-Olivares, M.; Porras, N.; Abuín-Fernández, J.; Bravo-Bardají, M.F.; García-de-Quevedo, D.; Olveira, G. Global Subjective Assessment and Mini Nutritional Assessment Short Form Better Predict Mortality Than GLIM Malnutrition Criteria in Elderly Patients with Hip Fracture. *Nutrients* **2023**, *15*, 1828. [CrossRef] [PubMed]
12. De Luis, D.; Primo, D.; Izaola, O.; Gómez Hoyos, E.; López Gómez, J.J. Relationship of circulating resistin levels with muscle mass determined by bioelectrical impedance in females with obesity. *Endocrinol. Diabetes Nutr. (Engl. Ed.)* **2023**, *70*, 468–475. [CrossRef] [PubMed]

13. Primo, D.; Izaola, O.; Gomez, J.J.L.; Luis, D. Anthropometric, muscle and serum myokine levels effects of physical exercise with an online platform in female patients with obesity. *Endocrinol. Diabetes Nutr. (Engl. Ed.)* **2023**, *70*, 484–491. [PubMed]
14. López-Gómez, J.J.; García-Beneitez, D.; Jiménez-Sahagún, R.; Izaola-Jauregui, O.; Primo-Martín, D.; Ramos-Bachiller, B.; Gómez-Hoyos, E.; Delgado-García, E.; Pérez-López, P.; Luis-Román, D.; et al. Nutritional Ultrasonography, a method to evaluate Muscle Mass and Quality in Morphofunctional Assessment of Disease Related Malnutrition. *Nutrients* **2023**, *15*, 3923. [CrossRef]

nutrients

MDPI

Article

Global Subjective Assessment and Mini Nutritional Assessment Short Form Better Predict Mortality Than GLIM Malnutrition Criteria in Elderly Patients with Hip Fracture

Francisco José Sánchez-Torralvo [1,2,3,*], Verónica Pérez-del-Río [3,4], María García-Olivares [1], Nuria Porras [1], Jose Abuín-Fernández [1], Manuel Francisco Bravo-Bardají [4], David García-de-Quevedo [4] and Gabriel Olveira [1,2,3,5]

1 Unidad de Gestión Clínica de Endocrinología y Nutrición, Hospital Regional Universitario de Málaga, 29007 Malaga, Spain
2 Instituto de Investigación Biomédica de Málaga (IBIMA), Plataforma Bionand, 29010 Malaga, Spain
3 Departamento de Medicina y Dermatología, Facultad de Medicina, University of Malaga, 29010 Malaga, Spain
4 Unidad de Gestión Clínica de Cirugía Ortopédica y Traumatología, Hospital Regional Universitario de Málaga, 29010 Malaga, Spain
5 Centro de Investigación Biomédica en Red de Diabetes y Enfermedades Metabólicas Asociadas (CIBERDEM), Instituto de Salud Carlos III, 28029 Madrid, Spain
* Correspondence: fransancheztorralvo@gmail.com

Abstract: The objective of our study is to determine the prevalence of malnutrition in elderly patients with fragility hip fractures through different diagnostic tools and to determine which nutritional assessment tool better predicts mortality. Methods: This is a prospective study in patients over 65 years of age hospitalized with a diagnosis of hip fracture. A nutritional assessment was performed using several tools: the Mini Nutritional Assessment Short Form (MNA-SF), the Subjective Global Assessment (SGA), and the GLIM criteria. For the definition of low muscle mass, four different methods were used: hand grip strength (HGS), calf circumference (CC), anthropometry, and bioelectrical impedance (BIA). Mortality was registered at three, six and twelve months. Results: 300 patients were included, 79.3% female, mean age 82.9 ± 7.1 years. The MNA-SF found 42% at risk of malnutrition, and 37.3% malnourished. Using SGA, there were 44% with moderate malnutrition, and 21.7% with severe malnutrition. In application of the GLIM criteria, 84.3%, 47%, 46%, and 72.7% of patients were malnourished when HGS, anthropometry, BIA, and CC were used, respectively. Mortality was 10%, 16.3% and 22% at 3, 6 and 12 months, respectively. In malnourished patients according to MNA-SF, mortality was 5.7 times greater [95%CI 1.3–25.4; $p = 0.022$] at 6 months and 3.8 times greater [95%CI 1.3–11.6; $p = 0.018$] at 12 months. In malnourished patients according to SGA, mortality was 3.6 times greater [95%CI 1.02–13.04; $p = 0.047$] at 3 months, 3.4 times greater [95%CI 1.3–8.6; $p = 0.012$] at 6 months and 3 times greater [95%CI 1.35–6.7; $p = 0.007$] at 12 months. Conclusion: The prevalence of malnutrition in patients admitted for fragility hip fracture is high. The SGA and MNA-SF are postulated as adequate tools to diagnose malnutrition in these patients, with predictive value for mortality at three, six, and twelve months.

Keywords: hip fracture; elderly; malnutrition; Mini Nutritional Assessment Short Form; Subjective Global Assessment; GLIM criteria

1. Introduction

Given the current aging of the population, there is an increasing incidence of osteoporosis. This has led to increased interest in the prevention and treatment of fragility fractures, which are those produced by low impact (such as a fall from a height corresponding to a standing position, mainly in the humerus, wrist, vertebrae, and hip) [1]. Specifically, hip fracture is the most important, due to its high risk of mortality and refracture, which also entails a large economic cost [2,3]. The global incidence of hip fracture stands at 1.7 million cases per year worldwide [4], of which around 620,000 are in Europe [5]. Since 2011, evidence has emerged of the usefulness of the existence of Fracture Coordination Units (UCF or FLS, Fracture Liaison Services), which focus their activity on the secondary prevention of fragility fractures [6]. These units evaluate in a multidisciplinary way various aspects of the process of secondary prevention of fractures [7] and application of its methods has shown a significant reduction of all-cause mortality [8].

In this context, the nutritional aspect of these patients is very important, since there is a positive association between the presence of malnutrition and the rate of hip fractures [9]. Current data shows great variability in the prevalence of malnutrition, probably due to the existence of non-standardized criteria. However, most of the existing literature refers to an approximate prevalence of 20–30% malnutrition and a 40–50% risk of malnutrition [9–14]. Other studies show higher figures [15]. Malnutrition relates to complications, lower functional recovery, and higher mortality. There is also an association between morbidity and mortality and nutritional status [9,12,16], although this association is not as established as it is with other pathologies closely related to malnutrition, such as oncological pathology [17]. A correct nutritional intervention in these patients can prevent complications [18] and, in addition, could reduce recovery times and mortality after the intervention [19,20].

The Global Leadership Initiative on Malnutrition (GLIM) criteria for malnutrition were introduced in 2018 [21], but to our knowledge few studies have included them in the assessment of the nutritional status of patients admitted for hip fracture [22,23]. Although some studies have explored the relationship between malnutrition and mortality in these patients [14,24,25], to date, we are not aware of studies that have used GLIM to verify the relationship between malnutrition and mortality, nor studies that compare the results of the application of different diagnostic tools for malnutrition.

Our hypothesis is that the prevalence of malnutrition in patients admitted for fragility hip fracture in the Trauma Unit could be high and be related to an increase in mortality.

The objective of our study is to determine the prevalence of malnutrition in elderly patients with fragility hip fracture through different diagnostic tools and to determine which nutritional assessment tool better predicts mortality at 3, 6, and 12 months.

2. Materials and Methods

This is a prospective study, in patients over 65 years of age hospitalized with a diagnosis of hip fracture in the Trauma Surgery Unit of the Regional Hospital of Malaga, between September 2019 and February 2021. Fracture type and the presence of a previous fracture were recorded. Medical comorbidities were measured by the Charlson Comorbidity Index (CCI) [26]. Pre-fracture functional status was assessed by means of the Barthel index [27] and the Functional Ambulation Category Scale (FAC) [28]. Analytical data for C-reactive protein and albumin were collected and the CRP/albumin ratio was calculated.

A nutritional assessment in the first 24–48 h after the intervention was performed. This assessment was carried out using several tools:

- the Mini Nutritional Assessment Short Form (MNA-SF) [29], replacing the body mass index (BMI) item with calf circumference (CC).
- the Subjective Global Assessment (SGA) [30], and
- the Global Leadership in Malnutrition (GLIM) criteria for diagnosis of malnutrition [21].

Height was calculated with a stadiometer (Holtain Limited, Crymych, UK) when possible and weight was calculated fasting with a scale set to 0.1 kg (SECA 665, Hamburg, Germany). When the determination of height and weight was not possible, data reported by the patient were used.

2.1. Malnutrition according to the GLIM Criteria

To diagnose malnutrition according to the GLIM criteria, at least one phenotypic criterion and one etiological criterion must be present [21]. All patients were considered to have at least one etiological criterion, due to the existence of an inflammatory response after having undergone surgery for a hip fracture in the previous days. This was confirmed by the CRP/albumin ratio.

The following phenotypic criteria were evaluated: unintentional weight loss (> 5% in 6 months), low BMI (for age < 70 years, a BMI $\geq$ 20 kg/m^2 was considered normal; for age $\geq$ 70, a BMI $\geq$ 22 kg/m^2 was established as normal), and/or reduction in muscle mass. For the definition of low muscle mass, four different methods were used: a low hand grip strength (represented by the fifth percentile population) [31], a low calf circumference (CC), or a low fat-free mass index (FFMI) according to ESPEN cut-off points [32], this being determined by anthropometry (triceps skinfold) and bioelectrical impedance (BIA).

BIA was performed with the Akern BIA-101/Nutrilab analyzer (Akern SRL, Pontassieve, 160 Florence, Italy). Measurements were taken in the supine position, with the upper (30°) and lower (45°) limbs abducted. Software (AKERN Bodygram Dashboard, Pontassieve, Florence, Italy) was used to determine the FFMI.

Measurement of the triceps skinfold was performed using a Holtain caliper (Holtain Limited). Measurements were taken in triplicate in the dominant arm and the mean was calculated. The percentages and kilograms of fat mass and fat-free mass (FFM) were estimated according to the Siri and Durnin and Womersley formulas [33,34]. For the FFMI, the cut-off points established by ESPEN were applied, considering low muscle mass for values <15 kg/m^2 in women and <17 kg/m^2 in men [32].

Calf circumference (CC) was measured using a non-elastic tape at the point of the greatest circumference. A low CC was defined using the cutoff points suggested in the GLIM criteria guidelines: 33 cm for men and 32 cm for women [35].

Hand grip strength was measured in the dominant hand with a Jamar dynamometer (Asimow Engineering Co., Los Angeles, CA, USA). The patients performed the test with the shoulder adducted and the forearm in neutral rotation, the elbow flexed to 90°, and the forearm and wrist in a neutral position. Patients were asked to perform three consecutive contractions one minute apart, and the mean value was calculated. Results were expressed in absolute terms, and scores below the fifth percentile of the population were considered to have low hand grip strength. [31].

2.2. Follow-Up

After discharge, a telematic follow-up was carried out (through a review of the clinical history) of the evolution of the patients, recording mortality at three, six and twelve months.

2.3. Statistical Analysis

Quantitative variables were expressed as mean $\pm$ standard deviation. The relationship between malnutrition diagnosis using different tools and mortality was estimated using the chi-square test, with Fisher's correction when necessary. For the concordance between diagnostic techniques, the kappa coefficient was used. The variables that showed an association with mortality in the chi-square test were included in a multivariate logistic regression model to assess the association between mortality and malnutrition, controlling for confounding variables such as sex, age and Charlson Comorbidity Index. For calculations, significance was set at $p < 0.05$ for two tails. Data analysis was performed using the SPSS 26.0 program (SPSS Inc., Chicago, IL, USA).

3. Results

A total of 300 patients were included (Figure 1), 62 men (20.7%) and 238 women (79.3%), with a mean age of 82.9 $\pm$ 7.1 years. The estimated mean BMI was 25.8 $\pm$ 5.1 kg/m^2.

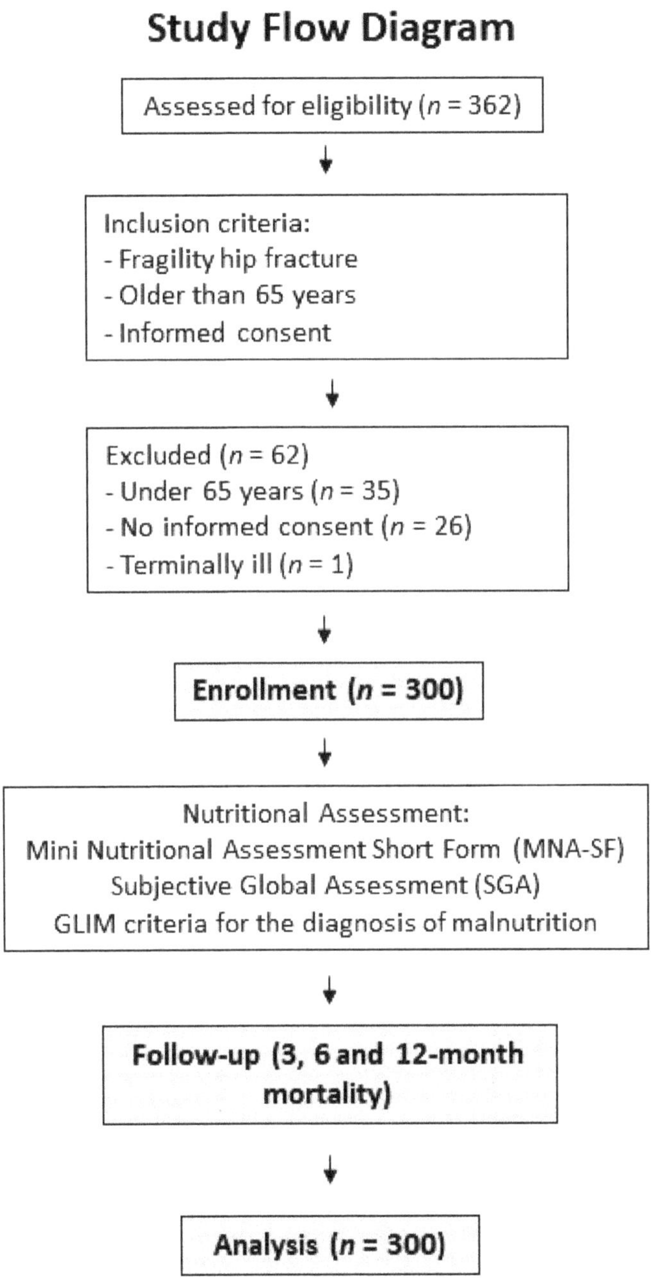

Figure 1. Study flow diagram and research methodology.

The general characteristics of the sample are shown in Table 1.

The mean triceps skinfold was 11.9 ± 4 mm for men, giving an FFMI by anthropometry of 19.4 ± 8.6 kg/m^2 (25.8% below 17 kg/m^2). In women, the mean triceps skinfold was 15.7 ± 6.1 mm, determining an FFMI of 17.4 ± 2.9 kg/m^2 (19.7% below 15 kg/m^2).

Table 1. General features.

		n = 300
Age (years)	mean ± SD	82.9 ± 7.1
Sex	n (%)	
Men		62 (20.7)
Women		238 (79.3)
Charlson Comorbidity Index	mean ± SD	5.67 ± 1.91
Barthel Index	mean ± SD	73.71 ± 27.72
Functional Ambulation Category Scale	n (%)	
0		78 (26.1)
1,2,3		206 (68.6)
4,5		16 (5.3)
Type of fracture	n (%)	
Pertrochanteric		135 (45)
Sub-capital		131 (43.7)
Sub-tronchanteric		18 (6)
Basi-cervical		15 (5)
Transcervical		1 (0.3)
Previous fracture	n (%)	34 (11.3)
C-reactive protein (CRP) (mg/l)	mean ± SD	115.4 ± 56.5
Albumin (g/dL)	mean ± SD	2.5 ± 0.4
CRP/Albumin ratio	mean ± SD	47.1 ± 25.5
Length of stay	mean ± SD	8.1 ± 5.4
3-month exitus	n (%)	30 (10)
6-month exitus	n (%)	49 (16.3)
12-month exitus	n (%)	66 (22)

Abbreviations: BMI = Body Mass Index; m = mean; SD = Standard Deviation.

The mean calf circumference was 32.4 ± 2.8 cm in men (54.8% below 33 cm) and 30.7 ± 3.8 cm in women (67.2% below 32 cm).

The FFMI by BIA was 20.9 ± 9.6 kg/m^2 for men (8.7% below 17 kg/m^2) and 17.5 ± 2.1 kg/m^2 for women (9.1% below 15 kg/m^2).

HGS showed a mean of 19.7 ± 9.7 kg for men (69.4% below the p5 population percentile) and 7.7 ± 6.4 kg for women (72.3% below the population percentile p5). Body composition parameters are shown in Table 2.

Regarding the prevalence of malnutrition (Figure 2), the MNA-SF found 20.7% normally nourished, 42% at risk of malnutrition, and 37.3% malnourished. Using SGA, 34.3% were found to be normally nourished, 44% with moderate malnutrition, and 21.7% with severe malnutrition (kappa coefficient of 0.53 with MNA-SF; $p < 0.001$).

In application of the GLIM criteria, 68 patients (22.7%) presented a low BMI and 113 (37.7%) a loss of more than 5% of body weight in the previous months. Considering the previous phenotypic criteria and using HGS as a determinant of muscle mass, we found 84.3% of patients undernourished; 47% when anthropometry was used, 46% when BIA was used, and 72.7% when CC was used (kappa coefficient of 0.39, 0.37, 0.41, 0.37 and with SGA respectively; $p < 0.001$). We found good agreement between GLIM with anthropometry and GLIM with anthropometry (kappa coefficient of 0.94; $p < 0.001$).

During follow-up, a total of 30 patients (10%) died in the first 3 months after the intervention, 49 patients (16.3%) at 6 months, and 66 patients (22%) at 12 months.

Table 3 shows the results of the analysis that relates 3-, 6- and 12-months mortality to the diagnosis of malnutrition according to the various nutritional assessment tools.

An association was found between age and the Charlson Comorbidity Index, and mortality at 3, 6, and 12 months ($p < 0.001$ at all times). For this reason, these variables were included in the logistic regression adjustment.

Malnutrition according to GLIM using HGS was not included in the regression, since the absence of positive events in the few normally nourished patients prevented a correct risk analysis. Table 4 shows the relationship between mortality at 3, 6 and 12 months, and the diagnosis of malnutrition using SGA and MNA SF, adjusted for age, sex and Charlson Comorbidity Index.

Table 2. Body composition parameters.

		n = 300
BMI (kg/m^2)	mean ± SD	
Men		25.9 ± 3.5
Women		25.8 ± 5.4
Triceps skinfold (mm)	mean ± SD	
Men		11.9 ± 4
Women		15.7 ± 6.1
Calf circumference (cm)	mean ± SD	
Men		32.4 ± 2.8
Women		30.7 ± 3.8
Fat-free mass (anthropometry) (kg)	mean ± SD	
Men		53.4 ± 8.3
Women		42.8 ± 7.3
FFMI (anthropometry) (kg/m^2)	mean ± SD	
Men		19.4 ± 8.6
Women		17.5 ± 2.1
Phase angle (°)	mean ± SD	
Men		5.18 ± 1.13
Women		4.5 ± 0.94
Fat-free mass (BIA) (kg)	mean ± SD	
Men		57.6 ± 7.8
Women		42.9 ± 5.4
FFMI (BIA) (kg/m^2)	mean ± SD	
Men		20.9 ± 9.6
Women		15.4 ± 1.5
Handgrip strength (kg)	mean ± SD	
Men		19.7 ± 9.7
Women		7.7 ± 6.4

BMI: body mass index; SD: standard deviation; FFMI: fat-free mass index; BIA: Bioelectrical impedance analysis.

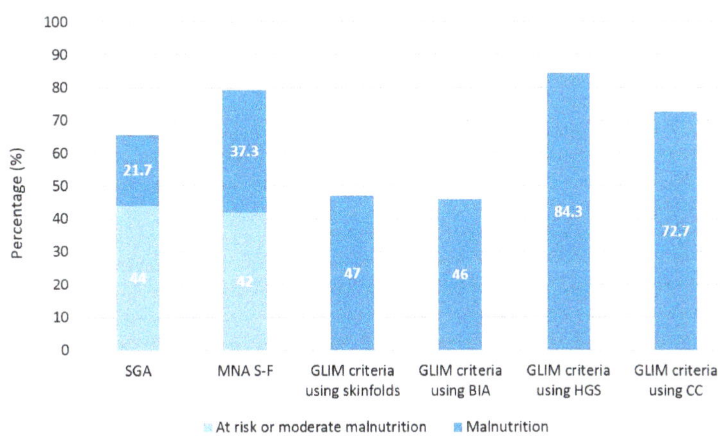

Figure 2. Malnutrition diagnosis according to the tool used. SGA: Subjective Global Assessment; MNA S-F: Mini Nutritional Assessment Short Form; GLIM: Global Leadership on Malnutrition; BIA: Bioelectrical impedance analysis; HGS: Handgrip Strength; CC: calf circumference.

Table 3. Relationship between malnutrition and mortality.

	3-Month Mortality			6-Month Mortality			12-Month Mortality		
	Malnourished	Normo-Nourished	*p* Value	Malnourished	Normo-Nourished	*p* Value	Malnourished	Normo-Nourished	*p* Value
Malnutrition according to SGA	23 (13.7%)	3 (2.9%)	0.002	43 (21.8%)	6 (5.8%)	<0.001	57 (29.9%)	9 (8.7%)	<0.001
Malnutrition according to MNA-SF	29 (12.2%)	1 (1.6%)	0.006	47 (19.7%)	2 (3.2%)	0.001	62 (26%)	4 (6.5%)	<0.001
Malnutrition according to GLIM using skinfolds	13 (9.2%)	17 (10.7%)	0.41	27 (19.1%)	22 (13.8%)	0.139	35 (24.8%)	31 (19.5%)	0.166
Malnutrition according to GLIM using BIA	11 (8.3%)	13 (7.7%)	0.527	26 (19%)	18 (11.3%)	0.056	32 (24.8%)	26 (16.2%)	0.057
Malnutrition according to GLIM using HGS	30 (11.8%)	0 (0%)	0.005	49 (19.4%)	0 (0%)	<0.001	65 (25.7%)	1 (2.1%)	<0.001
Malnutrition according to GLIM using CC	23 (10.6%)	7 (8.5%)	0.391	39 (17.9%)	10 (12.2%)	0.155	53 (24.3%)	13 (15.9%)	0.076

SGA: Subjective Global Assessment; MNA SF: Mini Nutritional Assessment Short Form; GLIM: Global Leadership on Malnutrition; BIA: Bioelectrical impedance analysis; HGS: Handgrip Strength; CC: calf circumference.

Table 4. Relationship between mortality and malnutrition according to SGA and MNA SF, adjusted for age, sex and Charlson Comorbidity Index.

	Crude				Adjusted			
	Odds Ratio	95% CI		*p* Value	Odds Ratio	95% CI		*p* Value
		Lower	Upper			Lower	Upper	
Malnutrition according to SGA								
3-month mortality	5.29	1.57	17.89	0.007	3.64	1.02	13.04	0.047
6-month mortality	4.51	1.85	11	0.001	3.35	1.31	8.58	0.012
12-month mortality	4.25	2	9	<0.001	3.02	1.35	6.72	0.007
Malnutrition according to MNA-SF								
3-month mortality	8.46	1.13	63.41	0.038	6.36	0.79	51.06	0.082
6-month mortality	7.38	1.74	31.29	0.007	5.71	1.28	25.36	0.022
12-month mortality	5.11	1.78	14.65	0.002	3.81	1.25	11.57	0.018

SGA: Subjective Global Assessment; MNA SF: Mini Nutritional Assessment Short Form; CI: Confidence interval.

4. Discussion

In our study, the prevalence of malnutrition in elderly patients operated on for fragility hip fracture is high, hovering between 45 and 85% depending on the nutritional assessment tool used. These figures agree with those previously presented by other authors [9–13,15,20].

Previously, the most commonly used diagnostic tool for the diagnosis of malnutrition has been the MNA-SF [9,11–13,15,20,25]. The use of MNA-SF as a tool for diagnosing malnutrition is supported by its ease of application and reproducibility, without the need for biochemical determinations. Although the "Short Form" version was designed as a screening test, it can also be used for nutritional assessment [29]. Its use is widespread in the geriatric population. In our work, we used calf circumference instead of BMI, since the exact weight could not be available in some cases. As an alternative to the MNA-SF, the use of SGA in the nutritional assessment of hospitalized patients is justified since it is a valid, sensitive tool with prognostic value and adequate concordance with other tools [36,37].

In our sample, mortality at 3, 6 and 12 months presented a risk up to 3–4 times higher in patients who were malnourished according to SGA than those who were normo-nourished. These data are consistent with those of the study of Miu et al., in which hospital mortality was higher in malnourished individuals compared to patients at risk of malnutrition and normally nourished patients, presenting this trend also at 6 months, although without reaching statistical significance [9]. The authors postulated that there could be certain limitations in the MNA for mortality prediction, such as the use of BMI or the absence of analytical parameters. This, however, differs from our results, in which malnourished patients according to MNA-SF presented a risk of mortality between 3 and 6 times higher than normally nourished patients. In this case, the different results could be justified by our decision to use the CC instead of the BMI when applying the MNA-SF.

Hand grip strength is a technique that correlates very well with lean mass and is an inexpensive tool that is easy to reproduce [31]. The prevalence of low hand grip strength values is very high in our sample, something that was described in similar populations, reaching over 90% [10,38]. In previous studies carried out on patients admitted to our hospital, we already found a high prevalence of low hand grip strength [38]. In the present study, patients with a recent hip intervention were included, so that in most of the cases, greater difficulty in sitting could determine lower values. A poor technique could have implied an artificially high prevalence of low hand grip strength, which could lead to an overestimation of malnourished patients when applying the GLIM criteria, something that has had a direct impact on the estimation of its association with mortality in the statistical analyses of our study. For this reason, HGS does not seem to be a reliable tool for these patients.

In recent years, the use of bioelectrical impedance analysis in nutritional assessment has spread. Some authors have included BIA in the assessment of elderly patients operated on for a hip fracture [10,22,38], including muscle mass parameters, such as the musculoskeletal index (SMI), although presenting disparate data. In our study, the FFMI was used as a determinant of muscle mass, presenting low values in 8–9% of the patients, which could be interpreted as an overestimation of muscle mass by the BIA. Nevertheless, a recent study has investigated the use of the GLIM criteria for malnutrition in patients with hip fractures, using BIA as determinant of muscle mass, determining that is useful for predicting gait ability at discharge during acute hospitalization [22].

The use of calf circumference in patients with hip fracture is common in estimating muscle mass [9,23]. In a recent study, CC was found to be a valuable tool in predicting sarcopenia risk compared with other screening tools [39]. Our study determined a low CC according to the cut-off points recommended in the GLIM criteria guidelines (33 cm for men and 32 cm for women) while, for applying the MNA-SF, a single cut-off point is used at 31 cm. With a lower cut-off point, the MNA-SF detected a lower percentage of patients with low muscle mass, but both the prevalence of malnutrition and the relationship with mortality were higher than when applying the GLIM criteria, possibly due to the use of other subjective parameters.

To date, only two studies have applied the GLIM criteria for the diagnosis of malnutrition in patients with fragility hip fractures [22,23]. In a retrospective Swedish study [23], phenotypic criteria were assessed, using calf circumference as a determinant of muscle mass, although the prevalence of malnutrition was not detailed. On the other hand, the study by Kobayashi et al. used the BIA as a determinant of muscle mass and found a prevalence of malnutrition of 73.9%. The fundamental difference to our study was the use of the skeletal muscle mass index (SMI) instead of the FFMI. In addition, mortality was not studied and non-weight bearing patients were excluded [22].

Although the prevalence of malnutrition determined using anthropometry and BIA in the application of the GLIM criteria was similar in our sample (good concordance), the low predictive value of mortality could place the use of the GLIM criteria one step below SGA and MNA-SF in this group of patients.

On the other hand, although the use of hand grip strength in the application of the GLIM criteria could have a good prognostic value for mortality according to our results [37], the great discrepancy found in the results, motivated by its difficulty in performance after a hip intervention, makes its use as a determinant of muscle mass in this case not recommended.

It is worth noting the greater concordance found in our study between SGA and MNA S-F than between SGA and the GLIM criteria, regardless of the technique used to measure muscle mass. This may be due to the fact that the GLIM criteria use BMI as one of sources of the phenotypic data, and in the case of our patients, this data was in most cases reported verbally. On the other hand, the difficulty in measuring muscle mass with the techniques used could also have led to a greater disparity in the estimation of the prevalence of malnutrition.

Based on other previously published studies [9–13,18,19,40], the implementation of a generalized nutritional screening for those patients with fragility hip fractures could reduce the incidence of refractures in the case of carrying out an appropriate nutritional intervention, as well as a possible reduction in the average stay and in complications. In our study, we have not evaluated a nutritional intervention, but our results indicate that the application of a systematic nutritional screening and assessment protocol to all those patients admitted for hip fragility fracture could be useful for the early detection of subjects at risk or malnourished.

Our study has several strengths. It is a prospective study with a large number of subjects and medium-term follow-up. In addition, it uses simple techniques for the measurement and definition of muscle mass loss and the presence of malnutrition, something that can be useful when other methods are not available.

In turn, there are several potential limitations. This is a single-center observational study, so the results need to be interpreted in the appropriate population context, particularly in populations with different surgical approaches to hip fracture, and no causal relationships can be established. On the other hand, patients underwent hip surgery in the hours before the assessment, so the results of some diagnostic techniques, such as hand grip strength and BIA, could be affected. In most cases, patients' height and weight were reported verbally due to their inability to stand. This can affect the calculations of techniques such as BIA. For this reason, we recommend using calf circumference instead of BMI when using the MNA-SF if weight and height cannot be measured correctly.

5. Conclusions

In conclusion, the prevalence of malnutrition in elderly patients admitted for fragility hip fracture is high. The SGA and MNA-SF are postulated as adequate tools for the diagnosis of malnutrition, with predictive value for mortality at 3, 6 and 12 months in elderly patients operated on for fragility hip fracture. Further studies are needed to analyze the role of the GLIM criteria in diagnosing malnutrition in these patients.

Author Contributions: Conceptualization, F.J.S.-T., V.P.-d.-R., J.A.-F. and G.O.; methodology, J.A.-F., N.P. and G.O.; formal analysis, F.J.S.-T.; investigation, V.P.-d.-R., N.P., M.G.-O., J.A.-F. and M.F.B.-B.; resources, V.P.-d.-R. and M.F.B.-B.; data curation, F.J.S.-T., N.P. and M.G.-O.; writing—original draft preparation, F.J.S.-T.; writing—review and editing, V.P.-d.-R. and G.O.; supervision, D.G.-d.-Q. and G.O.; project administration, D.G.-d.-Q. and G.O.; funding acquisition, G.O. All authors have read and agreed to the published version of the manuscript.

Funding: This study was partially funded by an unrestricted grant from Abbott Laboratories (Spain).

Institutional Review Board Statement: The study was conducted in accordance with the Declaration of Helsinki and approved by Re-search Ethics Committee of Malaga on 30 March 2021.

Informed Consent Statement: Informed consent was obtained from all subjects involved in the study.

Data Availability Statement: Not applicable.

Acknowledgments: The authors would like to thank all those who participated in this study for their willingness to cooperate.

Conflicts of Interest: The funders had no role in the design of the study; in the collection, analyses, or interpretation of data; in the writing of the manuscript; or in the decision to publish the results.

References

1. Tebé, C.; del Río, L.M.; Casas, L.; Estrada, M.D.; Kotzeva, A.; Di Gregorio, S.; Espallargues, M. Factores de riesgo de fracturas por fragilidad en una cohorte de mujeres españolas. *Gac. Sanit.* **2011**, *25*, 507–512. [CrossRef] [PubMed]
2. Rizzoli, R.; Biver, E.; Bonjour, J.P.; Coxam, V.; Goltzman, D.; Kanis, J.A.; Lappe, J.; Rejnmark, L.; Sahni, S.; Weaver, C.; et al. Benefits and safety of dietary protein for bone health—An expert consensus paper endorsed by the European Society for Clinical and Economical Aspects of Osteopororosis, Osteoarthritis, and Musculoskeletal Diseases and by the International Osteoporosis Foundation. *Osteoporos. Int.* **2018**, *29*, 1933–1948. [CrossRef] [PubMed]
3. Nikkel, L.E.; Fox, E.J.; Black, K.P.; Davis, C.; Andersen, L.; Hollenbeak, C.S. Impact of Comorbidities on Hospitalization Costs Following Hip Fracture. *J. Bone Jt. Surg.-Am. Vol.* **2012**, *94*, 9–17. [CrossRef] [PubMed]
4. Cummings, S.R.; Melton, L.J. Epidemiology and outcomes of osteoporotic fractures. *Lancet* **2002**, *359*, 1761–1767. [CrossRef]
5. Kanis, J.A.; Cooper, C.; Rizzoli, R.; Reginster, J.Y. European guidance for the diagnosis and management of osteoporosis in postmenopausal women. *Osteoporos. Int.* **2018**, *30*, 3–44. [CrossRef]
6. Eisman, J.A.; Bogoch, E.R.; Dell, R.; Harrington, J.T.; McKinney, R.E., Jr.; McLellan, A.; Mitchell, P.J.; Silverman, S.; Singleton, R.; Siris, E.; et al. Making the first fracture the last fracture: ASBMR task force report on secondary fracture prevention. *J. Bone Miner. Res.* **2012**, *27*, 2039–2046. [CrossRef]
7. Wu, C.H.; Tu, S.T.; Chang, Y.F.; Chan, D.C.; Chien, J.T.; Lin, C.H.; Singh, S.; Dasari, M.; Chen, J.F.; Tsai, K.S. Fracture liaison services improve outcomes of patients with osteoporosis-related fractures: A systematic literature review and meta-analysis. *Bone* **2018**, *111*, 92–100. [CrossRef]
8. González-Quevedo, D.; Pérez-Del-Río, V.; Moriel-Garceso, D.; Fernández-Arroyabe, N.; García-Meléndez, G.; Montañez-Ruiz, M.; Bravo-Bardají, M.; García-de-Quevedo, D.; Tamimi, I. A 2-year follow-up of a novel Fracture Liaison Service: Can we reduce the mortality in elderly hip fracture patients? A prospective cohort study. *Osteoporos. Int.* **2022**, *33*, 1695–1702. [CrossRef]
9. Miu, K.Y.D.; Lam, P.S. Effects of Nutritional Status on 6-Month Outcome of Hip Fractures in Elderly Patients. *Ann. Rehabil. Med.* **2017**, *41*, 1005–1012. [CrossRef]
10. Díaz de Bustamante, M.; Alarcón, T.; Menéndez-Colino, R.; Ramírez-Martín, R.; Otero, Á.; González-Montalvo, J.I. Prevalence of malnutrition in a cohort of 509 patients with acute hip fracture: The importance of a comprehensive assessment. *Eur. J. Clin. Nutr.* **2018**, *72*, 77–81. [CrossRef]
11. Olofsson, B.; Stenvall, M.; Lundström, M.; Svensson, O.; Gustafson, Y. Malnutrition in hip fracture patients: An intervention study. *J. Clin. Nurs.* **2007**, *16*, 2027–2038. [CrossRef] [PubMed]
12. Malafarina, V.; Reginster, J.Y.; Cabrerizo, S.; Bruyère, O.; Kanis, J.A.; Martinez, J.A.; Zulet, M.A. Nutritional Status and Nutritional Treatment Are Related to Outcomes and Mortality in Older Adults with Hip Fracture. *Nutrients* **2018**, *10*, 555. [CrossRef] [PubMed]
13. Pérez Durillo, F.T.; Ruiz López, M.D.; Bouzas, P.R.; Martín-Lagos, A. Nutritional status in elderly patients with a hip fracture. *Nutr. Hosp.* **2010**, *25*, 676–681. [PubMed]
14. Feng, L.; Chen, W.; Ping, P.; Ma, T.; Li, Y.; Xu, L.; Feng, Z.; Zhao, Y.; Fu, S. Preoperative malnutrition as an independent risk factor for the postoperative mortality in elderly Chinese individuals undergoing hip surgery: A single-center observational study. *Ther. Adv. Chronic Dis.* **2022**, *13*, 20406223221102739. [CrossRef]
15. Inoue, T.; Misu, S.; Tanaka, T.; Sakamoto, H.; Iwata, K.; Chuman, Y.; Ono, R. Pre-fracture nutritional status is predictive of functional status at discharge during the acute phase with hip fracture patients: A multicenter prospective cohort study. *Clin. Nutr.* **2017**, *36*, 1320–1325. [CrossRef]

16. Inoue, T.; Maeda, K.; Nagano, A.; Shimizu, A.; Ueshima, J.; Murotani, K.; Sato, K.; Tsubaki, A. Undernutrition, Sarcopenia, and Frailty in Fragility Hip Fracture: Advanced Strategies for Improving Clinical Outcomes. *Nutrients* **2020**, *12*, 3743. [CrossRef]
17. Muscaritoli, M.; Arends, J.; Bachmann, P.; Baracos, V.; Barthelemy, N.; Bertz, H.; Bozzetti, F.; Hütterer, E.; Isenring, E.; Kaasa, S.; et al. ESPEN Guideline ESPEN practical guideline: Clinical Nutrition in cancer. *Clin. Nutr.* **2021**, *40*, 2898–2913. [CrossRef]
18. Avenell, A.; Smith, T.O.; Curtain, J.P.; Mak, J.C.; Myint, P.K. Nutritional supplementation for hip fracture aftercare in older people. *Cochrane Database Syst Rev.* **2016**, *11*, CD001880. [CrossRef]
19. Bastow, M.D.; Rawlings, J.; Allison, S.P. Benefits of supplementary tube feeding after fractured neck of femur: A randomised controlled trial. *Br. Med. J. (Clin. Res. Ed.)* **1983**, *287*, 1589–1592. [CrossRef]
20. Wyers, C.E.; Reijven, P.L.; Breedveld-Peters, J.J.; Denissen, K.F.; Schotanus, M.G.; van Dongen, M.C.; Eussen, S.J.; Heyligers, I.C.; van den Brandt, P.A.; Willems, P.C.; et al. Efficacy of Nutritional Intervention in Elderly After Hip Fracture: A Multicenter Randomized Controlled Trial. *J. Gerontol. A Biol. Sci. Med. Sci.* **2018**, *73*, 1429–1437. [CrossRef]
21. Cederholm, T.; Jensen, G.L.; Correia, M.I.T.D.; Gonzalez, M.C.; Fukushima, R.; Higashiguchi, T.; Baptista, G.; Barazzoni, R.; Blaauw, R.; Coats, A.J.S.; et al. GLIM criteria for the diagnosis of malnutrition—A consensus report from the global clinical nutrition community. *J. Cachexia Sarcopenia Muscle* **2019**, *10*, 207–217. [CrossRef] [PubMed]
22. Kobayashi, H.; Inoue, T.; Ogawa, M.; Abe, T.; Tanaka, T.; Kakiuchi, M. Malnutrition diagnosed by the Global Leadership Initiative on Malnutrition criteria as a predictor of gait ability in patients with hip fracture. *Injury* **2022**, *53*, 3394–3400. [CrossRef] [PubMed]
23. Probert, N.; Lööw, A.; Akner, G.; Wretenberg, P.; Andersson, G. A Comparison of Patients with Hip Fracture, Ten Years Apart: Morbidity, Malnutrition and Sarcopenia. *J. Nutr. Health Aging* **2020**, *24*, 870–877. [CrossRef]
24. Millrose, M.; Schmidt, W.; Krickl, J.; Ittermann, T.; Ruether, J.; Bail, H.J.; Gesslein, M. Influence of Malnutrition on Outcome after Hip Fractures in Older Patients. *J. Pers. Med.* **2023**, *13*, 109. [CrossRef] [PubMed]
25. Chavarro-Carvajal, D.A.; Dueñas-Orejuela, M.F.; Aruachan-Torres, S.A.; Caicedo Correa, S.M.; Segura Valencia, A.I.; Cano-Gutierrez, C.A. Mortalidad al año y factores asociados en pacientes llevados a cirugía por fractura de cadera. *Rev. Esp. Cir. Ortop. Traumatol.* 2022; *in press*. [CrossRef]
26. Charlson, M.E.; Pompei, P.; Ales, K.L.; MacKenzie, C.R. A new method of classifying prognostic comorbidity in longitudinal studies: Development and validation. *J. Chronic. Dis.* **1987**, *40*, 373–383. [CrossRef] [PubMed]
27. Mahoney, F.I.; Barthel, D. Functional Evaluation: The Barthel Index. *Md. State Med. J.* **1965**, *14*, 61–65.
28. Holden, M.; Gill, K.; Magliozzi, M.; Nathan, J.; Piehl-Baker, L. Clinical gait assessment in the neurologically impaired. Reliability and meaningfulness. *Phys. Ther.* **1984**, *64*, 35–40. [CrossRef] [PubMed]
29. Kaiser, M.J.; Bauer, J.M.; Ramsch, C.; Uter, W.; Guigoz, Y.; Cederholm, T.; Thomas, D.R.; Anthony, P.; Charlton, K.E.; Maggio, M.; et al. Validation of the Mini Nutritional Assessment short-form (MNA-SF): A practical tool for identification of nutritional status. *J. Nutr. Health Aging* **2009**, *13*, 782–788. [CrossRef]
30. Detsky, A.S.; Baker, J.P.; Johnston, N.; Whittaker, S.; Mendelson, R.A.; Jeejeebhoy, K.N. What is subjective global assessment of nutritional status? *J. Parenter. Enter. Nutr.* **1987**, *11*, 8–13. [CrossRef]
31. Torralvo, F.J.S.; Porras, N.; Fernández, J.A.; Torres, F.G.; Tapia, M.J.; Lima, F.; Soriguer, F.; Gonzalo, M.; Martínez, G.R.; Olveira, G. Normative reference values for hand grip dynamometry in Spain. Association with lean mass. *Nutr. Hosp.* **2018**, *35*, 98–103.
32. Cederholm, T.; Bosaeus, I.; Barazzoni, R.; Bauer, J.; Van Gossum, A.; Klek, S.; Muscaritoli, M.; Nyulasi, I.; Ockenga, J.; Schneider, S.M.; et al. Diagnostic criteria for malnutrition—An ESPEN Consensus Statement. *Clin. Nutr.* **2015**, *34*, 335–340. [CrossRef] [PubMed]
33. Siri, W.E. Body composition from fluid spaces and density: Analysis of methods. *Nutrition* **1961**, *9*, 480–491; discussion 480, 492.
34. Durnin, J.V.; Womersley, J. Body fat assessed from total body density and its estimation from skinfold thickness: Measurements on 481 men and women aged from 16 to 72 years. *Br. J. Nutr.* **1974**, *32*, 77–97. [CrossRef] [PubMed]
35. Barazzoni, R.; Jensen, G.L.; Correia, M.I.T.; Gonzalez, M.C.; Higashiguchi, T.; Shi, H.P.; Bischoff, S.C.; Boirie, Y.; Carrasco, F.; Cruz-Jentoft, A.; et al. Guidance for assessment of the muscle mass phenotypic criterion for the Global Leadership Initiative on Malnutrition (GLIM) diagnosis of malnutrition. *Clin. Nutr.* **2022**, *41*, 1425–1433. [CrossRef] [PubMed]
36. Olveira, G.; Tapia, M.J.; Ocón, J.; Cabrejas-Gómez, C.; Ballesteros-Pomar, M.D.; Vidal-Casariego, A.; Arraiza-Irigoyen, C.; Olivares, J.; Conde-García, M.C.; García-Manzanares, Á.; et al. The subjective global assessment predicts in-hospital mortality better than other nutrition-related risk indexes in noncritically ill inpatients who receive total parenteral nutrition in Spain (prospective multicenter study). *J. Acad. Nutr. Diet.* **2013**, *113*, 1209–1218. [CrossRef] [PubMed]
37. Contreras-Bolívar, V.; Sánchez-Torralvo, F.J.; Ruiz-Vico, M.; González-Almendros, I.; Barrios, M.; Padín, S.; Alba, E.; Olveira, G. Glim criteria using hand grip strength adequately predict six-month mortality in cancer inpatients. *Nutrients* **2019**, *11*, 2043. [CrossRef]
38. Malafarina, V.; Malafarina, C.; Ugarte, A.B.; Martinez, J.A.; Goñi, I.A.; Zulet, M.A. Factors Associated with Sarcopenia and 7-Year Mortality in Very Old Patients with Hip Fracture Admitted to Rehabilitation Units: A Pragmatic Study. *Nutrients* **2019**, *11*, 2243. [CrossRef]

39. Borges, K.; Artacho, R.; Jodar-Graus, R.; Molina-Montes, E.; Ruiz-López, M.D. Calf Circumference, a Valuable Tool to Predict Sarcopenia in Older People Hospitalized with Hip Fracture. *Nutrients* **2022**, *14*, 4255. [CrossRef]
40. Ekinci, O.; Yanık, S.; Terzioğlu Bebitoğlu, B.; Yılmaz Akyüz, E.; Dokuyucu, A.; Erdem, Ş. Effect of Calcium β-Hydroxy-β-Methylbutyrate (CaHMB), Vitamin D, and Protein Supplementation on Postoperative Immobilization in Malnourished Older Adult Patients With Hip Fracture. *Nutr. Clin. Pract.* **2016**, *31*, 829–835. [CrossRef]

nutrients

MDPI

Article

Nutritional Ultrasonography, a Method to Evaluate Muscle Mass and Quality in Morphofunctional Assessment of Disease Related Malnutrition

Juan José López-Gómez [1,2,*], David García-Beneitez [3], Rebeca Jiménez-Sahagún [1,2], Olatz Izaola-Jauregui [1,2], David Primo-Martín [1,2], Beatriz Ramos-Bachiller [1,2], Emilia Gómez-Hoyos [1,2], Esther Delgado-García [1,2], Paloma Pérez-López [1,2] and Daniel A. De Luis-Román [1,2]

[1] Servicio de Endocrinología y Nutrición, Hospital Clínico Universitario de Valladolid, 47003 Valladolid, Spain; rebebel9@gmail.com (R.J.-S.); oizaolaj@saludcastillayleon.es (O.I.-J.); dprimoma@saludcastillayleon.es (D.P.-M.); bramosb@saludcastillayleon.es (B.R.-B.); emiliagomezhoyos@gmail.com (E.G.-H.); delgadogarciaesther@gmail.com (E.D.-G.); palomaperezz18@gmail.com (P.P.-L.); dadluis@yahoo.es (D.A.D.L.-R.)

[2] Centro de Investigación Endocrinología y Nutrición, Universidad de Valladolid, 47003 Valladolid, Spain

[3] Facultad de Medicina, Universidad de Medicina, 47003 Valladolid, Spain

* Correspondence: jjlopez161282@hotmail.com

Abstract: Nutritional ultrasonography is an emerging technique for measuring muscle mass and quality. The study aimed to evaluate the relationship between the parameters of body mass and quality of ultrasonography with other parameters of morphofunctional assessment in patients with disease-related malnutrition (DRM). Methods: A cross-sectional study was developed on 144 patients diagnosed with DRM according to the Global Leadership Initiative on Malnutrition (GLIM) criteria. Morphofunctional evaluation was assessed with anthropometric variables, handgrip strength and bioelectrical impedanciometry (BIA). Nutritional ultrasonography of quadriceps rectus femoris (QRF) was made (muscle mass (Muscle Area of Rectus Femoris index (MARFI)), Y axis and muscle quality (X-Y index and echogenicity). Results: The mean age of patients was 61.4 (17.34) years. The prevalence of sarcopenia in the sample was 33.3%. Patients with sarcopenia (S) had lower values of MARFI [(S: 1.09 (0.39) cm^2/m^2; NoS: 1.27 (0.45); $p = 0.02$), Y axis (S: 0.88 (0.27); NoS: 1.19 (0.60); $p < 0.01$) and X-Y index (S: 1.52 (0.61); NoS: 1.30 (0.53); $p < 0.01$)]. There was a correlation between BIA parameters (phase angle) and muscle mass ultrasonographic variables (MARFI) (r = 0.35; $p < 0.01$); there was an inverse correlation between muscle quality ultrasonographic variables (echogenicity) and handgrip strength (r = −0.36; $p < 0.01$). In the multivariate analysis adjusted by age, the highest quartile of the X-Y index had more risk of death OR: 4.54 CI95% (1.11–18.47). Conclusions: In patients with DRM and sarcopenia, standardized muscle mass and muscle quality parameters determined by ultrasonography of QRF are worse than in patients without sarcopenia. Muscle quality parameters had an inverse correlation with electric parameters from BIA and muscle strength. The highest quartile of the X-Y index determined by ultrasonography was associated with increased mortality risk.

Keywords: nutritional ultrasonography; disease-related malnutrition; morphofunctional assessment; echogenicity

1. Introduction

Disease-related malnutrition (DRM) is a highly prevalent pathology which has become a significant challenge in our health system. This disease has a prevalence between 20% and 50% in hospitalized patients [1,2]. The presence of this situation can be associated with an increase in complications and mortality. The EFFORT study showed that patients with malnutrition diagnosed by GLIM criteria had more risk for adverse clinical outcomes (OR: 1.53; 95%CI: 1.22–1.93) [3]. This condition may also increase the cost of hospitalization; in this way, the patients with the risk of malnutrition are supposed to have a high cost during hospitalization [4].

Malnutrition can be associated with other conditions, such as sarcopenia, defined by a loss of muscle mass and function. This disease was described as a primary condition associated with aging and frailty, but in 2019 the European Working Group on Sarcopenia in Older People (EWGSOP2) raised the secondary sarcopenia associated with several diseases [5]. This pathology can be present in up to 15% of patients with malnutrition and 32% of patients with cachexia in older adults [6]. The presence of sarcopenia also increases the risk of complications in surgical [7], medical patients [8,9] and older adults [10].

The main societies in nutrition worldwide, like the European Society of Clinical Nutrition and Metabolism (ESPEN) and the American Society of Parenteral and Enteral Nutrition (ASPEN), recommend starting medical nutrition treatment in medical and surgical patients at risk of malnutrition [2]. Therefore, an adequate and early diagnosis of malnutrition is very important to carry out an adapted Medical Nutrition Therapy to prevent complications [11].

The adequate diagnosis of malnutrition and sarcopenia is based on some tests to evaluate dietary intake, body composition, muscle strength and function, and biochemical parameters. This global approach to diagnose malnutrition has been called morphofunctional assessment of disease-related malnutrition [12]. Morphofunctional Assessment can help us evaluate patients at risk of malnutrition and an early diagnosis of disease-related malnutrition for personalized treatment.

The evaluation of body composition, especially muscle mass, is an important component of the diagnosis of malnutrition and sarcopenia, and it plays an essential role in monitoring the nutritional treatment of DRM. Nevertheless, the diagnosis of muscle quantity and quality is difficult. Some techniques are not as accurate as anthropometry with perimeters or estimative equations based on bioimpedanciometry. Besides, there are some tests like computerized tomography (CT), or magnetic resonance imaging (MRI) considered the gold standard but more expensive and not feasible in routine clinical practice [13].

Nutritional ultrasonography is an emerging technique in diagnosing DRM and sarcopenia to measure muscle mass and quality [14]. This probe allows a simple method to evaluate muscle mass in the consultation or bedside in hospitalized patients. It is an economical and not invasive test, and it helps us to determine several muscular groups. The main limitation of this technique is the scarce evidence of its relationship to the prognosis of DRM, the lack of use of a standardized muscle group and the need for validation with cutoff points for DRM and sarcopenia. Finally, this technique needs trained personnel capable of performing this ultrasound method and managing the data on the software [15].

Nutritional ultrasonography allows us to measure muscle mass as a quantitative method by determining muscle thickness and muscle area. A study by Fischer et al. in 2022 probed that ultrasound can predict CT L3 skeletal muscle area (SMA) [16]. On the other hand, muscle ultrasonography helps us to evaluate the quality of muscle by measuring its shape and echogenicity. A study in oncologic patients shows that ultrasonography correlates with body composition techniques with functional components such as bioimpedanciometry (phase angle) and handgrip strength [17].

Nutritional ultrasonography offers us an economical, feasible and not harmful technique to assess muscle mass and quality. This method of study of body composition allows us to make an early diagnosis of malnutrition to personalize medical nutrition therapy. Besides, the follow-up of changes in ultrasonography can help to monitor the effect on muscle of nutritional treatment.

This study aimed to evaluate the feasibility of nutritional ultrasonography in diagnosing malnutrition and sarcopenia and its relationship with the prognosis of patients with DRM. The main objectives of the study were to evaluate the relationship between the parameters of body mass and quality of ultrasonography with techniques of body composition such as bioimpedanciometry and muscle quality determined by handgrip strength, to describe the differences in muscle mass determined by ultrasonography in the function of diagnosis of sarcopenia and to characterize the prognosis of basic pathology related to the ultrasonography parameters.

2. Materials and Methods

2.1. Study Design

A cross-sectional study was developed in 144 patients diagnosed with disease-related malnutrition with GLIM criteria [18]. The patients were recruited in the Clinical Nutrition Unit of Clinic Universitary Hospital of Valladolid between January 2021 and September 2022.

After signing informed consent, patients were interviewed about medical history, disease progression and nutritional anamnesis. It was done anthropometry, electric bioimpedanciometry, handgrip strength and muscle mass and quality were evaluated by nutritional ultrasonography.

The study was approved by the ethics committee of East Valladolid Area with code PI 22-907 and carried out following the principles of the Helsinki Declaration.

2.2. Study Subject

The selected patients had the following inclusion criteria: community patients with a diagnosis of disease-related malnutrition with GLIM criteria; over 18 years. The exclusion criteria were: Uncontrolled hepatopathy, chronic kidney disease over the IV stage, and patients who didn't sign informed consent.

2.3. Variables

Anthropometry: The anthropometric variables measured were weight (kg), height (m); body mass index (BMI) as weight/height × height (kg/m^2); percentage of weight loss (%TWL): (Usual weight (kg) − Actual weight (kg))/Usual weight (kg) × 100). Arm Circumference (AC) (cm) and calf circumference (CC) cm were measured using the guideline of "Anthropometric variables of the Spanish sports population", which uses a modified version of the International Society for the Advancement Kinanthropometry (ISAK) protocol. The arm circumference was made at the middle point between the acromium and radium head with a relaxed arm. The calf circumference was made with the patient standing at the maximum perimeter between the knee and ankle [19]. One was taken measured at the right member (arm and calf). The person who did anthropometry was a dietitian-nutritionist formed in anthropometric measurement with skills in nutritional assessment and anthropometry. The measurements were always taken by the same operator.

Muscle Function: The muscle function was obtained with handgrip strength (JAMAR® dynamometer, Preston, Jackson, Missouri, MO, USA). The measure was taken with the patient sitting with the dominant arm at a straight angle with the body. We made three determinations, and we chose the highest value.

Body composition:

- Bioelectrical Impedanciometry (BIA): The BIA measure the hydration and cell density of the body by the determination of electric parameters such as resistance, reactance, and phase angle. The use of validated estimative equations allows us to define the compartments of body composition [20]. Bioimpedanciometry (BIA NutriLab; EFG Akern, Akern, Pisa, Italy) was performed between 8:00 and 9:15, after an overnight fast and after a time of 15 min in the supine position. The BIA measured the parameters of impedance (Z), resistance (R) and capacitance (X). The phase angle (PhA) is calculated with: PhA = ((X/R) × 180°/π). It was calculated by estimative equation fat mass (FM), fat-free mass (FFM), fat-free mass index (FFMI) and percentage of skeletal muscle mass (%MM) [20]. We estimated the appendicular skeletal muscle mass (ASMI) by Sergi Formula: −3.964 + (0.227 × RI) + (0.095 × weight) + (1.384 × sex) + (0.064 × Z), where RI resistivity index (sex: Male = 1; Female = 0) [21].
- Nutritional Ultrasonography: We made a muscular ultrasonography of the quadriceps rectus femoris (QRF) of the dominant lower extremity with a 10 to 12 MHz probe and

a multifrequency linear matrix (Mindray Z60, Madrid, Spain). The measurement was made with the patient in the supine position. The probe was aligned perpendicular to the longitudinal and transverse axis of QRF. The determination was performed without compression at the level of the lower third from the superior pole of the patella and the anterior superior iliac spine [14].

The variables that we measured to assess muscle mass were the anteroposterior (Y) and transversal muscle thickness (X), cross-sectional muscle area (MARF) and muscle circumference (MCRF) [15]. The area was standardized by height (muscle area (cm^2)/height × height (m^2) and is named the muscle area rectus femoris index (MARFI). The variables used to assess muscle quality were X-Y index ((Xaxis/Yaxis)/height^2) that relate transversal and anteroposterior muscle thickness; on the other hand, we measured muscle echogenicity with Image J software, version 1.52p (National Institutes of Health (NIH), Bethesda, MD, USA) [22]; to display echogenicity, we consider 0 as complete black color and 255 as complete white color, we selected a region of interest (ROI) centered in QRF, and we take the median of the values. We standardize by the formula: (Median/255) × 100 (see Figure 1).

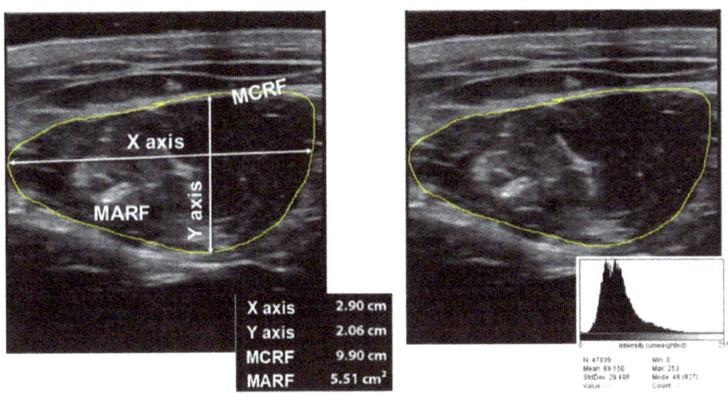

Figure 1. Parameters of muscle ultrasonography of quadriceps rectus femoris ((**right**) muscle mass measures; (**left**) echogenicity). MARF: Muscular Area Rectus Femoris; MCRF: Muscular Circumference Rectus Femoris.

Diagnostic test: Severity GLIM criteria: It was used to determine the severity GLIM criteria of severity to characterize the type of malnutrition (mild or severe). We considered severe malnutrition for those with phenotypic criteria of more than 10% weight loss in the last six months or >20% in one year or a BMI < 18.5 kg/m^2 in <70 years or <20 kg/m^2 in >70 years [18].

EWGSOP2 criteria: To determine the diagnosis of sarcopenia, we used the EWGSOP2 criteria [5]. Low muscle strength (or dynapenia) was considered as a handgrip strength <16 kg in women and <27 kg in men; low muscle mass was considered with appendicular skeletal mass index (ASMI) determined by BIA (ASMI < 5.5 kg/m^2 in women and ASMI < 7 kg/m^2 in men).

Comorbidity and mortality:

We consider the morbidity of disease, the number of visits to emergency service, the number of hospitalization episodes and the death.

2.4. Statistical Analysis

The database has been registered with permission of the National Data Protection Agency. The collected data was stored in a database using the statistical software SPSS 23.0 (SPSS Inc., Chicago, IL, USA).

Continuous variables were presented as mean and standard deviation, while parametric variables were analyzed using the unpaired Student's *t*-test. For non-parametric variables, tests such as Friedman, Wilcoxon and Mann-Whitney U test will be used. To compare variables in more than two groups, the ANOVA U test was applied with the Bonferroni post-hoc test. The analysis of the variables at different times of the study was carried out using multivariate analysis of variance (MANOVA). Qualitative variables were expressed as percentages and analyzed using the Chi-square test, with Fisher and Yates adjustments when necessary. Statistical significance was considered as a *p*-value with a value below 0.05.

3. Results

3.1. Sample Description

It analyzed 144 patients diagnosed with disease-related malnutrition (DRE). 60.4% of patients were women, and the average age was 61.4 (17.34). The pathologies which cause malnutrition are represented in Figure 2.

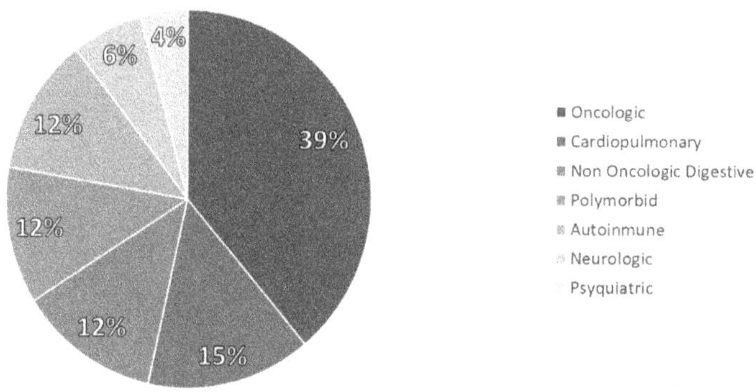

Figure 2. Distribution of pathologies.

The prevalence of sarcopenia with EWGSOP2 criteria was 33.30%. The low muscle mass criterion was fulfilled in 45.8% of patients, and the low muscle strength (dynapenia) was fulfilled in 51.4%. There were no differences in sarcopenia ($p = 0.72$) or dynapenia ($p = 0.12$) between sexes, but there were differences in low muscle mass criteria ($p < 0.01$) (Figure 3).

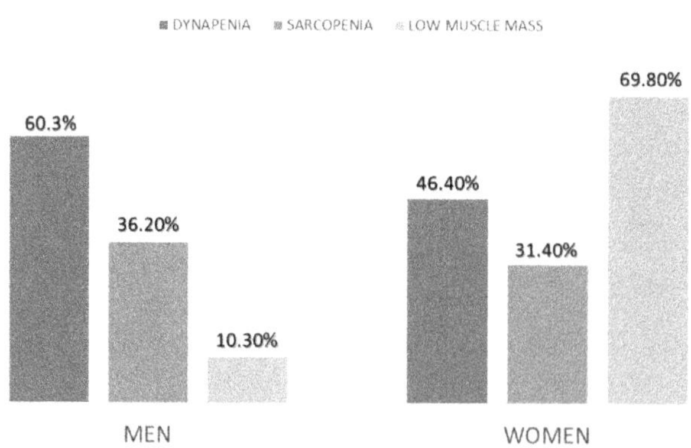

Figure 3. Differences in the diagnosis of sarcopenia, low muscle mass and dynapenia between sexes.

Morphofunctional assessment variables and the differences between sexes are represented in Table 1.

Table 1. Morphofunctional assessment variables and differences between sexes.

	Total	Men	Women	p-Value
	Anthropometry			
BMI (kg/m^2)	21.79 (4.61)	23.99 (4.62)	20.31 (4.01)	<0.01
Age (years)	61.4 (17.34)	64.91 (14.70)	60.71 (18.80)	0.15
%weight loss	11.84 (9.44)	10.42 (7.38)	12.88 (10.63)	0.15
Arm Circumference (cm)	23.07 (2.98)	24.73 (2.92)	21.97 (2.47)	<0.01
Calf circumference (cm)	31.03 (3.42)	32.47 (3.69)	30.06 (2.86)	<0.01
	Bioelectrical Impedanciometry			
Resistance (ohm)	595.81 (110.42)	531.03 (98.38)	638.73 (96.51)	<0.01
Reactance (ohm)	50.58 (11.76)	46.46 (12.17)	53.32 (10.69)	<0.01
Phase Angle (°)	4.86 (0.83)	4.99 (0.88)	4.78 (0.79)	0.15
ASMI (kg/m^2)	5.88 (1.09)	6.77 (0.96)	5.30 (0.71)	<0.01
MMI (kg/m^2)	9.69 (1.78)	10.75 (1.73)	9.02 (1.47)	<0.01
	Nutritional Ultrasonography			
MCRFI (cm/m^2)	3.33 (0.61)	3.19 (0.63)	3.41 (0.59)	0.03
MARFI (cm^2/m^2)	1.21 (0.43)	1.22 (0.51)	1.21 (0.38)	0.81
X-Y index	3.56 (1.35)	3.46 (1.37)	3.61 (1.35)	0.54
Echogenicity (%)	36.68 (9.70)	32.79 (9.42)	39.16 (9.09)	<0.01
	Muscle Strength			
Handgrip strength (kg)	20.28 (7.57)	24.82 (7.93)	17.15 (0.59)	<0.01

BMI: body mass index; ASMI: appendicular skeletal mass index; MMI: muscle mass index; MCRFI: muscle circumference rectus femoris index (cm/m^2); MARFI: muscle area rectus femoris index (cm/m^2). X: transversal rectus femoris axis; Y: anteroposterior rectus femoris axis.

The morbidity registered at three months was nine deaths (6.3%), 40 patients (27.8%) were hospitalized at least one time, and 70 patients (48.7%) went to emergency services at least one time. Between admitted patients, the median of admissions was 1 (1–2) times, and the days of admission were 10 (5–18.75) days. Between those who were admitted, the median of visits to emergency services was 1 (1–2.25) times.

3.2. Morphofunctional Assessment and Diagnosis of Sarcopenia

We compared the variables of morphofunctional assessment in the function of diagnosis of sarcopenia. We observed significant differences in anthropometry and bioimpedanciometry parameters except for reactance (Table 2). If we compare the ultrasonography parameters, we observe differences in muscle area as a measure of muscle mass and X-Y index as a quality measure (Table 2).

Table 2. Morphofunctional assessment variables related to diagnosis of sarcopenia.

	Sarcopenia	No Sarcopenia	p-Value
SEX (%M/%W)	36.2%/32.1%	63.8%/67.9%	0.72
	Anthropometry		
BMI (kg/m^2)	20.07 (3.49)	22.73 (4.89)	<0.01
Age (years)	67.92 (13.56)	59.62 (18.59)	<0.01
%weight loss	13.83 (11.14)	10.76 (8.35)	0.09
Arm Circumference (cm)	22.31 (2.08)	23.49 (3.28)	0.03
Calf circumference (cm)	29.57 (2.69)	31.83 (3.53)	<0.01
	Bioelectrical Impedanciometry		
Resistance (ohm)	641 (0.49)	569.53 (110.39)	<0.01
Reactance (ohm)	50.06 (9.07)	50.94 (13.02)	0.68
Phase Angle (°)	4.47 (0.79)	5.09 (0.84)	<0.01
ASMI (kg/m^2)	5.40 (0.76)	6.16 (1.13)	<0.01
MMI (kg/m^2)	8.69 (1.29)	10.26 (1.75)	<0.01

Table 2. *Cont.*

	Sarcopenia	No Sarcopenia	*p*-Value
	Nutritional Ultrasonography		
MCRFI (cm/m^2)	3.31 (0.55)	3.34 (0.64)	0.82
MARFI (cm^2/m^2)	1.09 (0.39)	1.27 (0.45)	0.02
X-Y index	4.12 (1.28)	3.29 (1.32)	<0.01
Echogenicity (%)	38.13 (10.72)	36.07 (9.12)	0.27
	Muscle Strength		
Handgrip strength (kg)	15.07 (5.85)	22.94 (6.96)	<0.01

BMI: body mass index; ASMI: appendicular skeletal mass index; MMI: muscle mass index; MCRFI: muscle circumference rectus femoris index (cm/m^2); MARFI: muscle area rectus femoris index (cm/m^2). X: transversal rectus femoris axis; Y: anteroposterior rectus femoris axis.

After the stratification in the function of components of sarcopenia (dynapenia and low muscle mass), we have observed differences in lower values of MARFI in those patients with dynapenia and higher values of echogenicity in these patients. We didn't observe these differences in patients with low muscle mass; the only difference observed is a lower value of echogenicity in patients with low muscle mass (Table 3). If we compare BIA parameters, the differences were in functional parameters such as reactance and phase angle in those patients with dynapenia, and there were differences in all parameters of BIA in those with low muscle mass (Table 3).

Table 3. Differences in morphofunctional assessment variables in the function of components of sarcopenia (dynapenia and low muscle mass).

	Dynapenia	No Dynapenia	*p*-Value	Low Muscle Mass	No Low Muscle Mass	*p*-Value
		Anthropometry				
BMI (kg/m^2)	22.29 (4.69)	21.34 (4.55)	0.22	19.76 (3.68)	25.61 (3.69)	<0.01
Age (years)	68.19 (14.27)	56.15 (18.52)	<0.01	59.66 (18.33)	67.56 (14.08)	<0.01
%weight loss	11.93 (10.01)	11.52 (8.78)	0.81	13.23 (9.68)	9.55 (8.64)	0.03
Arm Circumference (cm)	23.53 (3.01)	22.64 (2.89)	0.08	21.94 (2.39)	25.16 (2.83)	<0.01
Calf circumference (cm)	30.91 (3.58)	31.23 (3.28)	0.57	29.87 (2.99)	33.22 (3.12)	<0.01
		Bioelectrical Impedanciometry				
Resistance (ohm)	589.58 (110.45)	597.81 (108.62)	0.64	647.66 (89.31)	499.36 (75.92)	<0.01
Reactance (ohm)	47.37 (10.16)	54.17 (12.53)	<0.01	53.51 (11.21)	45.14 (10.88)	<0.01
Phase Angle (°)	4.61 (0.74)	5.17 (0.81)	<0.01	4,71 (0.77)	5.14 (0.88)	<0.01
ASMI (kg/m^2)	5.94 (1.13)	5.87 (1.03)	0.68	5.35 (0.71)	6.88 (0.98)	<0.01
MMI (kg/m^2)	9.63 (1.84)	9.85 (1.69)	0.47	8.77 (1.21)	11.40 (1.36)	<0.01
		Nutritional Ultrasonography				
MCRFI (cm/m^2)	3.31 (0.61)	3.36 (0.62)	0.62	3.27 (0.61)	3.43 (0.61)	0.13
MARFI (cm^2/m^2)	1.15 (0.45)	1.29 (0.41)	0.04	1.17 (0.42)	1.30 (0.45)	0.08
X-Y index	3.76 (1.41)	3.35 (1.28)	0.08	3.69 (1.30)	3.31 (1.43)	0.12
Echogenicity (%)	38.70 (10.35)	34.59 (8.49)	0.02	34.94 (9.58)	39.83 (9.21)	<0.01
		Muscle Strength				
Handgrip strength (kg)	16.02 (6.02)	24.91 (6.29)	<0.01	19.78 (7.72)	21.19 (7.28)	0.29

BMI: body mass index; ASMI: appendicular skeletal mass index; MMI: muscle mass index; MCRFI: muscle circumference rectus femoris index (cm/m^2); MARFI: muscle area rectus femoris index (cm/m^2). X: transversal rectus femoris axis; Y: anteroposterior rectus femoris axis.

3.3. Comparison of Parameters of Muscle Mass and Quality of Nutritional Ultrasonography

We considered muscle mass parameters in nutritional ultrasonography, the muscle area of the rectus femoris index (MARFI) and the muscle circumference of the rectus femoris index (MCRFI). We also considered muscle quality parameters, echogenicity, and X-Y index. It was observed a positive correlation between quality parameters (X-Y index and echogenicity) ($r = 0.27$; $p = 0.03$) and between muscle mass parameters (MARFI and MCRFI) (r = 0.75; $p < 0.01$) (Figure 4). When we compared quality and muscle mass parameters, we observed a positive correlation between MCRFI and the X-Y index (r = 0.22; $p = 0.01$) and a negative correlation between the MARFI and X-Y index (r = −0.30; $p < 0.01$).

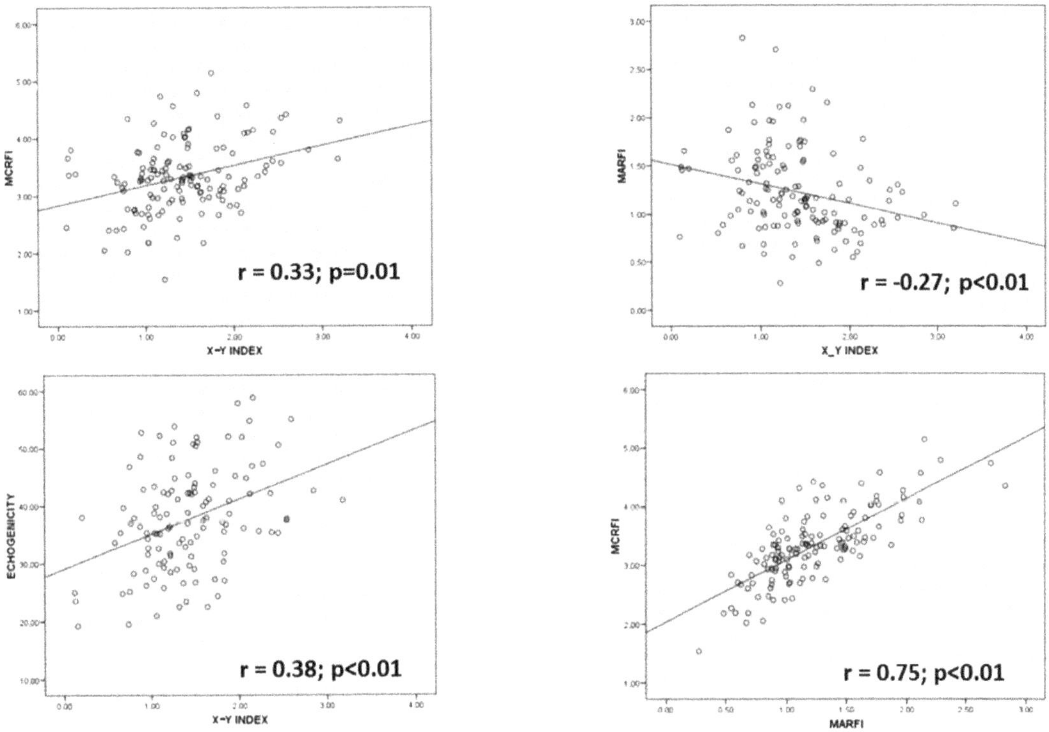

Figure 4. Regression graphics comparing ultrasonography variables. MARFI: muscle area of rectus femoris index; MCRFI: muscle circumference of rectus femoris index; X: transversal axis; Y: anteroposterior axis.

3.4. Comparison of Parameters of Muscle Mass and Quality of Nutritional Ultrasonog-Raphy

We compare variables obtained from nutritional ultrasonography with variables of body composition (BIA), muscle strength (handgrip strength) and anthropometry (braquial and calf circumferences). A positive correlation was observed between muscle mass parameter MARFI and body composition parameters such as ASMI, MMI and Phase Angle; a negative correlation was observed between MARFI and electric parameters from BIA (resistance and phase angle) (Table 4). If we compare muscle quality parameters (echogenicity and X-Y index), we find a negative correlation between these parameters and resistance, reactance, and phase angle (Table 4).

3.5. Relationship of Nutritional Ultrasonography with Morbidity

We compared the differences in ultrasonography parameters between those who suffered complications and those who did not. There were no differences between admitted patients and those who were not. There were no differences between patients who went to emergency services. Nevertheless, patients who suffered death had a higher X-Y index (4.67 (1.43) vs. 3.48 (1.32); $p = 0.02$) and a higher MCRFI than those who did not (3.86 (0.70) vs. 3.29 (0.59); $p < 0.01$). In the multivariate analysis adjusted by age, the highest quartile of the X-Y index has more risk of death OR: 4.54 CI95% (1.11–18.47); $p = 0.03$ (Figure 5).

Table 4. Correlation of ultrasonography with parameters of morphofunctional assessment.

	Echogenicity	Marfi	X-Y Index
Arm Circumference (cm)	r = 0.05; p = 0.55	r = 0.05; p = 0.55	r = −0.03; p = 0.75
Calf Circumference (cm)	r = 0.07; p = 0.41	r = 0.13; p = 0.12	r = −0.04; p = 0.62
ASMI (kg/m^2)	r = −0.05; p = 0.56	r = 0.17; p = 0.04 *	r = −0.11; p = 0.19
MMI (kg/m^2)	r = −0.03; p = 0.76	r = 0.25; p < 0.01 *	r = −0.23; p < 0.01 *
Resistance (ohm)	r = −0.03; p = 0.71	r = −0.17; p = 0.04 *	r = −0.03; p = 0.74
Reactance (ohm)	r = −0.21; p = 0.02 *	r = 0.12; p = 0.15	r = −0.31; p < 0.01 *
Phase Angle (°)	r = −0.23; p = 0.01 *	r = 0.35; p < 0.01 *	r = −0.42; p < 0.01 *
Handgrip Strength (kg)	r = −0.36; p < 0.01 *	r = 0.13; p = 0.13	r = −0.18; p = 0.04 *

MARFI: Muscular Area of Rectus Femoris Index; ASMI: appendicular skeletal muscle index; MMI: muscle mass index, * $p < 0.05$.

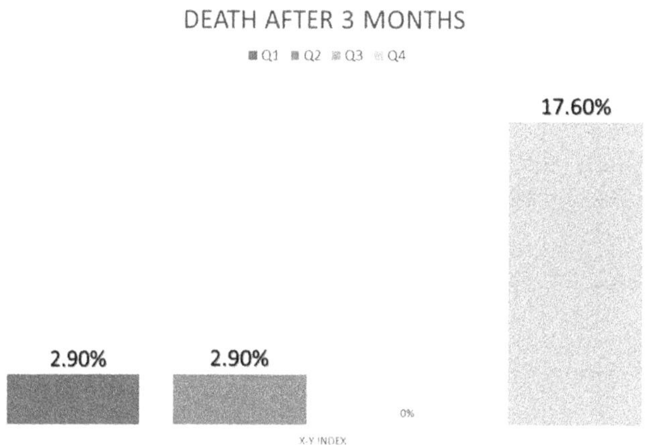

Figure 5. Percent of deaths related to quartile of X-Y index.

4. Discussion

Nutritional ultrasonography is a novel technique that allows us to measure muscle mass and muscle quality. This study has shown that muscle mass parameters of ultrasonography as MARFI are higher in patients with sarcopenia and have a positive correlation with parameters of body composition like ASMI, MMI and phase angle. On the other hand, muscle quality parameters like muscle echogenicity and X-Y index show differences in strength criteria from sarcopenia (dynapenia) and have a negative correlation with parameters related to muscle function like handgrip strength and phase angle and reactance from BIA.

4.1. Use of Nutritional Ultrasonography in Disease-Related Malnutrition

Patients analyzed had a varied distribution of pathologies that cause disease-related malnutrition, with a predominance of oncologic patients. These diseases and malnutrition can produce sarcopenia, as we have seen in 30% of patients in our sample. These results are higher than those observed in a study developed in 2021 in admitted patients, with 10.5% of patients with sarcopenia and disease-related malnutrition [23]. This difference can be related to the type of patients. In our study, patients are predominantly oncologic, while in the study referred are cardiorespiratory patients. Another study by Riesgo et al. in older patients with COVID-19 showed a higher prevalence of risk of sarcopenia due to the type of disease and method of diagnosis [24].

The body composition has differences between men and women. This condition explains the changes in anthropometry, BIA, and handgrip strength that we have seen in the function of sex [25]. Ultrasonography showed differences between genders in absolute values but did not show differences if the values were standardized by height. These data are similar to those of the study of Arts et al. that showed a difference between males and females in muscular ultrasonography [26].

4.2. Nutritional Ultrasonography and Diagnosis of Sarcopenia

There were age differences when we compared patients with and without sarcopenia. Primary sarcopenia is a frequent disease in patients with more than 70 years. This condition relates to the reduction from 3 to 8% of muscle mass each decade since the age of 30, more marked in patients with more than 60 years [27]. DRM is related to sarcopenia, but the association with age can increase the risk of this pathology. A Pekin Union Medical College hospital study showed that the patients with risk of malnutrition and sarcopenia had a higher age than those who do not have sarcopenia, as we have reported in our study [28]. In our study, the correlation analysis pointed out that the measures from ultrasonography have values related to loss of mass and quality in relation to the increase in age. These alterations in ultrasonographic parameters are related to a decline in function. This condition has been seen in community patients with older age in a study from Albacete, where dynapenia had a higher prevalence in patients over 75 years (59.7% vs. 35.7%) [29].

Sarcopenia is defined as reduced mass and function of muscle. The usefulness of ultrasonography in the diagnosis and staging of sarcopenia can be used mostly to evaluate muscle mass. We have seen low values in structural measures of the muscle as MARF, MARFI and Y axis. The use of ultrasonography has been planted in patients with primary sarcopenia in older adults [30], but the use in secondary sarcopenia and disease-related malnutrition is still unclear. Some studies have shown low values of muscle mass measured by ultrasonography, such as Sánchez-Torralvo et al., in patients with cistyc fibrosis [31]. Another study in patients from the internal medicine department of the University Hospital of Siena showed significantly lower values of muscle thickness measured by ultrasonography in patients with sarcopenia [32]. However, if we compared the values of nutritional ultrasonography related to the low muscle mass criterion, we did not find any difference. This situation can be produced in relation to conditions that can increase the mass of muscle but decrease the function of myoesteatosis or inflammation. In a study by Bot et al. in patients with end-stage liver disease, low SMI was not related to muscle function in a 6-min walking distance, but myoesteatosis showed a relation to an altered 6-min walking distance [33].

The parameters of muscle quality as an X-Y index showed differences in sarcopenia. This marker indicates the relationship between transversal and anteroposterior axis. Low values relate to better muscle quality due to the predominance of the Y axis, which demonstrates a harder muscle. Considering only the dynapenia criterion, we observe differences in the X-Y index and echogenicity. These characteristics of muscle can help us to evaluate muscle quality and function. Muscle echogenicity has shown an inverse relationship with muscle strength, and it is related to density by CT [34].

4.3. Nutritional Ultrasonography in Morphofunctional Assessment

Morphofunctional assessment of DRE uses techniques of intake evaluation, body composition, muscle function and biochemical parameters to carry out a global approach to nutritional assessment. Ultrasonography plays an important role in this nutritional assessment. It is necessary to know the relationship between nutritional ultrasonography and other components of morphofunctional assessment.

Femoral muscle ultrasonography can be adequate to assess muscle mass compared to CT at the third lumbar vertebra (CT L3 MM), as described in a study by Arai et al. developed in Intensive Care Unit Admission patients. This study reported a r = 0.48 for rectus femoris, which had the discriminative power to assess low muscularity [35]. Another study by Fischer et al. observed that ultrasound measures at the tight can predict CT L3 MM in different populations with non-critical illness [16]. In our study, the assessment of muscle mass by ultrasonography using MARFI correlated with muscle mass measures determined by BIA like ASMI and MMI, and it correlated also with cellularity measures like phase angle determined by BIA. The evaluation of phase angle and its correlation with muscle mass by ultrasonography has been proposed in obese females [36] and oncological patients [37]. In this study (AnyVida trial), phase angle and ultrasonography were prognostic factors for 12-month mortality [37].

Muscle quality measurement of ultrasonography was assessed by echogenicity and X-Y index. These parameters correlated with muscle strength determined by handgrip strength. The quality measures from ultrasonography as echogenicity have demonstrated a relation to muscle strength, as in the study from Bunout et al., where the lowest muscle echogenicity is related to a higher quadriceps torque and a higher handgrip strength in older adults [34]. In another study by Mañago et al., echogenicity was inversely correlated with muscle strength ($r = -0.46$, $p < 0.01$) and power ($r = -0.50$, $p = 0.006$) in patients with multiple sclerosis.

Muscle ultrasonography quality parameters are also correlated with electric parameters from BIA, like reactance and phase angle that are related to body cell mass. Body composition assessed by BIA is based on electrical characteristics of the human body to estimate components such as muscle mass, hydration, or fat mass. However, in BIA, the direct measure from electric parameters can help us know body cell mass as a body composition variable and functional parameters. The electrical parameters from BIA can be related to disease-related malnutrition and body function or inflammation and are related to disease prognosis [20]. Correlation between ultrasound quality measures and electrical parameters from BIA leads to nutritional ultrasonography as a useful determination of muscle function, body function and disease prognosis. Phase angle has demonstrated the relationship with muscle mass and density studied with TC in a study from Gen et al. [38]; in this study, in elderly patients, lower values of phase angle are associated with low density of muscle determined by CT [38]. Another study by Bourgeois et al. showed a relationship between muscular echogenicity and phase angle in healthy individuals [39].

4.4. Nutritional Ultrasonography and Complications in DRE

Muscle mass parameters (MARF, muscle thickness) in ultrasonography have a relationship with prognosis in some pathologies in acute and chronic patients. A study from Málaga showed that muscle thickness is a prognostic factor for mortality in patients with cancer [37]. A systematic review conducted by Casey et al. demonstrated that cross-sectional area and muscle thickness are associated with readmission, length of stay and survival; it was done with 37 studies (22 of them are in patients in ICU) [40]. Our study did not show differences in muscle mass parameters except MCRF. Nevertheless, this parameter could have more of a relationship with muscle quality than muscle mass. Muscle size can be influenced by myoesteatosis and edema with higher values. On the other hand, the high variability of pathologies analyzed can interfere with no differences in the events analyzed.

Muscle quality parameters showed differences in the X-Y index and MCRF for mortality. X-Y index can offer us an information about muscle stiffness that cannot be done by other measures. Casey's systematic review showed the relationship between muscle quality parameters such as echogenicity and prognosis. Conversely, muscle thickness is related to Y-axis size, which is also associated with a patient's prognosis [40]. Echogenicity did not show differences in prognosis, but it could be related to variability in the type of patients and its relationship with hydration and the effect of treatment of the primary disease [41].

4.5. Strengths and Limitations

The main strength of this study is the use of a novel technique, such as nutritional ultrasonography, in a large sample of patients diagnosed with disease-related malnutrition. This condition can help us to understand the behavior of this diagnostic method in ill patients. On the other hand, this is a study in community patients. Most of the studies done with ultrasonography are in critical or non-critic hospitalized patients. At last, using the technique inside a morphofunctional assessment planning allows us to better understand the utility of ultrasonography in studying muscle mass and function of patients with DRM.

The limitations of this study were the selection of different pathologies which cause DRM are associated with a high variability in morphofunctional assessment to find differences but also gives more statistical power to the differences obtained. The lack of cutoff points to standardize ultrasonography prevents us from evaluating sarcopenia or evaluation of prognosis. Using a correlation test limits our comparison to one with the techniques, and the lack of gold standard techniques such as CT or MRI hinders an adequate validation of the test. The age of patients can interfere with an adequate interpretation of data related to the influence of age and disease over muscle mass and function.

4.6. Future Lines of Investigation

Nutritional ultrasonography is an emerging technique for nutritional assessment of patients since it is an inexpensive and easy-to-perform method. The morphofunctional assessment associated with ultrasonography could help us to make an easy diagnosis and follow-up of sarcopenia, disease-related malnutrition and its treatment. However, scientific evidence on disease-related malnutrition is still scarce. It is needed the categorization of cutoff points to help in the diagnosis of nutrition-related pathologies (sarcopenia and DRM). On the other hand, validation of nutritional ultrasonography is needed in the pathologies that cause sarcopenia and disease-related malnutrition. It is important to consider ultrasonography as a method to evaluate muscle mass and quality and standardize the technique to determine the measurements of variables and the most adequate muscle to use in each pathology.

5. Conclusions

In community patients with DRM, the prevalence of sarcopenia was 33.3%. This prevalence was superior in women than men. In patients with sarcopenia, muscle mass parameters determined by nutritional ultrasonography of the rectus femoris muscle (muscle area, muscle thickness (Y axis)) are lower than in patients without sarcopenia. Muscle quality parameters (X-Y index) showed the worst values in patients with sarcopenia; echogenicity only showed differences (higher values) in patients with dynapenia criterion of sarcopenia.

Muscle mass ultrasonography parameters were correlated with electrical parameters (resistance and phase angle), and estimated muscle parameters (ASMI, MMI) were assessed by BIA. Muscle quality parameters (echogenicity and X-Y index) had a higher correlation with electric parameters from BIA than muscle mass parameters; they correlated with muscle strength assessed by handgrip strength. Ultrasonography X-Y index (highest quartile) is associated with an increase in the risk of mortality in patients with disease-related malnutrition assessed by ultrasonography.

Muscle mass assessment by ultrasonography is a good and easy method to evaluate muscle mass and quality in patients with disease-related malnutrition. We need to develop studies to complete the evidence about this technique, standardize it, and integrate it into usual clinical practice to diagnose disease-related malnutrition and monitor medical nutrition therapy.

Author Contributions: Conceptualization, J.J.L.-G. and D.A.D.L.-R.; Data curation, J.J.L.-G., D.G.-B., O.I.-J., D.P.-M. and P.P.-L.; Formal analysis, J.J.L.-G.; Funding acquisition, D.A.D.L.-R.; Investigation, J.J.L.-G., D.G.-B., R.J.-S., O.I.-J., D.P.-M., B.R.-B., E.G.-H., E.D.-G. and P.P.-L.; Methodology, J.J.L.-G. and D.A.D.L.-R.; Project administration, J.J.L.-G. and D.A.D.L.-R.; Resources, J.J.L.-G., E.G.-H., E.D.-G. and D.A.D.L.-R.; Software, J.J.L.-G. and D.A.D.L.-R.; Supervision, J.J.L.-G. and D.A.D.L.-R.; Validation, J.J.L.-G. and D.A.D.L.-R.; Visualization, J.J.L.-G. and D.A.D.L.-R.; Writing—original draft, J.J.L.-G. and D.G.-B.; Writing—review & editing, J.J.L.-G. and D.A.D.L.-R. All authors have read and agreed to the published version of the manuscript.

Funding: This research received no external funding.

Institutional Review Board Statement: The study was conducted in accordance with the Declaration of Helsinki and approved by the Institutional Review Board (or Ethics Committee) of Comité Ética en Investigación con Medicamentos (Valladolid Área Este) (protocol code 22-907 date of approval: 13 October 2022).

Informed Consent Statement: Informed consent was obtained from all subjects involved in the study.

Data Availability Statement: Data is unavailable due to privacy or ethical restrictions.

Conflicts of Interest: The authors declare no conflict of interest.

References

1. Álvarez Hernández, J.; Planas Vila, M.; León-Sanz, M.; García de Lorenzo, A.; Celaya-Pérez, S.; García-Lorda, P.; Araujo, K.; Sarto Guerri, B.; on behalf of the PREDyCES® Researches. Prevalencia y costes de la malnutrición en pacientes hospitalizados; estudio predyces. *Nutr. Hosp.* **2012**, *27*, 1049–1059. [CrossRef] [PubMed]
2. Merker, M.; Felder, M.; Gueissaz, L.; Bolliger, R.; Tribolet, P.; Kägi-Braun, N.; Gomes, F.; Hoess, C.; Pavlicek, V.; Bilz, S.; et al. Association of Baseline Inflammation with Effectiveness of Nutritional Support Among Patients with Disease-Related Malnutrition: A Secondary Analysis of a Randomized Clinical Trial. *JAMA Netw. Open* **2020**, *3*, e200663. [CrossRef] [PubMed]
3. Kaegi-Braun, N.; Boesiger, F.; Tribolet, P.; Gomes, F.; Kutz, A.; Hoess, C.; Pavlicek, V.; Bilz, S.; Sigrist, S.; Brändle, M.; et al. Validation of modified GLIM criteria to predict adverse clinical outcome and response to nutritional treatment: A secondary analysis of a randomized clinical trial. *Clin. Nutr.* **2022**, *41*, 795–804. [CrossRef] [PubMed]
4. León-Sanz, M.; Brosa, M.; Planas, M.; García-de-Lorenzo, A.; Celaya-Pérez, S.; Hernández, J.Á. PREDyCES study: The cost of hospital malnutrition in Spain. *Nutrition* **2015**, *31*, 1096–1102. [CrossRef]
5. Cruz-Jentoft, A.J.; Bahat, G.; Bauer, J.; Boirie, Y.; Bruyère, O.; Cederholm, T.; Cooper, C.; Landi, F.; Rolland, Y.; Sayer, A.A.; et al. Sarcopenia: Revised European consensus on definition and diagnosis. *Age Ageing* **2019**, *48*, 16–31. [CrossRef]
6. Gingrich, A.; Volkert, D.; Kiesswetter, E.; Thomanek, M.; Bach, S.; Sieber, C.C.; Zopf, Y. Prevalence and overlap of sarcopenia, frailty, cachexia and malnutrition in older medical inpatients. *BMC Geriatr.* **2019**, *19*, 120. [CrossRef]
7. Park, B.; Bhat, S.; Xia, W.; Barazanchi, A.W.; Frampton, C.; Hill, A.G.; MacCormick, A.D. Consensus-defined sarcopenia predicts adverse outcomes after elective abdominal surgery: Meta-analysis. *BJS Open* **2023**, *7*, zrad065. [CrossRef]
8. Jensen, S.; Bloch, Z.; Quist, M.; Hansen, T.T.D.; Johansen, C.; Pappot, H.; Suetta, C.; Skjødt Rafn, B. Sarcopenia and loss of muscle mass in patients with lung cancer undergoing chemotherapy treatment: A systematic review and meta-analysis. *Acta Oncol.* **2023**, *62*, 318–328. [CrossRef]
9. Mazeaud, S.; Zupo, R.; Couret, A.; Panza, F.; Sardone, R.; Castellana, F. Prevalence of Sarcopenia in Liver Cirrhosis: A Systematic Review and Meta-Analysis. *Clin. Transl. Gastroenterol.* **2023**, *14*, e00584. [CrossRef]
10. Chan, H.C.N.; Fei, X.; Leung, E.L.Y.; Langston, K.; Marshall, S.; van der Meij, B.S. Post-discharge consequences of protein-energy malnutrition, sarcopenia, and frailty in older adults admitted to rehabilitation: A systematic review. *Clin. Nutr. ESPEN* **2023**, *54*, 382–397. [CrossRef]
11. Schuetz, P.; Fehr, R.; Baechli, V.; Geiser, M.; Deiss, M.; Gomes, F.; Kutz, A.; Tribolet, P.; Bregenzer, T.; Braun, N.; et al. Individualised nutritional support in medical inpatients at nutritional risk: A randomised clinical trial. *Lancet* **2019**, *393*, 2312–2321. [CrossRef]
12. García-Almeida, J.M.; García-García, C.; Ballesteros-Pomar, M.D.; Olveira, G.; Lopez-Gomez, J.J.; Bellido, V.; Bretón Lesmes, I.; Burgos, R.; Sanz-Paris, A.; Matia-Martin, P.; et al. Expert Consensus on Morphofunctional Assessment in Disease-Related Malnutrition. Grade Review and Delphi Study. *Nutrients* **2023**, *15*, 612. [CrossRef] [PubMed]
13. Barazzoni, R.; Jensen, G.L.; Correia, M.I.T.; Gonzalez, M.C.; Higashiguchi, T.; Shi, H.P.; Bischoff, S.C.; Boirie, Y.; Carrasco, F.; Cruz-Jentoft, A.; et al. Guidance for assessment of the muscle mass phenotypic criterion for the Global Leadership Initiative on Malnutrition (GLIM) diagnosis of malnutrition. *Clin. Nutr.* **2022**, *41*, 1425–1433. [CrossRef] [PubMed]
14. Hernández-Socorro, C.R.; Saavedra, P.; López-Fernández, J.C.; Ruiz-Santana, S. Assessment of Muscle Wasting in Long-Stay ICU Patients Using a New Ultrasound Protocol. *Nutrients* **2018**, *10*, 1849. [CrossRef] [PubMed]
15. García-Almeida, J.M.; García-García, C.; Vegas-Aguilar, I.M.; Pomar, M.D.B.; Cornejo-Pareja, I.M.; Medina, B.F.; de Luis Román, D.A.; Guerrero, D.B.; Lesmes, I.B.; Madueño, F.J.T. Nutritional ultrasound®: Conceptualisation, technical considerations and standardisation. *Endocrinol. Diabetes Nutr.* **2022**, *70*, 74–84. [CrossRef]
16. Fischer, A.; Hertwig, A.; Hahn, R.; Anwar, M.; Siebenrock, T.; Pesta, M.; Liebau, K.; Timmermann, I.; Brugger, J.; Posch, M.; et al. Validation of bedside ultrasound to predict lumbar muscle area in the computed tomography in 200 non-critically ill patients: The USVALID prospective study. *Clin. Nutr.* **2022**, *41*, 829–837. [CrossRef]
17. LóLópez-Gómez, J.J.; Benito-Sendín Plaar, K.; Izaola-Jauregui, O.; Primo-Martín, D.; Gómez-Hoyos, E.; Torres-Torres, B.; De Luis-Román, D.A. Muscular Ultrasonography in Morphofunctional Assessment of Patients with Oncological Pathology at Risk of Malnutrition. *Nutrients* **2022**, *14*, 1573. [CrossRef]
18. Cederholm, T.; Jensen, G.L.; Correia, M.I.T.D.; Gonzalez, M.C.; Fukushima, R.; Higashiguchi, T.; Baptista, G.; Barazzoni, R.; Blaauw, R.; Coats, A.J.S.; et al. GLIM criteria for the diagnosis of malnutrition—A consensus report from the global clinical nutrition community. *Clin. Nutr.* **2019**, *38*, 207–217. [CrossRef]

19. Canda, A.S. *Variables Antropométricas de la Población Deportista Española*; Consejo Superior de Deportes, Servicio de Documentación y Publicaciones: Madrid, Spain, 2012.
20. Bellido, D.; García-García, C.; Talluri, A.; Lukaski, H.C.; García-Almeida, J.M. Future lines of research on phase angle: Strengths and limitations. *Rev. Endocr. Metab. Disord.* **2023**, *24*, 563–583. [CrossRef]
21. Sergi, G.; De Rui, M.; Veronese, N.; Bolzetta, F.; Berton, L.; Carraro, S.; Bano, G.; Coin, A.; Manzato, E.; Perissinotto, E. Assessing appendicular skeletal muscle mass with bioelectrical impedance analysis in free-living Caucasian older adults. *Clin. Nutr.* **2015**, *34*, 667–673. [CrossRef]
22. Schneider, C.A.; Rasband, W.S.; Eliceiri, K.W. NIH Image to ImageJ: 25 years of image analysis. *Nat. Methods* **2012**, *9*, 671–675. [CrossRef] [PubMed]
23. Ballesteros-Pomar, M.D.; Gajete-Martín, L.M.; Pintor-De-La-Maza, B.; González-Arnáiz, E.; González-Roza, L.; García-Pérez, M.P.; González-Alonso, V.; García-González, M.A.; de Prado-Espinosa, R.; Cuevas, M.J.; et al. Disease-Related Malnutrition and Sarcopenia Predict Worse Outcome in Medical Inpatients: A Cohort Study. *Nutrients* **2021**, *13*, 2937. [CrossRef] [PubMed]
24. Riesgo, H.; Castro, A.; Del Amo, S.; San Ceferino, M.J.; Izaola, O.; Primo, D.; Gomez Hoyos, E.; Lopez Gomez, J.J.; de Luis, D.A. Prevalence of Risk of Malnutrition and Risk of Sarcopenia in a Reference Hospital for COVID-19, Relationship with Mortality. *Ann. Nutr. Metab.* **2021**, *77*, 324–329. [CrossRef]
25. Campa, F.; Coratella, G.; Cerullo, G.; Stagi, S.; Paoli, S.; Marini, S.; Grigoletto, A.; Moroni, A.; Petri, C.; Andreoli, A.; et al. New bioelectrical impedance vector references and phase angle centile curves in 4367 adults: The need for an urgent update after 30 years. *Clin. Nutr.* **2023**, *42*, 1749–1758. [CrossRef]
26. Arts, I.M.P.; Pillen, S.; Schelhaas, H.J.; Overeem, S.; Zwarts, M.J. Normal values for quantitative muscle ultrasonography in adults. *Muscle Nerve* **2010**, *41*, 32–41. [CrossRef]
27. Cannataro, R.; Carbone, L.; Petro, J.L.; Cione, E.; Vargas, S.; Angulo, H.; Forero, D.A.; Odriozola-Martínez, A.; Kreider, R.B.; Bonilla, D.A. Sarcopenia: Etiology, Nutritional Approaches, and miRNAs. *Int. J. Mol. Sci.* **2021**, *22*, 9724. [CrossRef] [PubMed]
28. Li, C.-W.; Yu, K.; Shyh-Chang, N.; Li, G.-X.; Jiang, L.-J.; Yu, S.-L.; Xu, L.-Y.; Liu, R.-J.; Guo, Z.-J.; Xie, H.-Y.; et al. Circulating factors associated with sarcopenia during ageing and after intensive lifestyle intervention. *J. Cachexia Sarcopenia Muscle* **2019**, *10*, 586–600. [CrossRef]
29. Sáez Moreno, M.Á.; Jiménez Lorenzo, R.; Lueso Moreno, M.; López-Torres Hidalgo, J. Prevalence of dynapenia in patients over 65 years. *Aten Primaria* **2018**, *50*, 567–568. [CrossRef]
30. Nijholt, W.; Scafoglieri, A.; Jager-Wittenaar, H.; Hobbelen, J.S.M.; van der Schans, C.P. The reliability and validity of ultrasound to quantify muscles in older adults: A systematic review. *J. Cachexia Sarcopenia Muscle* **2017**, *8*, 702–712. [CrossRef] [PubMed]
31. Sánchez-Torralvo, F.J.; Porras, N.; Ruiz-García, I.; Maldonado-Araque, C.; García-Olivares, M.; Girón, M.V.; Gonzalo-Marín, M.; Olveira, C.; Olveira, G. Usefulness of Muscle Ultrasonography in the Nutritional Assessment of Adult Patients with Cystic Fibrosis. *Nutrients* **2022**, *14*, 3377. [CrossRef]
32. Rustani, K.; Kundisova, L.; Capecchi, P.L.; Nante, N.; Bicchi, M. Ultrasound measurement of rectus femoris muscle thickness as a quick screening test for sarcopenia assessment. *Arch. Gerontol. Geriatr.* **2019**, *83*, 151–154. [CrossRef] [PubMed]
33. BBot, D.; Lucassen, C.; Werkman, M.; van Dijk, S.; Feshtali, S.S.; Tushuizen, M.E.; van Hoek, B. Skeletal muscle mass in patients with end-stage liver disease: Not only muscle size but especially muscle quality matters in relation to physical fitness. *Clin. Nutr. ESPEN* **2023**, *55*, 407–413. [CrossRef]
34. Bunout, D.; Gonzalez, S.; Canales, M.; Barrera, G.; Hirsch, S. Ultrasound assessment of rectus femoris pennation angle and echogenicity. Their association with muscle functional measures and fat infiltration measured by CT scan. *Clin. Nutr. ESPEN* **2023**, *55*, 420–424. [CrossRef] [PubMed]
35. Arai, Y.; Nakanishi, N.; Ono, Y.; Inoue, S.; Kotani, J.; Harada, M.; Oto, J. Ultrasound assessment of muscle mass has potential to identify patients with low muscularity at intensive care unit admission: A retrospective study. *Clin. Nutr. ESPEN* **2021**, *45*, 177–183. [CrossRef] [PubMed]
36. Primo, D.; Izaola, O.; Gómez, J.J.L.; de Luis, D. Correlation of the Phase Angle with Muscle Ultrasound and Quality of Life in Obese Females. *Dis. Markers* **2022**, *2022*, 7165126. [CrossRef]
37. García-García, C.; Vegas-Aguilar, I.M.; Rioja-Vázquez, R.; Cornejo-Pareja, I.; Tinahones, F.J.; García-Almeida, J.M. Rectus Femoris Muscle and Phase Angle as Prognostic Factor for 12-Month Mortality in a Longitudinal Cohort of Patients with Cancer (AnyVida Trial). *Nutrients* **2023**, *15*, 522. [CrossRef]
38. Geng, J.; Wei, Y.; Xue, Q.; Deng, L.; Wang, J. Phase angle is a useful bioelectrical marker for skeletal muscle quantity and quality in hospitalized elderly patients. *Medicine* **2022**, *101*, e31646. [CrossRef]
39. Bourgeois, B.; Fan, B.; Johannsen, N.; Gonzalez, M.C.; Ng, B.K.; Sommer, M.J.; Shepherd, J.A.; Heymsfield, S.B. Improved strength prediction combining clinically available measures of skeletal muscle mass and quality. *J. Cachexia Sarcopenia Muscle* **2019**, *10*, 84–94. [CrossRef]

40. Casey, P.; Alasmar, M.; McLaughlin, J.; Ang, Y.; McPhee, J.; Heire, P.; Sultan, J. The current use of ultrasound to measure skeletal muscle and its ability to predict clinical outcomes: A systematic review. *J. Cachexia Sarcopenia Muscle* **2022**, *13*, 2298–2309. [CrossRef]
41. Stock, M.S.; Thompson, B.J. Echo intensity as an indicator of skeletal muscle quality: Applications, methodology, and future directions. *Eur. J. Appl. Physiol.* **2021**, *121*, 369–380. [CrossRef]

nutrients

MDPI

Article

Influence of the Results of Control of Intakes, Proteins and Anthropometry Nutritional Screening, Sarcopenia and Body Composition on the Clinical Evolution of Hospitalized Patients

Elena Márquez Mesa [1,*], José Pablo Suárez Llanos [1], Patricia Mercedes Afonso Martín [2], Carla Brito Negrín [2], María García Ascanio [2], Samuel González González [2] and Ignacio Llorente Gómez de Segura [1]

[1] Endocrinology and Nutrition Department, Hospital Universitario Nuestra Señora de Candelaria, Ctra. Del Rosario 145, 38010 Santa Cruz de Tenerife, Spain; psuarezllanos@gmail.com (J.P.S.L.)
[2] Faculty of Health Sciences, University of La Laguna, Calle Padre Herrera, 38200 La Laguna, Spain
* Correspondence: elenamqz@hotmail.com; Tel.: +34-922602972

Abstract: (1) Background: Hospital malnutrition and sarcopenia are common in inpatients and are associated with worse prognosis. Our objective is to determine the association of the positivity of CIPA (Control of Intakes, Proteins and Anthropometry) nutrition screening tool and sarcopenia and evaluate its prognostic implications (length of stay, readmissions and mortality) as well as different components of body composition. (2) Methodology: Cross-sectional single-center study and prospective six months follow-up for prognostic variables. On admission, CIPA and EWGSOP2 criteria were assessed. (3) Results: Four hundred inpatients, a median of 65.71 years old and 83.6% with high comorbidity, were evaluated. In total, 34.8% had positive CIPA and 19.3% sarcopenia. Positive CIPA and sarcopenia had worse results in body composition (fat mass (FM), fat-free mass (FFM) and appendicular skeletal muscle mass index (ASMI)) and dynamometry. Positive CIPA is significantly associated with worse prognosis (mortality (OR = 1.99), readmissions (OR = 1.86) and length of stay (B = 0.19)). Positive CIPA and sarcopenia combined are associated with a tendency to higher mortality (OR = 2.1, $p = 0.088$). Low hand grip strength (HGS) is significantly related to a higher length of stay (B = −0.12). (4) Conclusions: In hospitalized patients, malnutrition independently and combined with sarcopenia is associated with a worse prognosis but not body composition. Low HGS is related to a higher length of stay.

Keywords: disease-related malnutrition; CIPA; sarcopenia; EWGSOP2; hand grip strength; appendicular skeletal muscle index; body composition; phase angle; hospital stay; mortality

1. Introduction

Malnutrition is a poor prognostic factor for inpatients, but numerous research papers corroborate that nutritional intervention can improve the clinical evolution of hospitalized malnourished patients [1]. The development of the GLIM (Global Leadership Initiative on Malnutrition) criteria has made it possible to have a common strategy for nutritional evaluation. It is made up of two steps: first, a validated nutritional screening test is carried out, and then the nutritional evaluation itself, analyzing phenotypic and etiological criteria, including the evaluation of reduced muscle mass [2].

Hospital malnutrition is a frequent problem in patients admitted to a hospital. Prevalences ranging between 10% and 50% have been observed. In Spain, the multicenter PREDYCES study found that 23.7% of hospitalized patients were malnourished or at nutritional risk [3], while the seDREno study, using the GLIM malnutrition criteria, observed that 29.7% of hospitalized patients were malnourished [4].

A nutritional screening method called CIPA (Control of Intakes, Proteins and Anthropometry) was designed at Hospital Universitario Nuestra Señora de Candelaria (HUNSC) in Tenerife. In this tool, different items are evaluated: (a) decrease in intake < 50% in the first 72 h of admission; (b) plasma albumin < 3 g/dL; and (c) BMI < 18.5 kg/m^2 or mid-upper arm circumference (MUAC) $\leq$ 22.5 cm (if the BMI cannot be determined). Positivity of at least one of these items translates into a positive CIPA nutritional screening and identifies the patient with malnutrition or at risk of suffering from it. Since 2015, it has been implemented in the HUNSC and has been evaluated by different validation, optimization and cost-effectiveness studies [5,6].

In addition, the importance of assessing body composition is being increasingly recognized. The European Working Group on Sarcopenia in Older People 2 (EWGSOP2) has established new criteria for the diagnosis of sarcopenia, evaluating muscle mass and muscle function [7]. These parameters can be measured in daily clinical practice by bioimpedance analysis (BIA) and hand grip strength (HGS), respectively.

The BIA is the most widespread instrumental method in the study of body composition. It is a non-invasive, low-cost and easily accessible technique. The most frequently applied model to evaluate body composition is two-compartmental, dividing the body into fat mass (FM) and fat-free mass (FFM) that includes bone mineral content, extracellular water, intracellular water and visceral protein [8]. In the assessment of body composition, the BIA is based on the principle of the resistance that the body offers to an electric current, and the FFM can be estimated using predictive equations [9]. Different studies have shown that altered results of these items are associated with worse prognostic outcomes [10,11].

Dynamometry is a functional muscle strength assessment method that measures the isometric strength of the hand and forearm. It is a cheap and easy measurement to perform, so its implementation in clinical practice is simple. Furthermore, there are normality values with which to compare in numerous populations. Hand dynamometry tends to adequately reflect the body's muscle strength and correlates well with the body lean mass determined by different techniques such as BIA, densitometry (DXA) and computed tomography (CT) and with analytical measures of inflammation such as the decrease in plasma albumin [12,13]. Likewise, HGS has clinical and prognostic value, being associated with greater morbidity and mortality, worse quality of life and functional limitations [14–16].

Loss of muscle mass and muscle function are common in inpatients, especially in older and malnourished ones, and have potentially serious adverse effects. Different studies have shown that the presence of sarcopenia was associated with a worse quality of life, higher readmission rate and mortality [17–19].

For this reason, it is important to detect malnourished patients early, or those at risk of malnutrition, as well as those with sarcopenia, in order to implement appropriate therapeutic measures to reduce the associated side effects and improve the prognosis. Therefore, we investigate whether the malnutrition or risk of malnutrition determined by the CIPA nutrition screening tool and/or the presence of sarcopenia determined by the EWGSOP2 criteria is associated with changes in body composition as well as worse prognostic evolution (death, length of stay and readmissions at six months).

2. Materials and Methods

2.1. Type of Study and Ethical Aspects

Cross-sectional single-center study carried out in patients > 18 years old admitted in HUNSC evaluating the presence of malnutrition or risk of presenting it using de CIPA screening tool and sarcopenia determined by EWGSOP2 criteria and subsequent prospective follow-up of patients for up to six months. The ethics committee of HUNSC gave its approval to carry out this study on 17 December 2020 (project code CHUNSC_2020_105). The study was carried out in accordance with the requirements expressed in the Declaration of Helsinki [revision of Fortaleza (Brazil), October 2013] and the Laws and Regulations in force in Europe and Spain. The information sheet was delivered to the participating subjects. The investigator explained to the patient the objectives and procedures of the study and requested the signing of the informed consent form. Once the consent was signed, the researcher began the explorations and data collection necessary for the study.

The investigator did not initiate any investigation corresponding to the study until the consent of the patient had been obtained.

2.2. Inclusion and Exclusion Criteria

The inclusion criteria included adult subjects of both sexes with a hospital stay of more than three days who were attached to one of the following departments: general surgery, internal medicine, vascular surgery, digestive system, hematology, nephrology, pneumology, oncology, neurology, traumatology or cardiology. The exclusion criteria included subjects not eligible for CIPA nutritional screening at the HUNSC with a prognosis of hospital stay of less than or equal to three days; admission to a department with a low incidence of malnutrition (ophthalmology, dermatology, obstetrics ...); pediatric patient or critical care unit and palliative care; or patients already receiving artificial nutritional treatment. Patients with edemo-ascitic overload were also excluded. Written informed consent was requested from patients who met all the inclusion criteria and none of the exclusion criteria, and in the case of minors or disabled patients, that of their parents or legal guardians was collected.

2.3. Collected and Analyzed Data

The malnutrition screening that is usually used in the hospital (CIPA) was performed, to which the EWGSOP2 criteria were added. The evaluation of malnutrition and functionality was carried out after three days of hospital stay. The scores of both were recorded together with the data collection via the clinical history. For the CIPA test, BMI, albumin levels and percentage of decreased intake were recorded. Positivity of at least one of these items was considered a positive CIPA nutritional screening result: (a) decrease in intake < 50% in 72 h; (b) plasma albumin < 3 g/dL; and (c) BMI < 18.5 kg/m^2, MUAC $\leq$ 22.5 cm (if the BMI could not be determined) [20].

For the EWGSOP2 criteria, muscle mass and function were determined by BIA and HGS, respectively, and for de the diagnosis of sarcopenia, it was necessary that both items were diminished. Body composition was estimated by electrical bioimpedance (BIA 101® Akern Anniversary, Akern SRL, Pontassieve, Florence, Italy) using electrical values to determine appendicular skeletal muscle mass (ASM). Raw measurements produced by the device were used along with the Sergi equation for ASM estimation in elderly patients (>65 years) [21] and the Kyle equation in patients between 18 and 65 years [22]. ASM index (=ASM/height^2) values below 7 kg/m^2 in men and 5.5 kg/m^2 in women were considered as low muscle mass [7]. HGS was measured using a validated dynamometer Jamar® (JLW Instrumets, Chicago, IL, USA); the patient was seated with the arm adducted at the side, with the elbow flexed to 90° and the forearm in a mid-prone position. Hand grip duration had to be of at least 3 s with the dominant hand, and the maximum strength of three repeated grips was used as the test score. Values under 27 kg in men and 16 kg in women were considered abnormal [7].

Together with the usual work protocols and data depending on the pathology under treatment, the variables collected were age, sex, cause of admission, comorbidity (Charlson comorbidity index (CCI)) and functionality. Subsequently, the sample of patients with a positive CIPA result received therapeutic interventions according to the usual protocol [20]. The patients were followed up for the study of prognostic factors that also were recorded: length of stay, readmissions in the next 30 days and mortality in the following 6 months. Patients were included in the period between February 2021 and April 2023.

2.4. Statistical Analysis

Qualitative variables were summarized as frequency distribution, and normally distributed quantitative variables as mean $\pm$ standard deviation (SD). The continuous, non-normally distributed variables were summarized as median and interquartile range (IQR). To assess the skewness of quantitative variables, a graphical inspection of histograms and box plots, together with quantile-quantile normality plots, was performed.

For the analysis, a new variable was generated based on the combination of the positive results of sarcopenia and/or malnutrition (normal, CIPA positive, Sarcopenia positive and CIPA+ Sarcopenia positive). Qualitative variables were compared with the Pearson chi-square test. The comparison of normally distributed quantitative variables between two groups was performed using the Student's t-test or analysis of variance (ANOVA) for more than two groups.

The relationship of outcome variables (6-month mortality and readmission for 30 days) with the diagnosis of malnutrition and/or sarcopenia and body composition variables was assessed using binary logistic regression. For the outcome variable length of stay, a linear regression model was fitted. As the length of stay was not normally distributed, this data was log-transformed. Each model was adjusted by age, sex, CCI and department of admission. Statistical significance was assumed as $p < 0.05$. All analyses were performed using SPSS 26.0 (IBM Corp., Armonk, NY, USA).

3. Results

3.1. Characteristics of the Sample

A total of 400 patients who met the inclusion criteria during the study period and agreed to participate were recruited for the study. The most frequent admission departments were Digestive (13.8%), Traumatology (13.5%), Internal Medicine (12%), Pneumology (11.5%) and Neurology (10.3%). A percentage of 72.5% of the admissions were in a medical service and 27.5% in a surgical one. In total, 51.5% of the patients were male, the mean age was 65.71 ± 14.69 years and 83.6% had a CCI > 3, which is considered indicative of high comorbidity. Table 1 shows the baseline clinical characteristics and body composition.

Table 1. Baseline clinical characteristics and body composition data of the included patients.

	n = 400 Mean (SD)
Age (years)	65.71 (27.23)
Sex (% men)	51.5
CCI	7.63 (5.33)
BMI (kg/m^2)	27.23 (6.39)
HGS (kg)	19.17 (10.64)
ASMI (kg/m^2)	7.36 (1.68)
FFM (kg)	52.22 (11.58)
FM (kg)	21.98 (13.45)
Albumin (g/dL)	3.54 (0.62)

SD: standard deviation. CCI = Charlson comorbidity index. BMI = body mass index. HGS = hand grip strength. ASMI = appendicular skeletal muscle mass index. FFM = fat-free mass. FM = fat mass.

3.2. Malnutrition and Sarcopenia Screening and Diagnosis

In total, 34.8% presented a positive CIPA, determining malnutrition or risk of suffering from it. A percentage of 20.5% presented plasma albumin < 3 g/dL, 15.8% decrease in oral intake < 50% and 5.8% BMI < 18.5 kg/m^2. The CIPA was positive for presenting one altered item in 28.5% of the patients, two in 5.3% and three items in 1%. The parameters that were the most frequent cause of the CIPA positive result were plasma albumin < 3 g/dL (14.8%) and a decrease in oral intake < 50% in the first 72 h of admission (10%), both without alteration of the other items.

Probable sarcopenia was observed in 62.5% of the patients with low HGS. Of the patients, 24.8% had low muscle mass by ASMI. Finally, sarcopenia was confirmed in 19.3% of the patients according to the EWGSOP2 criteria.

The combination of positive CIPA and sarcopenia occurred in 11% of the patients. Table 2 shows the characteristics of the patients based on the diagnosis of malnutrition or risk of malnutrition, and sarcopenia. Patients with sarcopenia and positive CIPA were older, had worse results in body composition (low BMI, HGS, muscle mass, FFM and muscle function) and had higher comorbidity.

Table 2. Characteristics of the patients depending on the diagnosis of malnutrition or risk of malnutrition by CIPA screening and/or diagnosis of sarcopenia by EWGSOP2 criteria.

	Normal	Positive CIPA	Sarcopenia	Positive CIPA + Sarcopenia	*p*
n (%)	228 (57)	139 (34.8)	77 (19.3)	44 (11)	-
Age (years) *	63.45 (14.51)	65.77 (15.51)	74.3 (10.85)	70.84 (12.89)	<0.01
Sex (% men)	50.99	45.3	57.9	63.6	0.204
BMI (kg/m^2) *	29.12 (6.03)	27.41 (6.06)	23.06 (3.03)	20.12 (4.09)	<0.01
Admission service (% surgical)	29.4	27.4	27.3	18.2	0.508
CCI *	6.93 (5.07)	8.42 (5.66)	8.28 (5.04)	9.02 (5.68)	0.023
Albumin < 3 g/dL (%)	3.81 (0.45)	3.03 (0.63)	3.57 (0.44)	3.19 (0.58)	<0.01
Low HGS (%)	48.2	65.2	100	100	<0.01
Low muscle mass (%)	6.6	7.4	100	100	<0.01
FFM (kg) *	54.7 (11.04)	53.66 (12.03)	43.97 (7.46)	42.04 (6.81)	<0.01
FM (kg) *	24.93 (14.3)	20.67 (12.03)	17.68 (8.6)	12.79 (8.75)	<0.01

* data expressed as mean and standard deviation. CCI = Charlson comorbidity index. BMI = body mass index. HGS = hand grip strength. FFM = fat-free mass. FM = fat mass.

3.3. Association between Prognostic Clinical Outcomes and CIPA Results, Sarcopenia and Body Composition

A mortality of 17.3% of the total sample was observed at 6 months, 7.5% of early readmission and a median stay of 14 (8–24) days.

Positive CIPA alone and also a positive CIPA with sarcopenia were associated with higher mortality (24.4% and 29.5%, respectively) than normal patients (12.3%); $p = 0.008$. However, patients with a diagnosis of sarcopenia alone did not present higher mortality than patients without it and negative CIPA. Regarding early readmission rate (<30 days), a trend toward significance was observed with a higher readmission rate in the CIPA positive group vs. the negative group (21.1% vs. 11.8%; $p = 0.083$) (Figure 1).

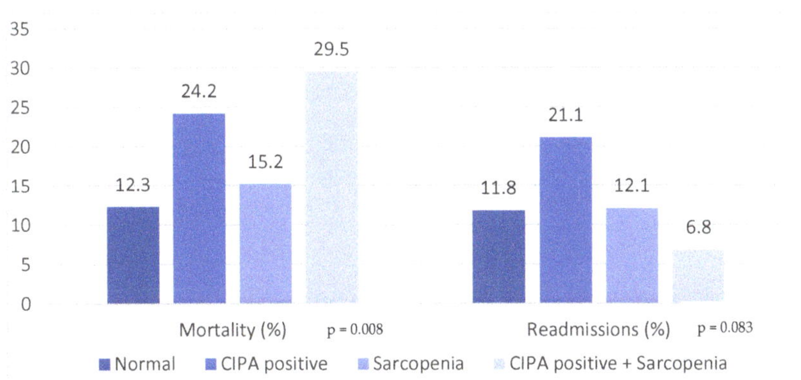

Figure 1. Percentage of mortality and readmissions by groups.

An analysis of the relationship between other body composition variables and worse prognosis was performed, but no significant differences were observed regarding mortality or readmissions (Table 3).

Table 4 shows the results of the multivariate analysis of the relationship between the body composition variables and the diagnosis of malnutrition and/or sarcopenia with the outcome variables. These results were adjusted for age, sex, CCI and admission service (medical/surgical).

Table 3. Association of body composition variables and prognostic evolution (readmissions and mortality).

	No Readmissions	Readmissions	*p*	No Mortality	Mortality	*p*
BMI (kg/m^2)	27.27 (6.58)	26.98 (5.03)	0.755	27.2 (6.43)	26.33 (6.18)	0.202
HGS (kg)	19.23 (10.94)	18.74 (8.47)	0.757	19.54 (10.71)	17.37 (10.19)	0.132
ASMI (kg/m^2)	7.32 (1.7)	7.67 (1.5)	0.150	7.38 (1.69)	7.28 (1.63)	0.654
FFM (kg)	51.97 (11.75)	53.84 (10.47)	0.270	52.34 (11.57)	51.67 (11.75)	0.663
FM (kg)	22.38 (13.76)	19.49 (11.02)	0.143	22.38 (13.77)	20.09 (11.67)	0.197

Data expressed as mean and standard deviation (SD). BMI = body mass index. HGS = hand grip strength. ASMI = appendicular skeletal muscle mass index. FFM = fat-free mass. FM = fat mass.

Table 4. Risk of worse prognostic evolution (mortality, readmissions, length of stay) with respect to diagnostic groups (malnutrition and/or sarcopenia) and body composition variables.

	Mortality (<6 Months)		Readmissions (<30 Days)		Length of Stay (Log-Transformed)	
	OR_a (IC 95%)	*p*	OR_a (IC 95%)	*p*	B_a (IC 95%)	*p*
Normal	Ref		Ref		Ref	
Positive CIPA	1.99 (1.02–3.91)	0.043	1.86 (0.94–3.65)	0.073	0.19 (0.01;0.38)	0.040
Sarcopenia	1.01 (0.33–3.08)	0.9	1.16 (0.35–3.79)	0.805	0.21 (−0.08;0.49)	0.159
Positive CIPA + Sarcopenia	2.10 (0.90–4.92)	0.088	0.43 (0.12–1.58)	0.205	0.19 (−0.05;0.45)	0.126
BMI	0.98 (0.94–1.03)	0.466	0.99 (0.95–1.04)	0.901	−0.01 (−0.02;0.003)	0.130
HGS	0.97 (0.93–1.01)	0.097	0.98 (0.94–1.02)	0.372	−0.012 (−0.02;−0.002)	0.015
ASMI	0.94 (0.78–1.13)	0.510	1.10 (0.92–1.31)	0.295	0.009 (−0.04;−0.057)	0.727
FFM	0.97 (0.95–1.01)	0.115	1.00 (0.97–1.04)	0.798	−0.005 (−0.01;0.003)	0.208
FM	0.99 (0.97–1.01)	0.483	0.98 (0.96–1.01)	0.141	−0.004 (−0.01;0.01)	0.126

OR_a (IC); B_a (IC). BMI = body mass index. HGS = hand grip strength. ASMI = appendicular skeletal muscle mass index. FFM = fat-free mass. FM = fat mass.

The CIPA-positive group had a higher mortality risk (OR = 1.99; $p = 0.043$). This was also observed in the CIPA positive and sarcopenia group, with close to statistical significance (OR = 2.1; $p = 0.088$). An increase in early readmissions rate was observed in the CIPA group, also close to statistical significance (OR = 1.8; $p = 0.073$), with no differences observed in the rest of the variables. A longer length of stay was observed in the CIPA-positive group (B = 0.19; $p = 0.04$). Also, a significant decrease in length of stay was observed as HGS increased (B = −0.012; $p = 0.015$) (Table 4).

4. Discussion

Our study evaluated the clinical prognostic value of malnutrition (or risk of presenting it via the CIPA nutrition screening tool), the presence of sarcopenia, and different body composition components.

A prevalence of malnutrition or risk of it of 34.8% was detected, similar to that described in previous studies with this nutritional screening tool, 35.8% in no surgical patients [23] and 35.4% in surgical patients [5]. This prevalence is slightly higher than described in the PREDYCES study, 23.7% with Nutritional Risk Screening (NRS-2002) [3] and more similar to the 29.7% described in the seDREno study with the GLIM criteria [4]. However, we must take into account that in the PREDYCES study, the prevalence of malnutrition in the group of patients over 70 years of age increased to 37%. This could be related to the average age of our sample, close to 70 years, as well as the inclusion of other markers of malnutrition, such as albumin.

The clinical evolution of patients detected as malnourished or at risk of malnutrition was worse than in patients with negative nutritional screening, presenting higher mortality and average length of stay and a trend toward a higher rate of early readmissions. This data is consistent with the previous results obtained in other studies in which CIPA has been used as the nutritional screening tool. CIPA detected that surgical patients had a greater risk of mortality during hospitalization (5% vs. 0%, $p = 0.006$), higher median length of stay (21 days [IQR 14–34 days] vs. 14.5 days [IQR 9–27 days], $p = 0.002$) and rate of early readmissions (25.3% vs. 8.2%, $p < 0.001$) [5]. In other studies, such as PREDyCES, it was also observed that malnutrition increased hospital stay (11.5 ± 7.5 versus 8.5 ± 5.8 d; $p < 0.001$) as well as costs [3]. More recently, the EFFORT Trial has shown that intensive nutritional treatment during hospitalization allows a 21% reduction in serious adverse effects that include mortality, admissions to the intensive care unit, readmissions after 30 days, major complications, functional impairment and mortality (OR = 0.65 (0.47–0.91); $p = 0.011$) [24]. These data reveal the importance of detecting malnutrition and its early management.

The sample analyzed had a high rate of comorbidities, being representative of the population of developed countries with a high rate of polymorbidity that is associated with a higher rate of complications, making an early evaluation of malnutrition and sarcopenia important [25].

The prevalence of sarcopenia was 19.3%, similar to that described in previous studies. Ballesteros et al. [18] evaluated the presence of sarcopenia in 200 hospitalized patients, presenting 33% of them with probable sarcopenia and 22.5% confirmed sarcopenia on admission, increasing to 53.3% at discharge. Cerri et al. [19] described the presence of sarcopenia in 21.4% of hospitalized patients with malnutrition or risk of malnutrition. The GLISTEN (Gruppo Lavoro Italiano Sarcopenia—Trattamento e Nutrizione) determined that 34.7% of 600 hospitalized elderly people presented sarcopenia at admission. This higher prevalence could be related to an older sample of patients (mean age 81.0 ± 6.8 years) [26].

Sarcopenia itself has been shown to be a negative prognostic factor in multiple pathologies. It increases the risk of falls and fractures, impairs the ability to perform activities of daily living, is associated with cardiac disease, respiratory disease and cognitive impairment, leads to mobility disorders and contributes to lowered quality of life, loss of independence or need for long term care placement and death [7]. Ballesteros et al. [18] found that patients with sarcopenia had a worse prognosis with a worse quality of life, higher readmission rate (OR = 2.25) and mortality (OR = 8.16). They independently analyzed the prognostic implications of HGS and muscle mass, finding that patients with higher HGS had a higher quality of life, fewer readmissions and less mortality adjusted for age, sex and comorbidities but not with low muscle mass alone. Also, the GLISTEN group [17] reported that patients with dynapenia had a longer hospital stay. These results are consistent with ours, in which we have observed that patients with altered HGS have a longer average stay and a trend toward higher mortality, but we have not observed an association of confirmed sarcopenia with worse prognostic evolution. This could be related to the difficulty in determining muscle mass since the pathologies themselves, as well as the treatments used in hospitalized patients (fluid therapy, hydroelectrolyte replacement and depletive therapies), can alter the results obtained via BIA. Other more accurate methods could be used, such as DXA, CT or magnetic resonance imaging (MRI), but their limited availability and the emission of ionizing radiation limit their use in clinical practice. The standardization and use of muscle ultrasound in the evaluation of sarcopenia could be of interest and is currently being developed in different populations [26]. On the other hand, dynamometry can be implemented easily and at a low cost, presenting a good correlation with body muscle strength. Numerous studies have described its association with higher mortality and complication rates in different pathologies, reinforcing its role as a prognostic marker [27], being recommended in the latest expert consensus on morphofunctional assessment of malnutrition related to the disease [28]. However, it must be evaluated whether the established cut-off points are the most appropriate. Some studies, such as that of Westbury et al., use more lax cut-off points that allow the identification of a greater prevalence of sarcopenia while maintaining a strong association with mortality [29].

Furthermore, in recent years, interest has grown in the study of different components of body composition, such as FM and FFM, as well as ASMI, being these two last parameters of phenotypic criteria of malnutrition in the GLIM malnutrition criteria [2]. Body composition has been studied in many pathologies, but not so much in heterogeneous hospitalized patients of different ages. In the study by Ji et al. [11], they found that reduced muscle mass determined by ASMI in cancer patients was associated with worse survival. Cereda et al. [10] analyzed the FFM index (FFMI) in a cohort of cancer patients, observing that patients with a decreased FFMI had higher mortality and lower quality of life. In our study, an association of worse results in the body composition values of the different compartments with a higher prevalence of malnutrition and sarcopenia was evident. However, it was not observed that patients with altered body composition data had a worse prognostic outcome.

The results obtained in our study, showing a worse clinical evolution in patients with decreased muscle function (determined by HGS) but not in patients with low muscle mass, could be related to the fact that the decrease in muscle strength can appear even before changes in the measurements of muscle mass are observed. Furthermore, this alteration in functionality could be more related to the alteration of muscle quality than to the quantity. Roberti et al. [30] found that the amount of intermuscular fat deposits induces alterations of muscle quality without alterations of muscle quantity influencing the patient prognosis. Pereira et al. [31] did not identify a correlation between sarcopenia and the rate of adverse surgical outcomes in patients with early-stage breast cancer. Also, we must take into consideration that the use of predictive equations is necessary to estimate the different body compartments. Normally, these equations have been developed in healthy populations, but the age of the patients, the different pathologies, as well as the ethnic origin, can affect these estimates. This is why the evaluation of raw physical parameters is increasingly used in clinical practice, and its inclusion in the evaluation criteria for sarcopenia and malnutrition has been suggested [32].

As a limitation of this study, it should be noted that it is a single-center study with a limited number of patients, so the data must be extrapolated with caution to the general population. No functional tests were performed that would allow for the grading of the severity of sarcopenia. It was not recorded which patients received nutritional or rehabilitation therapy, so it was not possible to evaluate whether those who were treated had a better prognostic outcome.

5. Conclusions

In summary, we found that patients with malnutrition or at risk of suffering from it, as well as those who associate sarcopenia with malnutrition, have worse clinical outcomes. These groups of patients also present worse results in FM, FFM and ASMI. Special attention should be paid to muscle functionality, as, like in other works, low HGS appears to be a marker of a worse clinical prognosis. This is an interesting issue on the one hand because this evaluation is easy to perform, and on the other because muscle functionality impairment appears before the muscle mass is affected, so it can be an early marker.

Therefore, we consider early detection of malnutrition and sarcopenia (and especially muscle function) to be of great importance in order to early predict patients with worse clinical evolution.

Author Contributions: Conceptualization, E.M.M., J.P.S.L. and I.L.G.d.S.; methodology, E.M.M. and J.P.S.L.; validation, E.M.M. and J.P.S.L.; formal analysis, E.M.M. and J.P.S.L.; investigation, E.M.M. and J.P.S.L.; resources, E.M.M. and J.P.S.L.; writing—original draft preparation, E.M.M., P.M.A.M., C.B.N., M.G.A. and S.G.G.; writing—review and editing, E.M.M. and J.P.S.L.; supervision, J.P.S.L. and I.L.G.d.S.; project administration, J.P.S.L. All authors have read and agreed to the published version of the manuscript.

Funding: This research received no external funding.

Institutional Review Board Statement: The study was conducted in accordance with the Declaration of Helsinki and approved by the University Hospital Nuestra Señora de Candelaria (project code: CHUNSC_2020_105; approval date: 17 December 2020).

Informed Consent Statement: Informed consent was obtained from all subjects involved in the study. Written informed consent has been obtained from the patients to publish this paper.

Data Availability Statement: Data supporting the reported results are available upon request.

Acknowledgments: To Manuel Enrique Fuentes Ferrer for his methodological and statistics help.

Conflicts of Interest: The authors declare no conflict of interest.

References

1. Gomes, F.; Baumgartner, A.; Bounoure, L.; Bally, M.; Deutz, N.E.; Greenwald, J.L.; Stanga, Z.; Mueller, B.; Schuetz, P. Association of Nutritional Support With Clinical Outcomes Among Medical Inpatients Who Are Malnourished or at Nutritional Risk: An Updated Systematic Review and Meta-analysis. *JAMA Netw. Open* **2019**, *2*, e1915138. [CrossRef] [PubMed]
2. Cederholm, T.; Jensen, G.L.; Correia, M.I.T.D.; Gonzalez, M.C.; Fukushima, R.; Higashiguchi, T.; Baptista, G.; Barazzoni, R.; Blaauw, R.; Coats, A.J.; et al. GLIM criteria for the diagnosis of malnutrition—A consensus report from the global clinical nutrition community. *Clin. Nutr.* **2019**, *38*, 1–9. [CrossRef] [PubMed]
3. Álvarez-Hernández, J.; Planas Vila, M.; León-Sanz, M.; García de Lorenzo, A.; Celaya-Pérez, S.; García-Lorda, P.; Araujo, K.; Sarto Guerri, B. Prevalence and costs of malnutrition in hospitalized patients; the PREDyCES Study. *Nutr. Hosp.* **2012**, *27*, 1049–1059. [CrossRef] [PubMed]
4. Zugasti-Murillo, A.; Petrina-Jáuregui, M.E.; Ripa-Ciáurriz, C.; Sánchez-Sánchez, R.; Villazón-González, F.; Faes, Á.G.D.; Fernández-López, C.; Calles-Romero, L.; Martín-Palmero, M.Á.; Riestra-Fernández, M.; et al. SeDREno study—Prevalence of hospital malnutrition according to GLIM criteria, ten years after the PREDyCES study. *Nutr. Hosp.* **2021**, *38*, 1016–1025. [CrossRef] [PubMed]
5. Mora Mendoza, A.; Suárez Llanos, J.P.; Sánchez Morales, A.; Lorenzo González, C.; Zambrano Huerta, Y.; Llorente Gómez de Segura, I. Validation of CIPA nutritional screening through prognostic clinical variables in hospitalized surgical patients. *Endocrinol. Diabetes Nutr.* **2020**, *67*, 304–309. [CrossRef] [PubMed]
6. Suárez-Llanos, J.P.; Rosat-Rodrigo, A.; García-Niebla, J.; Vallejo-Torres, L.; Delgado-Brito, I.; García-Bello, M.A.; Pereyra-García-Castro, F.; Barrera-Gómez, M.A. Comparison of Clinical Outcomes in Surgical Patients Subjected to CIPA Nutrition Screening and Treatment versus Standard Care. *Nutrients* **2019**, *11*, 889. [CrossRef] [PubMed]
7. Cruz-Jentoft, A.J.; Bahat, G.; Bauer, J.; Boirie, Y.; Bruyère, O.; Cederholm, T.; Cooper, C.; Landi, F.; Rolland, Y.; Sayer, A.A.; et al. Sarcopenia: Revised European consensus on definition and diagnosis. *Age Ageing* **2019**, *48*, 16–31. [CrossRef]
8. Marra, M.; Sammarco, R.; De Lorenzo, A.; Iellamo, F.; Siervo, M.; Pietrobelli, A.; Donini, L.M.; Santarpia, L.; Cataldi, M.; Pasanisi, F.; et al. Assessment of Body Composition in Health and Disease Using Bioelectrical Impedance Analysis (BIA) and Dual Energy X-Ray Absorptiometry (DXA): A Critical Overview. *Contrast Media Mol. Imaging* **2019**, *2019*, 3548284. [CrossRef]
9. Patil, B.R.; Patkar, D.P.; Mandlik, S.A.; Kuswarkar, M.M.; Jindal, G.D. Single prediction equation for bioelectrical impedance analysis in adults aged 22–59 years. *J. Med. Eng. Technol.* **2011**, *35*, 109–114. [CrossRef]
10. Cereda, E.; Pedrazzoli, P.; Lobascio, F.; Masi, S.; Crotti, S.; Klersy, C.; Turri, A.; Stobäus, N.; Tank, M.; Franz, K.; et al. The prognostic impact of BIA-derived fat-free mass index in patients with cancer. *Clin. Nutr.* **2021**, *40*, 3901–3907. [CrossRef]
11. Ji, W.; Liu, X.L.; Liu, P.; He, Y.W.; Zhao, Y.X.; Zheng, K.; Cui, J.; Li, W. The efficacy of fat-free mass index and appendicular skeletal muscle mass index in cancer malnutrition: A propensity score match analysis. *Front. Nutr.* **2023**, *10*, 1172610. [CrossRef] [PubMed]
12. Bohannon, R.W. Muscle strength: Clinical and prognostic value of hand-grip dynamometry. *Curr. Opin. Clin. Nutr. Metab. Care* **2015**, *18*, 465–470. [CrossRef] [PubMed]
13. Sánchez Torralvo, F.J.; Porras, N.; Abuín Fernández, J.; García Torres, F.; Tapia, M.J.; Lima, F.; Soriguer, F.; Gonzalo, M.; Martínez, G.R.; Olveira, G.; et al. Normative reference values for hand grip dynamometry in Spain. Association with lean mass. *Nutr. Hosp.* **2018**, *35*, 98–103. [CrossRef] [PubMed]
14. Jochem, C.; Leitzmann, M.; Volaklis, K.; Aune, D.; Strasser, B. Association Between Muscular Strength and Mortality in Clinical Populations: A Systematic Review and Meta-Analysis. *J. Am. Med. Dir. Assoc.* **2019**, *20*, 1213–1223. [CrossRef] [PubMed]
15. Hwang, S.H.; Lee, D.H.; Min, J.; Jeon, J.Y. Handgrip Strength as a Predictor of All-Cause Mortality in Patients With Chronic Kidney Disease Undergoing Dialysis: A Meta-Analysis of Prospective Cohort Studies. *J. Ren. Nutr.* **2019**, *29*, 471–479. [CrossRef]
16. Mauricio, S.F.; Ribeiro, H.S.; Correia, M.I.T.D. Nutritional Status Parameters as Risk Factors for Mortality in Cancer Patients. *Nutr. Cancer* **2016**, *68*, 949–957. [CrossRef]
17. Rossi, A.P.; Fantin, F.; Abete, P.; Bellelli, G.; Bo, M.; Cherubini, A.; Corica, F.; Di Bari, M.; Maggio, M.; Manca, G.M.; et al. Association between hospitalization-related outcomes, dynapenia and body mass index: The Glisten Study. *Eur. J. Clin. Nutr.* **2019**, *73*, 743–750. [CrossRef]
18. Ballesteros-Pomar, M.D.; Gajete-Martín, L.M.; Pintor-De-la-maza, B.; González-Arnáiz, E.; González-Roza, L.; García-Pérez, M.P.; González-Alonso, V.; García-González, M.A.; de Prado-Espinosa, R.; Cuevas, M.J.; et al. Disease-Related Malnutrition and Sarcopenia Predict Worse Outcome in Medical Inpatients: A Cohort Study. *Nutrients* **2021**, *13*, 2937. [CrossRef]
19. Cerri, A.P.; Bellelli, G.; Mazzone, A.; Pittella, F.; Landi, F.; Zambon, A.; Annoni, G. Sarcopenia and malnutrition in acutely ill hospitalized elderly: Prevalence and outcomes. *Clin. Nutr.* **2015**, *34*, 745–751. [CrossRef] [PubMed]

20. Suárez-Llanos, J.P.; Benítez-Brito, N.; Vallejo-Torres, L.; Delgado-Brito, I.; Rosat-Rodrigo, A.; Hernández-Carballo, C.; Ramallo-Fariña, Y.; Pereyra-García-Castro, F.; Carlos-Romero, J.; Felipe-Pérez, N.; et al. Clinical and cost-effectiveness analysis of early detection of patients at nutrition risk during their hospital stay through the new screening method CIPA: A study protocol. *BMC Health Serv. Res.* **2017**, *17*, 292. [CrossRef]
21. Sergi, G.; De Rui, M.; Veronese, N.; Bolzetta, F.; Berton, L.; Carraro, S.; Bano, G.; Coin, A.; Manzato, E.; Perissinotto, E. Assessing appendicular skeletal muscle mass with bioelectrical impedance analysis in free-living Caucasian older adults. *Clin. Nutr.* **2015**, *34*, 667–673. [CrossRef] [PubMed]
22. Kyle, U.G.; Genton, L.; Hans, D.; Pichard, C. Validation of a bioelectrical impedance analysis equation to predict appendicular skeletal muscle mass (ASMM). *Clin. Nutr.* **2003**, *22*, 537–543. [CrossRef] [PubMed]
23. Suárez-Llanos, J.P.; Mora-Mendoza, A.; Benítez-Brito, N.; Pérez-Méndez, L.; Pereyra-García-Castro, F.; Oliva-García, J.G.; Palacio-Abizanda, J.E. Validity of the new nutrition screening tool Control of Food Intake, Protein, and Anthropometry (CIPA) in non-surgical inpatients. *Arch. Med. Sci.* **2018**, *14*, 1020–1024. [CrossRef] [PubMed]
24. Schuetz, P.; Fehr, R.; Baechli, V.; Geiser, M.; Deiss, M.; Gomes, F.; Kutz, A.; Tribolet, P.; Bregenzer, T.; Braun, N.; et al. Individualised nutritional support in medical inpatients at nutritional risk: A randomised clinical trial. *Lancet* **2019**, *393*, 2312–2321. [CrossRef] [PubMed]
25. Gomes, F.; Schuetz, P.; Bounoure, L.; Austin, P.; Ballesteros-Pomar, M.; Cederholm, T.; Fletcher, J.; Laviano, A.; Norman, K.; Poulia, K.-A.; et al. ESPEN guidelines on nutritional support for polymorbid internal medicine patients. *Clin. Nutr.* **2018**, *37*, 336–353. [CrossRef] [PubMed]
26. Perkisas, S.; Bastijns, S.; Baudry, S.; Bauer, J.; Beaudart, C.; Beckwée, D.; Cruz-Jentoft, A.; Gasowski, J.; Hobbelen, H.; Jager-Wittenaar, H.; et al. Application of ultrasound for muscle assessment in sarcopenia: 2020 SARCUS update. *Eur. Geriatr. Med.* **2021**, *12*, 45–59. [CrossRef] [PubMed]
27. Kaegi-Braun, N.; Tribolet, P.; Baumgartner, A.; Fehr, R.; Baechli, V.; Geiser, M.; Deiss, M.; Gomes, F.; Kutz, A.; Hoess, C.; et al. Value of handgrip strength to predict clinical outcomes and therapeutic response in malnourished medical inpatients: Secondary analysis of a randomized controlled trial. *Am. J. Clin. Nutr.* **2021**, *114*, 731–740. [CrossRef] [PubMed]
28. García-Almeida, J.M.; García-García, C.; Ballesteros-Pomar, M.D.; Olveira, G.; Lopez-Gomez, J.J.; Bellido, V.; Lesmes, I.B.; Burgos, R.; Sanz-Paris, A.; Matia-Martin, P.; et al. Expert Consensus on Morphofunctional Assessment in Disease-Related Malnutrition. Grade Review and Delphi Study. *Nutrients* **2023**, *15*, 612. [CrossRef]
29. Westbury, L.D.; Beaudart, C.; Bruyère, O.; Cauley, J.A.; Cawthon, P.; Cruz-Jentoft, A.J.; Curtis, E.M.; Ensrud, K.; Fielding, R.A.; Johansson, H.; et al. Recent sarcopenia definitions-prevalence, agreement and mortality associations among men: Findings from population-based cohorts. *J. Cachexia Sarcopenia Muscle* **2023**, *14*, 565–575. [CrossRef]
30. Roberti, E.; Merlano, M.; Ravanelli, M.; Alberti, A.; Esposito, A.; Gili, R.; Spinazzé, S.; Baré, C.; Jocollé, G.; Benasso, M.; et al. Muscle quality and not quantity as a predictor of survival in head and neck squamous cell carcinoma. *Oral. Oncol.* **2023**, *145*, 106540. [CrossRef]
31. Aleixo, G.F.P.; Valente, S.A.; Wei, W.; Moore, H.C.F. Association of body composition and surgical outcomes in patients with early-stage breast cancer. *Breast Cancer Res. Treat.* **2023**, *202*, 305–311. [CrossRef] [PubMed]
32. Sheean, P.; Gonzalez, M.C.; Prado, C.M.; McKeever, L.; Hall, A.M.; Braunschweig, C.A. American Society for Parenteral and Enteral Nutrition Clinical Guidelines: The Validity of Body Composition Assessment in Clinical Populations. *JPEN J. Parenter. Enteral Nutr.* **2020**, *44*, 12–43. [CrossRef] [PubMed]

nutrients

MDPI

Article

Bioelectrical Impedance Vector Analysis, Nutritional Ultrasound®, and Handgrip Strength as Innovative Methods for Monitoring Critical Anorexia Nervosa Physical Recovery: A Pilot Study

Jose M. Romero-Márquez [1,2,*,†], María Novo-Rodríguez [1,2,†], Cristina Novo-Rodríguez [1,3], Víctor Siles-Guerrero [1], Isabel Herrera-Montes [1], Francisco Garzón Navarro-Pelayo [4], Martín López-de-la-Torre-Casares [1,3,‡] and Araceli Muñoz-Garach [1,3,5,*,‡]

1 Department of Endocrinology and Nutrition, Virgen de las Nieves University Hospital, 18014 Granada, Spain; marianovor@correo.ugr.es (M.N.-R.); cristina.novo.sspa@juntadeandalucia.es (C.N.-R.); victor.siles.sspa@juntadeandalucia.es (V.S.-G.); isabel.herrera.montes.sspa@juntadeandalucia.es (I.H.-M.); martin.lopeztorre.sspa@juntadeandalucia.es (M.L.-d.-l.-T.-C.)
2 Foundation for Biosanitary Research of Eastern Andalusia—Alejandro Otero (FIBAO), 18012 Granada, Spain
3 Granada Biosanitary Research Institute (Ibs. Granada), 18014 Granada, Spain
4 Eating Disorders Hospital Unit, Virgen de las Nieves University Hospital, 18014 Granada, Spain; francisco.garzon.n.sspa@juntadeandalucia.com
5 Network Biomedical Research Center Physiopathology of Obesity and Nutrition (CiberOBN), Carlos III Health Institute, 28029 Madrid, Spain
* Correspondence: romeromarquez@ugr.es (J.M.R.-M.); araceli.munoz.garach.sspa@juntadeandalucia.es (A.M.-G.); Tel.: +34-958-020-365 (J.M.R.-M. & A.M.-G.)
† These authors contributed equally to this work.
‡ These authors share senior position.

Abstract: Eating disorders (EDs) manifest as persistent disruptions in eating habits or related behaviors, significantly impacting physical health and psychosocial well-being. Nutritional assessment in ED patients is crucial for monitoring treatment efficacy. While dual-energy X-ray absorptiometry (DEXA) remains standard, interest in alternative methods such as bioelectrical impedance vector analysis (BIVA) and Nutritional Ultrasound® (NU) has risen due to their affordability and portability. Additionally, hand dynamometry offers a user-friendly approach to assessing grip strength (HGS), indicative of nutritional status. A prospective study was carried out to evaluate the utility of BIVA, NU®, and HGS in 43 female AN patients. Measurements were taken at baseline and hospital discharge. A total of 41 patients completed the study. After the intervention, numerous BIVA-related parameters such as fat (3.5 ± 2 kg vs. 5.3 ± 2.7 kg, $p < 0.001$) and free fat mass (33.9 ± 3.8 kg vs. 37.5 ± 4.1 kg, $p < 0.001$) were partially restored. Similarly, Nutritional Ultrasound® showed promising results in assessing body composition changes such as total abdominal fat tissue (0.5 ± 0.3 cm vs. 0.9 ± 0.3 cm, $p < 0.05$). In the same way, rectus femoris cross-sectional area values correlated with clinical outcomes such as free fat mass (0.883, $p < 0.05$) and appendicular muscle mass (0.965, $p < 0.001$). HGS reached the normality percentile after the intervention (21.6 ± 9.1 kg vs. 25.9 ± 12.3 kg, $p < 0.05$), demonstrating a significant association between grip strength and body composition parameters such as free fat mass (0.658, $p < 0.001$) and appendicular muscle mass (0.482, $p < 0.001$). Incorporating BIVA-, NU®-, and HGS-enhanced nutritional assessment into the treatment of AN patients offers cost-effective, portable, and non-invasive alternatives to DEXA. These techniques offer valuable insights into changes in body composition and nutritional status, which, in turn, facilitate treatment monitoring and contribute to improved patient outcomes.

Keywords: anorexia nervosa; body composition; anthropometric; BIVA; HGS; dynamometer; muscle mass; fat mass; rectus femoris; adipose tissue; nutrition

1. Introduction

EDs manifest as persistent disruptions in eating habits or related behaviors, significantly impacting physical health and psychosocial well-being. EDs typically emerge during adolescence, carrying significant implications for both physical and mental well-being. Addressing these disorders involves a multifaceted therapeutic approach, necessitating the involvement of various medical specialties [1]. Among these disorders, anorexia nervosa (AN) is characterized by severe dietary restriction leading to a dangerously low body weight, driven by an intense fear of weight gain and a distorted body image [2]. AN predominantly affects girls and young women, with the highest risk occurring between ages 10 and 24. The incidence and prevalence of AN have surged within this demographic, particularly since the onset of the COVID-19 pandemic [3]. Surprisingly, a recent cross-sectional study conducted on 730 adolescents from Murcia (Spain) demonstrated that 30% of the adolescents presented with disordered eating patterns, which were associated with female sex, immigrant status, and excess weight [3]. Despite concerted therapeutic efforts, treatment efficacy remains modest, with remission rates fluctuating between 40% and 60% for AN and eating disorders not otherwise specified [1,4]. This variance in remission rates is partly ascribed to the heterogeneous definition of remission, which should encompass psychological, cognitive, behavioral (such as binge eating episodes or purging behaviors), and physical aspects (classically, body mass index [BMI]) [5]. Furthermore, relapses are frequent, particularly post-hospital discharge, underscoring the importance of suitable follow-up strategies. Therefore, international guidelines [6] recommend both psychological and physical interventions for monitoring the effectiveness of the treatment for individuals with AN. Historically, anthropometric measurements have served as the primary method for assessing nutritional status and body composition in AN patients. However, these measurements (such as BMI or only weight) may not adequately differentiate between key body compartments, reflecting methodological limitations [2]. In fact, in a meta-analysis with AN patients, the primary outcome considered was solely body weight. The study revealed that adolescents experienced faster weight gain compared to adults, but this was not associated with psychological findings in treating adults with AN [7].

Currently, DEXA, magnetic resonance imaging (MRI), and computed tomography (CT) are considered the gold standard techniques for body composition analysis [8]. However, numerous constraints continue to impede their widespread adoption in routine practice. Firstly, these techniques incur significant costs and demand skilled professionals for their administration and interpretation, often requiring specialized post-processing procedures [9]. Additional challenges include patient compliance issues, such as the hyperactivity frequently observed in AN patients [10], potentially compromising the quality of scanned images and subsequent analysis. Moreover, these patients may undergo multiple evaluations, leading to heightened exposure to ionizing radiation owing to the increased radiation doses associated with these imaging modalities.

These limitations have sparked interest in alternative methods such as BIVA. BIVA offers advantages such as affordability, portability, speed, and the absence of radiation exposure, analyzing impedance vectors and phase angle data to assess body water distribution, body cell mass, and cellular integrity, serving as indicators of nutritional status [11]. Similarly, NU® employs ultrasound technology to target fat-free mass and fat mass, presenting an emerging, cost-effective, portable, and non-invasive solution. With linear, broadband, multifrequency probes capable of assessing the musculoskeletal area in-depth, it quantifies muscle modifications associated with malnutrition, providing valuable insights into functional changes within the body [12]. Additionally, the hand dynamometer provides a quick, user-friendly, and cost-effective method for assessing grip strength and, consequently, nutritional status. In fact, clinical studies across various patient populations have linked reduced grip strength, measured by hand dynamometry, with prolonged hospital stays, higher mortality rates, and increased complications [13].

The present research integrates the three aforementioned methods to conduct an in-depth characterization of body composition, specifically targeting muscle and body fat composition, as well as muscle function, in hospitalized AN patients. This research supplements these methods with laboratory parameters to elucidate the relationships among them. Therefore, the hypothesis of the present study is that the combined use of these methods will enable comprehensive monitoring of weight homeostasis recovery and enhance follow-up strategies for assessing the physical status of AN patients.

2. Materials and Methods

2.1. Study Design

This clinical practice study included 43 patients with a mean age of 28.7 ± 13.5 years who had been admitted to the Eating Disorders Hospitalization Unit (EDHU) of Virgen de las Nieves University Hospital from 2020 to 2023. Prior to admission, all female patients were diagnosed with anorexia nervosa (41) or eating disorders not otherwise specified (2) (EDNOS) according to DSM-V [14]. The inclusion criteria were the following: aged 16 years or older, a BMI of 14 or below, demonstrating genuine motivation for change and awareness of their illness, a confirmed diagnosis of AN, bulimia nervosa, or EDNOS with the severity not classified as mild, exhibiting a negative response to outpatient treatment, experiencing overwhelming or conflictive family dynamics, and displaying a tendency towards social isolation stemming from the illness.

2.2. Psychiatric and Nutritional Intervention in EDHU

Some outcomes were monitored during the EDHU hospitalization program, including the normalization of eating patterns, food exposure, intervention on compensatory behaviors such as compulsive physical exercise, vomiting, or the use of laxatives, acquisition and improvement of disease awareness, and restructuring of the main beliefs, thoughts, and attitudes, as well as basic altered emotions, about diet, weight, and body image. The psychiatric and nutritional care comprised a therapeutic dining room to restore eating patterns, with the goal of recovering from physical and environmental problems. Similarly, an eating behaviors intervention was implemented with the goal of normalizing eating behavior and aiding the transition to an outpatient setting. The idea was to offer tailored attention to each disorder's most defining eating patterns in the present moment. A thorough inspection of the tray prepared for the event was conducted, including all of the things previously established on the menu (sugar, oil, etc.). A registered dietitian prescribed a diet based on each patient's calorie and protein requirements. The diet was validated by medical indication (psychiatry and endocrinology units) and monitored by nursing personnel. Additionally, the EDHU presents a reliable protocol to prevent refeeding syndrome, which involves the administration of vitamins B1, B6, and B12, along with serum therapy recommendations. The decision to include or exclude potassium chloride, monosodium phosphate, and magnesium sulfate in serum therapy was determined by analytical findings.

2.3. Anthropometric Measurements

At baseline, a stadiometer was used to measure height, and weight was calculated using a calibrated weighing scale set (certified test weights ± 0.1 kg) (SECA 665, Hamburg, Germany). Calf (CC) and arm circumferences (AC), as well as triceps skinfold thickness (TST), were measured according to recommendations [15]. All measurements were taken during hospital admission and release. The procedure, performed by experienced professionals, aimed to minimize measurement variability at hospital admission and discharge.

2.4. Bioelectrical Impedance Vector Analysis

Whole-body BIVA measurements were conducted using a 50 kHz phase-sensitive impedance analyzer (BIA 101 AKERN, Pontassieve, Italy) with tetrapolar 800 mA wearable electrodes on the right hand and foot as previously reported [16]. The body's complex circuits, involving resistance (Rz) and reactance (Xc) elements, were stimulated with an alternating current to determine phase angle (PhA). According to standard protocol [17], one impedance adhesive electrode (Biatrodes Akern Srl, Florence, Italy) was placed on the back of the right hand (center of the third proximal phalanx) and the other electrode on the neck of the corresponding foot (proximal to the second and third metatarsophalangeal joints). BIVA interpretation, introduced by Piccoli et al. [18], involves plotting standardized Rz and Xc values on a resistance—reactance graph, enabling direct assessment of impedance without relying on body weight, equations, or models. Bioelectrical parameters were analyzed to estimate body composition, including fat mass (FM), fat-free mass (FFM), body cell mass (BMC), total muscle mass (TMM), appendicular skeletal muscle mass (ASMM), total body water (TBW), and extracellular body water (ECW). The procedure, performed by experienced professionals, aimed to minimize measurement variability at hospital admission and discharge.

2.5. Nutritional Ultrasound®

NU was carried out as previously reported [16]. Briefly, a HITACHI ALOKA F37 ultrasound scanner (Hitachi healthcare, Tokyo, Japan) and an Aloka UST-5413 Linear Array (10–12 MHz) transducer (Hitachi healthcare, Tokyo, Japan) were employed. Patients were positioned supine with a specified limb alignment and assessed by experienced specialists using water-soluble transmission gel. The pictures of the right rectus femoris (RF) muscle were taken one-third of the way between the patella and the iliac crest, beginning at the patella. The rectus femoris cross-sectional area (RF-CSA), RF axis (-X and -Y axes), and leg subcutaneous fat (L-SAT) were all measured as presented in Figure 1A. Rectus femoris was selected due to the correlation with metabolically active FFM [12]. The examination extended at the abdominal level, measuring at the midway between the xiphoid appendix and the navel. Measures comprised total subcutaneous abdominal adipose tissue (T-SAT), superficial subcutaneous abdominal fat (S-SAT), and total visceral adipose tissue (VAT), which were associated with the amount of fat deposits and their distribution (Figure 1B) [12]. The procedure, performed by experienced professionals, aimed to minimize measurement variability at hospital admission and discharge.

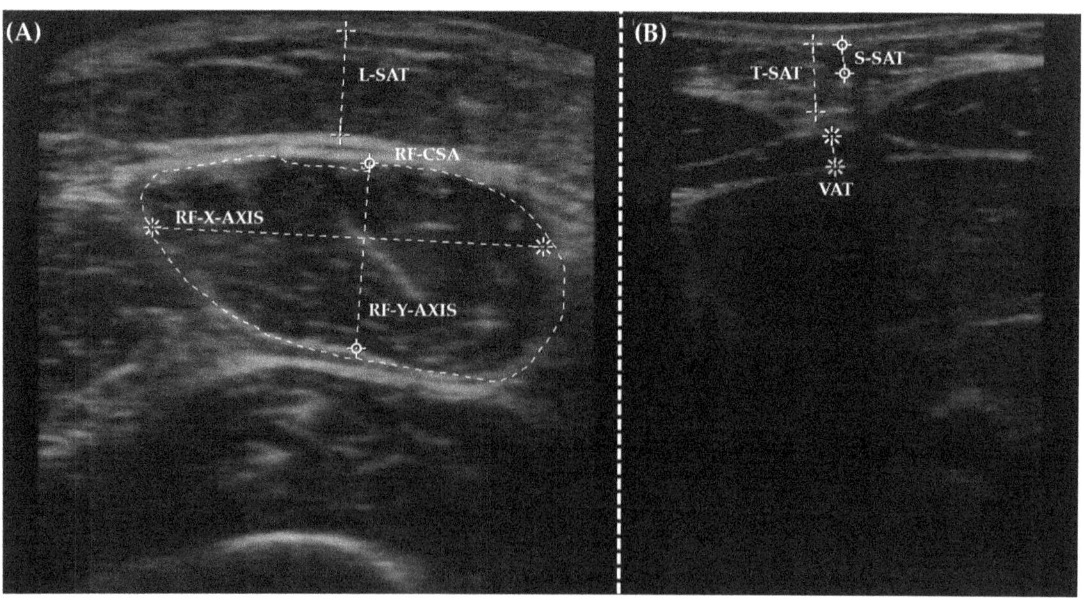

Figure 1. Illustrative captures of Nutritional Ultrasound® in the (**A**) rectus femoris and (**B**) abdomen.

2.6. Handgrip Strength Analysis

The measurement of hand grip strength (HGS) in the dominant hand was performed using a Jamar dynamometer (Asimow Engineering Co., Los Angeles, CA, USA). Patients were positioned in a seated posture with the wrist and forearm in a neutral position, the elbow bent at a 90-degree angle, the forearm neutrally rotated, and the shoulder adducted. To ensure accuracy, the mean value was calculated by instructing patients to perform three consecutive contractions spaced one minute apart as previously reported [16]. The procedure, performed by experienced professionals, aimed to minimize measurement variability at hospital admission and discharge.

2.7. Biochemical Analysis

Biomolecular markers were assessed to analyze nutrition and inflammation status, including glucose, creatinine, proteins, albumin, prealbumin, phosphorus, calcium, magnesium, potassium, C-reactive protein (CRP), total cholesterol (TC), and triglycerides levels.

2.8. Statistical Analysis

The statistical program IBM SPSS 25 (Chicago, IL, USA) was used to examine normality, variance homogeneity, and Pearson's correlation. Physical recovery results were analyzed using paired sample *t*-tests, with *p*-values < 0.05 indicating significance. In addition, the MetaboAnalyst V5.0 software was used to perform Partial Least Squares Discriminant Analysis (PLS-DA). PLS-DA was used to assess the normalized and autoscaled mean values of the 32 variables collected from the patients. In this PLS-DA, the variables of significance in projection (VIP) score selection criteria were values greater than one, equivalent to $p < 0.05$. The current study used an intention-to-treat analysis, with two patients who did not complete therapy included in the first analysis.

3. Results and Discussion

3.1. Body Composition Analysis in Critical AN Patients

A total of 41 patients completed the study, spending a mean of 49 $\pm$ 20.2 days in the unit. The patients had a mean age of 28 $\pm$ 13.2 years. Table 1 details the population characteristics upon hospital admission and discharge. As anticipated, the nutritional and psychiatric interventions led to an increase in body weight and BMI, aligning with the standard physical monitoring protocol for AN patients, as outlined previously [2,19]. Interestingly, the AC values increased after the intervention. This finding is corroborated by the TST value, which was higher at discharge, suggesting increased body fat deposition in the upper extremities. Although not statistically significant, there was a noticeable trend towards an increase in CC, suggesting a potential recovery of tissue in this region.

According to BIVA parameters, the PhA values did not change after the intervention. However, three studies have suggested that PhA improved following nutritional intervention in AN patients. Interestingly, these studies, which assessed the physical recovery of AN patients, reported significantly higher body weight and BMI compared to those presented in this study [2,19,20]. Indeed, the presented PhA was lower than that reported in the scientific literature [2,19], likely attributable to the critical condition of AN patients upon hospital admission. Notably, in 2012, Haas et al. demonstrated that short-term multidisciplinary interventions did not alter PhA in AN patients with comparable body weight and BMI to those in this study [21]. These results suggest that in cases of extremely low body weight, PhA might not serve as a reliable predictive tool for physical recovery in critical AN patients. In contrast, the FM and FFM values increased after the intervention, aligning with the reported body weight gain [2,19,20]. Likewise, the intervention resulted in increased ASMM values, as corroborated by the AC and CC values. This increase in muscle mass was accompanied by rises in extracellular and total body water content, consistent with findings from previously published studies that monitored changes in body composition during refeeding of patients with AN [2,19,22,23]. In recent years, there has been a growing focus on muscle gain as part of AN recovery efforts. Indeed, a recent systematic review demonstrated that therapeutic exercise led to an increase in muscle mass and was associated with improvements in anorexia symptoms, as well as physical and mental health [24]. Consequently, prioritizing muscle regain should be a central aspect of physical recovery for these patients.

Table 1. Population characteristics before and after psychiatric and nutritional intervention.

	EDHU Admission	95% CI Admission	EDHU Discharge	95% CI Discharge	*p*-Value
Anthropometry					
Weight (kg)	37.4 (4.5)	28–47.1	42.8 (4.5)	32.1–51.9	<0.001
BMI (kg/m^2)	14.3 (1.5)	11.4–17.3	16.3 (1.1)	13.1–18.6	<0.001
AC (cm)	18.2 (6.1)	14.18–21.5	19.9 (9.2)	16–23	<0.001
CC (cm)	27.8 (11.2)	20–31	29.1 (14.3)	23–33	0.052
TST (mm)	4.4 (2.7)	1.2–8.5	5.7 (3.3)	1.5–11	<0.01
BIVA					
PhA (°)	4.8 (0.7)	3.3–6	4.7 (0.5)	3.5–5.9	0.972
FM (kg)	3.5 (2)	1.7–10	5.3 (2.7)	1.7–12.6	<0.001
FFM (kg)	33.9 (3.8)	26.2–42.6	37.5 (4.1)	25.8–47.9	<0.001
TBW (L)	26.1 (2.7)	19.6–31.9	29.2 (7.3)	21.4–71.6	<0.05
ECW (L)	13.3 (2.0)	9.6–18	15 (4.4)	8.9–38.4	<0.05
BCM (kg)	15.8 (2.5)	10.2–20.9	17.4 (2.2)	11.3–21.8	<0.01
TMM (kg)	18.1 (2.5)	13.3–23	19.2 (2.8)	14.2–27.6	0.110
ASMM (kg)	12.5 (1.7)	9–16.2	13.4 (1.9)	10–18	<0.05
Functional measurement					
HGS max (kg)	21.6 (9.1)	8–35	25.9 (12.3)	14–37	<0.05
Nutritional Ultrasound®					
RF-CSA (cm^2)	3.2 (1.5)	1.4–4.0	3.7 (1.3)	3–4.4	0.284
RF-X-axis (cm)	3.4 (1.6)	2.9–4.0	3.2 (1.1)	2.9–3.4	0.750
RF-*Y*-axis (cm)	1.2 (0.55)	0.8–1.7	1.5 (0.5)	1.3–1.7	0.413
L-SAT (cm)	0.4 (0.26)	0.1–1.1	0.7 (0.27)	0.4–1.3	0.270
T-SAT (cm)	0.5 (0.3)	0.2–1.1	0.9 (0.3)	0.7–1.3	<0.05
S-SAT (cm)	0.3 (0.2)	0.1–0.8	0.4 (0.2)	0.3–0.6	0.074
VAT (cm)	0.3 (0.1)	0.1–0.5	0.4 (0.1)	0.2–0.6	0.154
Biochemical analysis					
Glucose (mg/dL)	69.4 (27.5)	41–85	76.7 (14.5)	56–93	<0.01
Creatinine (mg/dL)	0.7 (0.3)	0.5–1.1	0.6 (0.2)	0.5–0.9	0.051
Proteins (g/dL)	6.6 (2.7)	4.5–8.5	6.8 (2.2)	4–8.4	0.541
Albumin (mg/dL)	4.3 (1.7)	3.1–5.7	4.4 (1.2)	3.3–5.7	0.731
Prealbumin (mg/dL)	29.8 (21.0)	16–101	27.3 (7.2)	20–37	0.488
CPR (mg/L)	4.3 (8.6)	0.2–32	0.5 (0.5)	0.2–3.2	<0.05
Total cholesterol (mg/dL)	160.9 (98.4)	0.2–403	174.1 (60.2)	1.5–269	0.373
Triglycerides (mg/dL)	96.6 (59)	30–280	70 (41.5)	21–205	<0.05
Calcium (mg/dL)	9 (3.4)	7.8–10.4	9.1 (2.4)	7.7–9.9	0.455
Phosphorus (mg/dL)	3.6 (1.6)	1.9–5.3	4.3 (0.8)	3.5–5.2	<0.001
Magnesium (mg/dL)	2.0 (0.8)	1.8–2.9	1.9 (0.5)	1.6–2.3	0.099
Potassium (mg/dL)	4.2 (1.7)	3.6–5	4.2 (0.8)	1.4–5.3	0.790

Data are expressed as mean ± standard deviations. Abbreviations: AC: arm circumference; ASMM: appendicular skeletal muscle mass; BCM: body cell mass; CC: calf circumference; CI: confidence interval; CPR: C-reactive protein concentration; ECW: extracellular water volume; FFM: fat-free mass; FM: fat mass; HGS max: maximum handgrip strength; PhA: phase angle; RF-CSA: Rectus femoris cross-sectional area; RF-*X*-axis: rectus femoris *X*-axis length; RF-*Y*-axis: rectus femoris *Y*-axis length; SAT: Subcutaneous adipose fat of leg (L), and superficial (S) and total (T) abdominal; TST: triceps skinfold thickness; TBW: total body water volume; TMM: total muscle mass; VAT: visceral adipose tissue.

The ultrasound adipose-related parameters indicated an increase in T-SAT values, mirroring the observed increase in FM and supporting adipose tissue gain, particularly in the trunk. These results were supported by Lackner et al., who showed similar upper abdominal SAT values in AN patients using a linear probe (L8-18i RS) with similar conditions (8–16 MHz) [25]. Similarly, although not statistically significant, a slight trend was observed in S-SAT and L-SAT values. These findings align with studies that assessed body fat distribution using the DEXA method in AN patients. These studies demonstrated that following partial weight restoration, body fat deposition was more pronounced in the trunk region compared to the legs [26–28].

In contrast, the ultrasound muscle-related parameter did not detect slight variations in muscle gain. This could be attributed to the small variation in ASMM gain during the stay, which may not have been sufficient to manifest in the spatial muscle distribution of RF. These results are consistent with findings by Franzoni et al., who evaluated muscle content in the total body and lumbar spine (L1–L4) using the DEXA method in AN patients. Following a 12-month multidisciplinary intervention, an increase in body weight was observed but was not associated with local or total skeletal muscle mass gain [26]. Indeed, a systematic review investigating muscle recovery in AN patients post-intervention suggests lower muscle mass despite weight regain in this population. While these differences often did not reach significance in individual studies, the general trend in the current literature points towards incomplete muscle recovery after AN [29]. These findings are particularly compelling due to the high replicability and correlation observed between NU and DEXA methods. The ultrasound approach is a swift and reliable procedure that enables the direct evaluation of muscular and adipose tissue distribution during medical consultations. Therefore, NU could serve as a valuable tool for assessing the location-specific distribution of adipose and muscular tissue, potentially reducing healthcare costs and time spent on body composition evaluation for these patients.

According to body strength, limited evidence suggests that AN patients exhibit lower strength in both their legs [30,31] and arms [30] compared to healthy BMI-matched individuals in these studies. In this study, the mean initial HGS values were 21.6 $\pm$ 9.1 kg, which corresponds to the 25th percentile of the Andalusian population as reported using a validated Jamar dynamometer [13]. To the best of our knowledge, this is the first study to utilize HGS for monitoring physical recovery in AN patients. Interestingly, following multidisciplinary intervention, AN patients demonstrated an increase in mean HGS values (25.9 $\pm$ 12.3 kg), reaching the 50th percentile [13]. The hand dynamometer provides a swift, easy-to-use, and economical approach with which to evaluate grip strength, which can indicate the nutritional health of patients. Many clinical investigations involving various patient groups (such as those undergoing surgery, elderly individuals, cancer patients, etc.) have demonstrated that lower grip strength, assessed via hand dynamometry, is linked to longer hospital stays, elevated mortality rates, and heightened complications [13]. Therefore, potential rehabilitation programs or interventions should include physical activity, focused on strengthening muscle mass.

Most of the AN patients were admitted to the EDHU in a hypoglycemic state, which is a common feature in this population [32,33]. Interestingly, the multidisciplinary intervention successfully restored blood glucose levels to normal values, thereby reducing the potential occurrence of associated clinical comorbidities. In contrast, markers related to protein metabolism (creatinine, proteins, albumin, and prealbumin) were not affected by the multidisciplinary intervention. It is worth noting that all parameters remained within the normal range according to the Andalucía Health System (AHS). These findings were supported by a systematic review conducted by Lee et al., which evaluated the modulation of serum protein levels in both pathological and non-calorically restricted patients [34]. In this study, the albumin and prealbumin ranges in AN patients, matched for BMI, were similar to those presented in this manuscript, with modifications only observed in cases of extremely low BMI (<10 kg/m^2) [34]. These findings suggest that in such cases, serum protein markers may not be optimal for monitoring physical recovery in AN patients.

On the other hand, lipid-related metabolism showed a reduction in triglyceride levels but not in TC levels after weight gain. A recent systematic review with meta-analysis revealed a lack of consistency in results regarding these parameters following partial weight restoration. The authors noted that serum lipid modification varies significantly depending on the initial status of AN patients, indicating the need for more evidence in this field to better understand the pathophysiology of AN [35].

CRP is an acute-phase protein commonly used in biochemical analysis to monitor inflammation or infectious processes [36]. In the case of AN patients, four cross-sectional studies [37–40] and one longitudinal study [41] have indicated that AN patients typically exhibit lower CRP serum levels compared to BMI-matched healthy controls. In this study, the mean CRP value of the AN patients before the multidisciplinary intervention fell within the range defined by the AHS, with some values skewing towards the upper limit, indicating a trend towards being elevated. Interestingly, after the intervention, the serum CRP decreased by 8.6 times, with minimal dispersion of the data. The only study that evaluated changes in serum CRP levels in AN patients demonstrated no significant difference in CRP levels before and after weight gain. Remarkably, the initial BMI (16.7 ± 1.2 kg/m^2) and serum CRP levels (0.32 ± 0.25 mg/L) were similar to those obtained after the intervention in this research [41]. Considering the critical condition of the presented AN patients, these results suggest that after partial weight gain, CRP levels might be partially restored and may not be sensitive to slight weight gain, as reported in other studies [41]. Interestingly, an elevation in inflammatory markers has been linked to appetite suppression [42]. While there is no direct evidence of the correlation between CRP levels and appetite reduction, lowering CRP levels may represent a significant goal to pursue during the physical recovery phase of AN.

Finally, phosphorus but not calcium, magnesium, or potassium serum levels were increased after the intervention. Maintaining phosphorus homeostasis is crucial in managing AN due to refeeding hypophosphatemia (RH), which is commonly observed in these patients and complicates treatment [43]. These findings suggest that the nutritional intervention, particularly the refeeding protocol, was effective in preventing refeeding hypophosphatemia (RH) in critical patients with AN and partially promoting physical recovery in this population.

3.2. Pearson's Correlation Matrix Analysis

To identify potential connections between the evaluated parameters, Pearson's correlation analysis was conducted by selecting the most significant variables identified by the paired t-test and VIP scores from PLS-DA.

As depicted in Table 2, weight showed a moderate positive association with AC (0.414, $p < 0.05$). According to BIVA, weight exhibited moderate associations with FM (0.424, $p < 0.001$), TBW (0.351, $p < 0.05$), and ECW (0.318, $p < 0.05$). Interestingly, a very strong correlation was observed with FFM (0.805, $p < 0.001$) and BCM (0.789, $p < 0.05$), suggesting the very lean status of AN patients upon admission, as expected. In terms of HGS values, weight demonstrated a moderate association (0.510, $p < 0.001$), implying that patients with a higher body weight may exhibit improved HGS measures. This finding is consistent with a recent review demonstrating significant muscle atrophy and functional loss in AN patients [44]. These findings suggest that improving HGS could be an important outcome to target during the process of weight regain.

The most significant evidence from the biochemical analysis revealed a negative-to-moderate correlation between weight and CRP (-0.373, $p < 0.05$), indicating that extremely low body weight is associated with higher serum CRP levels. In terms of BMI correlation, the most notable association was observed with FM (0.593, $p < 0.001$) and NU parameters. Interestingly, BMI exhibited a strong negative association with the RF-Y axis (-0.828, $p < 0.05$) and T-SAT (-0.842, $p < 0.05$). These findings suggest that upon admission, AN patients may not only present with reduced total muscle mass but also significant depletion of lower limb muscle and central adiposity, as previously reported [30,31]. Therefore, focusing on muscle regain must play a central role in the physical recovery of these patients.

Table 2. Pearson's correlation analysis of classical anthropometry, BIVA, handgrip strength, and nutritional ultrasound® with the rest of the parameters on admission time.

	Anthropometry		BIVA		Functional	Ultrasound	
	Weight	**BMI**	**FM**	**BCM**	**HGS Max**	**RF-CSA**	**T-SAT**
Anthropometry							
Weight (kg)	1 **	0.510 **	0.424 **	0.789 **	0.386 *	-	-
BMI (kg/m^2)	0.510 **	1 **	0.593 **	0.400 **	-	-	−0.842 *
AC (cm)	0.414 *	0.516 **	0.430 *	-	-	-	−0.937 **
CC (cm)	-	-	-	-	-	-	-
TST (mm)	-	0.430 *	0.589 **	-	−0.414 *	-	-
BIVA							
PhA (°)	-	0.491 **	0.424 **	0.554 **	-	-	-
FM (kg)	0.424 **	0.593 **	1 **	-	−0.372 *	-	-
FFM (kg)	0.805 **	-	-	0.818 **	0.658 **	0.883 *	-
TBW (L)	0.351 *	-	-	0.365 **	0.359 *	-	-
ECW (L)	0.318 *	-	−0.365 *	-	0.399 *	-	-
BCM (kg)	0.789 *	0.400 **	-	1 **	0.671 **	-	-
TMM (kg)	-	-	−0.435 **	0.356 **	0.473 **	0.966 **	-
ASMM (kg)	-	-	−0.406 **	0.387 **	0.482 **	0.965 **	-
Functional parameters							
HGS max (kg)	0.386 *	-	−0.372 *	0.671 **	1 **	-	-
Time spent on the unit (days)	-	-	−0.347 *	-	-	-	-
Nutritional Ultrasound®							
RF-CSA (cm^2)	-	-	-	-	-	1 **	-
RF-*X*-axis (cm)	-	-	-	-	-	-	-
RF-*Y*-axis (cm)	-	−0.828 *	-	-	-	-	0.933 **
L-SAT (cm)	-	-	-	-	-	-	-
T-SAT (cm)	-	−0.842 *	-	-	-	-	1 **
S-SAT (cm)	-	-	-	-	-	-	-
VAT (cm)	-	-	-	-	-	-	-
Biochemical analysis							
Glucose (mg/dL)	-	-	-	-	-	-	-
Creatinine (mg/dL)	-	-	-	-	-	-	0.918 **
Proteins (g/dL)	-	-	0.364 *	-	-	-	-
Albumin (mg/dL)	−0.351 *	-	-	−0.324 *	-	-	-
Prealbumin (mg/dL)	-	-	-	-	-	-	-
CPR (mg/L)	−0.424 **	−0.373 *	-	−0.460 **	-	-	-
Total cholesterol (mg/dL)	-	-	-	-	-	-	-
Triglycerides (mg/dL)	−0.369 *	−0.352 *	-	−0.365 **	-	-	-
Calcium (mg/dL)	-	-	0.331 *	-	-	-	-
Phosphorus (mg/dL)	-	-	-	-	-	-	-
Magnesium (mg/dL)	0.342 *	-	-	-	-	-	-
Potassium (mg/dL)	-	-	-	-	-	-	-

Pearson's Correlation Analysis was assumed significant with p-value < 0.05 (* means < 0.05 and ** means p < 0.001); "-" means absence of association. Abbreviations: AC: arm circumference; ASMM: appendicular skeletal muscle mass; BCM: body cell mass; CC: calf circumference; CPR: C-reactive protein concentration; ECW: extracellular water volume; FFM: fat-free mass; FM: fat mass; HGS max: maximum handgrip strength; PhA: phase angle; RF-CSA: Rectus femoris cross-sectional area; RF-*X*-axis: rectus femoris *X*-axis length; RF-*Y*-axis: rectus femoris *Y*-axis length; SAT: Subcutaneous adipose fat of leg (L), and superficial (S) and total (T) abdominal; TST: triceps skinfold thickness; TBW: total body water volume; TMM: total muscle mass; VAT: visceral adipose tissue.

According to BIVA-related parameters, the most significant association observed was the negative correlation between FM and the duration of hospital admission (−0.347, $p < 0.05$), suggesting that patients with higher body fat mass may have a shorter hospital stay. This result is extremely interesting as the early detection of eating disorders could lead to less severe physical consequences such as central adiposity depletion, resulting in shorter hospital stays and reduced healthcare costs. To the best of our knowledge, this is the first study to correlate body composition with the duration of hospital admission. These findings are particularly noteworthy as they allow for a focus not only on weight but also on body fat mass as a potential target for monitoring physical recovery. Additionally, FM exhibited a moderate association with calcium levels (0.331, $p < 0.05$), which may be related to bone metabolism. While this study did not investigate bone mineral density (BMD), it has been noted that gaining FM has been identified as a crucial element linked with BMD enhancement in individuals with AN [45,46]. Achamrah et al. underscored that attaining normal bone levels is not solely tied to weight gain, emphasizing the significance of acknowledging the contribution of fat mass to the underlying mechanisms of osteoporosis and osteopenia in AN [45].

On the other hand, BCM values were closely associated with weight (0.789, $p < 0.001$) and BMI (0.400, $p < 0.001$). Moreover, BCM exhibited a strong association with hand strength (0.671, $p < 0.001$), suggesting that active cellular mass contributes to strength in these patients. Similarly, an increase in BCM was negatively associated with higher markers of inflammation such as CRP (−0.460, $p < 0.001$). Furthermore, HGS was associated with most muscle-related BIVA parameters such as TMM (0.473, $p < 0.001$), ASMM (0.482, $p < 0.001$), and FFM (0.658, $p < 0.001$). These findings underscore the validity of BIVA and HGS for analyzing muscle status and its functionality. Likewise, HGS may serve as a valuable and efficient predictor during consultations to assess muscle deterioration.

Regarding muscle-related NU parameters, RF-CSA showed strong associations with FFM (0.883, $p < 0.05$), TMM (0.966, $p < 0.001$), and ASMM (0.965, $p < 0.001$). These results also confirm the validity of this method for analyzing body composition and its reliability compared to other methods such as BIVA. Importantly, RF-CSA was not associated with body weight, BMI, or hydration status, indicating that it could be a useful tool when certain AN-related behaviors occur, such as vomiting or purgative use, which can compromise body weight and its derived measures.

Finally, T-SAT exhibited a strong and negative association with BMI (−0.842, $p < 0.05$) and AC (−0.937, $p < 0.001$) values upon admission. Once more, NU appears to be a valuable tool for monitoring physical recovery in AN patients, indicating a significant reduction in body fat composition upon admission. Similarly, patients with higher central adiposity were associated with longer RF (0.933, $p < 0.001$), as demonstrated in Table 2. These findings are supported by a recent review that highlighted significant muscle atrophy during weight loss-related starvation in AN patients [44].

3.3. Partial Least Squares-Discriminant Analysis

PLS-DA stands out as a valuable algorithm used for both predictive and descriptive modeling, as well as for selecting discriminative variables. It has demonstrated notable efficacy in handling complex datasets across various fields, including public health [47]. In this research, a threshold higher than 1 (equivalent to $p < 0.05$) was set as the criterion for selecting the VIP score in PLS-DA, as shown by a dashed vertical line in Figure 2B. Similarly, Figure 1A illustrates the PLS-DA analysis focusing on patients' admission and discharge from the EDHU. The analysis revealed a slight overlap of the groups. Notably, the time to discharge for critical AN patients was approximately 50 days. However, there was an interesting trend in the spatial distribution towards the top-right part of the plot, indicating a tendency to differentiate between patients at admission and discharge times. The VIP score indicated that over 34% of the studied parameters might contribute to the observed effects. Notably, HGS values were identified by VIP score as the most significant variable for distinguishing between EDHU admission and discharge. As mentioned earlier, this parameter was also related to most of the BIVA muscular-related parameters. Similarly, body composition parameters such as FM, FFM, and ECW were also identified by VIP score as modulators of physical recovery, corroborated by Pearson's correlation analysis. Additionally, the reduction of CRP after the intervention was also identified as a contributor to these differences.

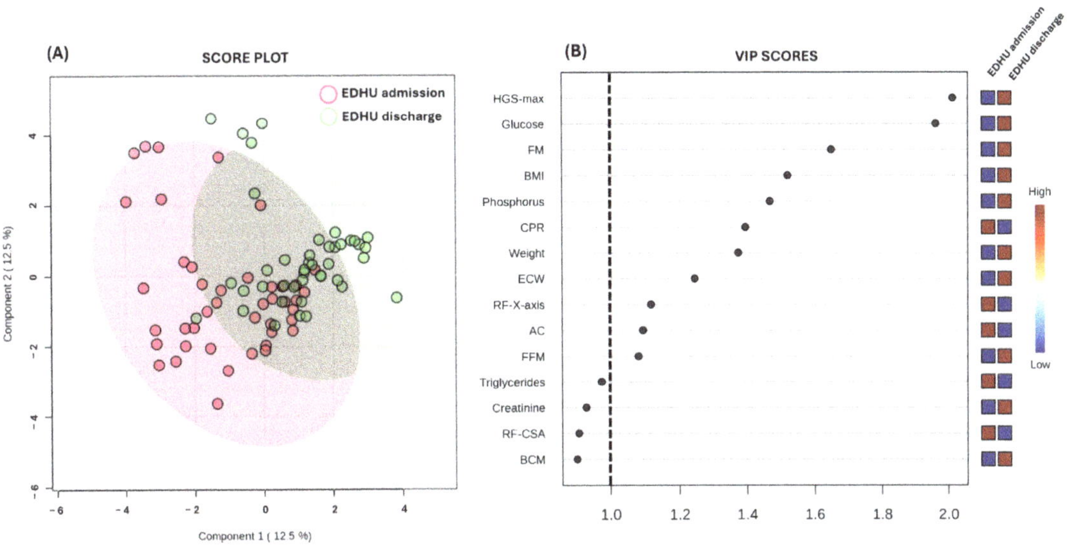

Figure 2. (**A**) PLS-DA score plot obtained from the mean values of the 32 parameters evaluated. (**B**) VIP score plots for the top 15 most important features by PLS-DA. The heatmap indicates the relative importance of the specific parameter in the different subpopulations and the dashed line represents statistical significance at $p < 0.05$. Abbreviations: AC: arm circumference; BCM: body cell mass; CPR: C-reactive protein concentration; ECW: extracellular water volume; FFM: fat-free mass; FM: fat mass; HGS max: maximum handgrip strength; RF-X-axis: rectus femoris X-axis length.

Interestingly, among the 11 parameters identified by VIP score as the main contributors before and after the intervention, 27% of the parameters were BIVA-related, 27% were from classical anthropometry, 27% were from biochemical analysis, and 18% were from HGS and NU. These findings are highly significant as they suggest that the rapid implementation of these nutritional assessment methods could enhance the screening for physical recovery in AN patients, thereby facilitating the provision of personalized therapeutic interventions.

4. Conclusions

In conclusion, this comprehensive study sheds light on the intricate interplay between various physiological parameters during the multidisciplinary intervention for patients with AN. Numerous BIVA-related parameters such as fat and free fat mass were partially restored. Similarly, NU showed results in assessing body composition changes such as total abdominal fat tissue, correlating with clinical outcomes such as free fat mass and appendicular muscle mass. Hand dynamometry reached the normality percentile, demonstrating a significant association between grip strength and body composition parameters such as free fat mass and appendicular muscle mass. Leveraging advanced techniques such as BIVA, NU, HGS, and biochemical analysis alongside classical anthropometry, the research reveals nuanced insights into the physical recovery process. Notably, the significant associations identified between body composition parameters, inflammatory markers, and functional indicators underscore the complexity of AN management and highlight the potential for personalized therapeutic approaches tailored to individual patient needs.

Furthermore, the integration of predictive modeling techniques such as PLS-DA offers valuable insights into the key contributors to physical recovery before and after intervention. With hand strength, BIVA-related parameters (extracellular water and fat and free fat mass), classical anthropometry (weight, BMI, and AC), biochemical markers (glucose, CPR, and phosphorus), and NU (RF-X-axis) emerging as significant predictors, the study emphasizes the importance of a multidimensional approach in monitoring and evaluating AN patients.

The limitation of the present research lies in the nature of the techniques employed. Although BIVA and NU serve as good alternatives to DEXA, they necessitate an initial outlay to acquire the equipment. Similarly, both methods rely on trained personnel, and interoperator variability may exist. Furthermore, while multivariate analysis can identify important variables, it does not establish causal associations. However, the utilization of both VIP scores and Pearson correlation enables the assignment of a specific marker's role in the observed effect.

These findings highlighted the potential for the rapid implementation of advanced nutritional assessment methods to enhance screening and optimize therapeutic strategies, ultimately improving outcomes for individuals undergoing treatment for anorexia nervosa.

Author Contributions: Conceptualization, I.H.-M.; methodology, M.N.-R. and I.H.-M.; validation, A.M.-G. and C.N.-R.; formal analysis, J.M.R.-M.; investigation, J.M.R.-M., M.N.-R., V.S.-G., F.G.N.-P. and I.H.-M.; resources, M.L.-d.-l.-T.-C.; data curation, J.M.R.-M.; writing—original draft preparation, J.M.R.-M.; writing—review and editing, J.M.R.-M., A.M.-G., C.N.-R. and M.L.-d.-l.-T.-C.; visualization, A.M.-G. and C.N.-R.; supervision, I.H.-M.; project administration, I.H.-M. and A.M.-G.; funding acquisition, M.L.-d.-l.-T.-C. and A.M.-G. All authors have read and agreed to the published version of the manuscript.

Funding: This research received no external funding.

Institutional Review Board Statement: The study was conducted in accordance with the Declaration of Helsinki. This prospective real clinical practice study was conducted in a double-blind fashion, ensuring the anonymity of participating patients. Informed consent was obtained orally from each patient. The local ethics committee waived approval because no personal data were utilized, and the study did not involve invasive procedures, extraction of biological samples, or testing new drugs, thus not requiring external committee review beyond approval from the hospital unit and management.

Informed Consent Statement: Informed consent was obtained from all subjects involved in the study. Written informed consent has been obtained from the patients to publish this paper.

Data Availability Statement: The original contributions presented in the study are included in the article, further inquiries can be directed to the corresponding authors.

Acknowledgments: Jose M. Romero-Márquez and María Novo-Rodríguez are researchers funded by the Foundation for Biosanitary Research of Eastern Andalusia—Alejandro Otero (FIBAO).

Conflicts of Interest: The authors declare no conflict of interest.

References

1. Monteleone, A.M.; Pellegrino, F.; Croatto, G.; Carfagno, M.; Hilbert, A.; Treasure, J.; Wade, T.; Bulik, C.; Zipfel, S.; Hay, P.; et al. Treatment of Eating Disorders: A Systematic Meta-Review of Meta-Analyses and Network Meta-Analyses. *Neurosci. Biobehav. Rev.* **2022**, *142*, 104857. [CrossRef] [PubMed]
2. Murray Hurtado, M.; Martín Rivada, Á.; Quintero Alemán, C.; Ruiz Alcántara, M.P.; Ramallo Fariña, Y. Body Composition and Nutritional Status Changes in Adolescents with Anorexia Nervosa. *An. Pediatría (Engl. Ed.)* **2023**, *99*, 162–169. [CrossRef] [PubMed]
3. López-Gil, J.F.; Jiménez-López, E.; Fernández-Rodríguez, R.; Garrido-Miguel, M.; Victoria-Montesinos, D.; Gutiérrez-Espinoza, H.; Tárraga-López, P.J.; Mesas, A.E. Prevalence of Disordered Eating and Its Associated Factors From a Socioecological Approach Among a Sample of Spanish Adolescents: The EHDLA Study. *Int. J. Public Health* **2023**, *68*, 1605820. [CrossRef] [PubMed]
4. Eddy, K.T.; Tabri, N.; Thomas, J.J.; Murray, H.B.; Keshaviah, A.; Hastings, E.; Edkins, K.; Krishna, M.; Herzog, D.B.; Keel, P.K.; et al. Recovery From Anorexia Nervosa and Bulimia Nervosa at 22-Year Follow-Up. *J. Clin. Psychiatry* **2017**, *78*, 184–189. [CrossRef] [PubMed]
5. Bardone-Cone, A.M.; Hunt, R.A.; Watson, H.J. An Overview of Conceptualizations of Eating Disorder Recovery, Recent Findings, and Future Directions. *Curr. Psychiatry Rep.* **2018**, *20*, 79. [CrossRef] [PubMed]
6. National Guideline Alliance (UK). *Eating Disorders: Recognition and Treatment*; National Institute for Health and Care Excellence: Guidelines; National Institute for Health and Care Excellence (NICE): London, UK, 2017.
7. Zeeck, A.; Herpertz-Dahlmann, B.; Friederich, H.-C.; Brockmeyer, T.; Resmark, G.; Hagenah, U.; Ehrlich, S.; Cuntz, U.; Zipfel, S.; Hartmann, A. Psychotherapeutic Treatment for Anorexia Nervosa: A Systematic Review and Network Meta-Analysis. *Front. Psychiatry* **2018**, *9*, 158. [CrossRef] [PubMed]

8. Plank, L.D. Dual-Energy X-Ray Absorptiometry and Body Composition. *Curr. Opin. Clin. Nutr. Metab. Care* **2005**, *8*, 305. [CrossRef] [PubMed]
9. Messina, C.; Albano, D.; Gitto, S.; Tofanelli, L.; Bazzocchi, A.; Ulivieri, F.M.; Guglielmi, G.; Sconfienza, L.M. Body Composition with Dual Energy X-Ray Absorptiometry: From Basics to New Tools. *Quant. Imaging Med. Surg.* **2020**, *10*, 1687–1698. [CrossRef]
10. Carrera, O.; Adan, R.A.H.; Gutierrez, E.; Danner, U.N.; Hoek, H.W.; van Elburg, A.A.; Kas, M.J.H. Hyperactivity in Anorexia Nervosa: Warming Up Not Just Burning-Off Calories. *PLoS ONE* **2012**, *7*, e41851. [CrossRef]
11. Silva, A.M.; Campa, F.; Stagi, S.; Gobbo, L.A.; Buffa, R.; Toselli, S.; Silva, D.A.S.; Gonçalves, E.M.; Langer, R.D.; Guerra-Júnior, G.; et al. The Bioelectrical Impedance Analysis (BIA) International Database: Aims, Scope, and Call for Data. *Eur. J. Clin. Nutr.* **2023**, *77*, 1143–1150. [CrossRef] [PubMed]
12. García-Almeida, J.M.; García-García, C.; Vegas-Aguilar, I.M.; Ballesteros Pomar, M.D.; Cornejo-Pareja, I.M.; Fernández Medina, B.; de Luis Román, D.A.; Bellido Guerrero, D.; Bretón Lesmes, I.; Tinahones Madueño, F.J. Nutritional Ultrasound®: Conceptualisation, Technical Considerations and Standardisation. *Endocrinol. Diabetes Nutr. (Engl. Ed.)* **2023**, *70* (Suppl. S1), 74–84. [CrossRef] [PubMed]
13. Sánchez-Torralvo, F.-J.; Porras, N.; Abuín-Fernández, J.; García-Torres, F.; Tapia, M.-J.; Lima, F.; Soriguer, F.; Gonzalo, M.; Rojo-Martínez, G.; Olveira, G.; et al. Valores de Normalidad de Dinamometría de Mano En España. Relación Con La Masa Magra. *Nutr. Hosp.* **2018**, *35*, 98–103. [CrossRef] [PubMed]
14. Smith, K.E.; Ellison, J.M.; Crosby, R.D.; Engel, S.G.; Mitchell, J.E.; Crow, S.J.; Peterson, C.B.; Le Grange, D.; Wonderlich, S.A. The Validity of DSM-5 Severity Specifiers for Anorexia Nervosa, Bulimia Nervosa, and Binge-Eating Disorder. *Int. J. Eat. Disord.* **2017**, *50*, 1109–1113. [CrossRef] [PubMed]
15. Rodríguez-Rodríguez, E.; López-Plaza, B.; López-Sobaler, A.M.; Ortega, R.M. Prevalencia de Sobrepeso y Obesidad En Adultos Españoles. *Nutr. Hosp.* **2011**, *26*, 355–363. [PubMed]
16. Prior-Sánchez, I.; Herrera-Martínez, A.D.; Zarco-Martín, M.T.; Fernández-Jiménez, R.; Gonzalo-Marín, M.; Muñoz-Garach, A.; Vilchez-López, F.J.; Cayón-Blanco, M.; Villarrubia-Pozo, A.; Muñoz-Jiménez, C.; et al. Prognostic Value of Bioelectrical Impedance Analysis in Head and Neck Cancer Patients Undergoing Radiotherapy: A VALOR® Study. *Front. Nutr.* **2024**, *11*, 1335052. [CrossRef] [PubMed]
17. Kyle, U.G.; Bosaeus, I.; De Lorenzo, A.D.; Deurenberg, P.; Elia, M.; Manuel Gómez, J.; Lilienthal Heitmann, B.; Kent-Smith, L.; Melchior, J.-C.; Pirlich, M.; et al. Bioelectrical Impedance Analysis-Part II: Utilization in Clinical Practice. *Clin. Nutr.* **2004**, *23*, 1430–1453. [CrossRef]
18. Piccoli, A.; Rossi, B.; Pillon, L.; Bucciante, G. A New Method for Monitoring Body Fluid Variation by Bioimpedance Analysis: The RXc Graph. *Kidney Int.* **1994**, *46*, 534–539. [CrossRef] [PubMed]
19. Dos Reis, T.O.; de Magalhães Oliveira, F.; Kattah, F.M.; Pena, N.F.; Soares, M.M.S.; da Gama Torres, H.O. Body Composition and Energy Expenditure in Anorexia Nervosa: Preliminary Data of Outpatients with Recovering and Active Disease. *J. Eat. Disord.* **2022**, *10*, 167. [CrossRef] [PubMed]
20. Abbaspour, A.; Reed, K.K.; Hübel, C.; Bulik-Sullivan, E.C.; Tang, Q.; Bulik, C.M.; Carroll, I.M. Comparison of Dual-Energy X-Ray Absorptiometry and Bioelectrical Impedance Analysis in the Assessment of Body Composition in Women with Anorexia Nervosa upon Admission and Discharge from an Inpatient Specialist Unit. *Int. J. Environ. Res. Public Health* **2021**, *18*, 11388. [CrossRef] [PubMed]
21. Haas, V.; Riedl, A.; Hofmann, T.; Nischan, A.; Burghardt, R.; Boschmann, M.; Klapp, B. Bioimpedance and Bioimpedance Vector Analysis in Patients with Anorexia Nervosa. *Eur. Eat. Disord. Rev.* **2012**, *20*, 400–405. [CrossRef] [PubMed]
22. Himmerich, H.; Dalton, B.; Patsalos, O.; Schmidt, U.; Campbell, I.C. Cytokines and Water Distribution in Anorexia Nervosa. *Mediat. Inflamm.* **2021**, *2021*, 8811051. [CrossRef] [PubMed]
23. Vaisman, N.; Corey, M.; Rossi, M.F.; Goldberg, E.; Pencharz, P. Changes in Body Composition during Refeeding of Patients with Anorexia Nervosa. *J. Pediatr.* **1988**, *113*, 925–929. [CrossRef]
24. Toutain, M.; Gauthier, A.; Leconte, P. Exercise Therapy in the Treatment of Anorexia Nervosa: Its Effects Depending on the Type of Physical Exercise-A Systematic Review. *Front. Psychiatry* **2022**, *13*, 939856. [CrossRef] [PubMed]
25. Lackner, S.; Mörkl, S.; Müller, W.; Fürhapter-Rieger, A.; Oberascher, A.; Lehofer, M.; Bieberger, C.; Wonisch, W.; Amouzadeh-Ghadikolai, O.; Moser, M.; et al. Novel Approaches for the Assessment of Relative Body Weight and Body Fat in Diagnosis and Treatment of Anorexia Nervosa: A Cross-Sectional Study. *Clin. Nutr.* **2019**, *38*, 2913–2921. [CrossRef] [PubMed]
26. Franzoni, E.; Ciccarese, F.; Di Pietro, E.; Facchini, G.; Moscano, F.; Iero, L.; Monaldi, A.; Battista, G.; Bazzocchi, A. Follow-up of Bone Mineral Density and Body Composition in Adolescents with Restrictive Anorexia Nervosa: Role of Dual-Energy X-ray Absorptiometry. *Eur. J. Clin. Nutr.* **2014**, *68*, 247–252. [CrossRef] [PubMed]
27. Misra, M.; Soyka, L.A.; Miller, K.K.; Grinspoon, S.; Levitsky, L.L.; Klibanski, A. Regional Body Composition in Adolescents with Anorexia Nervosa and Changes with Weight Recovery. *Am. J. Clin. Nutr.* **2003**, *77*, 1361–1367. [CrossRef] [PubMed]
28. de Alvaro, M.T.G.; Muñoz-Calvo, M.T.; Barrios, V.; Martínez, G.; Martos-Moreno, G.A.; Hawkins, F.; Argente, J. Regional Fat Distribution in Adolescents with Anorexia Nervosa: Effect of Duration of Malnutrition and Weight Recovery. *Eur. J. Endocrinol.* **2007**, *157*, 473–479. [CrossRef] [PubMed]
29. Rosa-Caldwell, M.E.; Eddy, K.T.; Rutkove, S.B.; Breithaupt, L. Anorexia Nervosa and Muscle Health: A Systematic Review of Our Current Understanding and Future Recommendations for Study. *Int. J. Eat. Disord.* **2023**, *56*, 483–500. [CrossRef] [PubMed]

30. Etemadi, S.; Sun, G.X.; Leung, S.-P.; Siddique, A.; Cooper, S.; Ezenwa, N.C.; Treasure, J.; Robinson, P. The Sit Up Squat Stand Test and Hand Grip Strength: What Is the Role of Tests of Muscle Power in Risk Assessment in Anorexia Nervosa? *Eur. Eat. Disord. Rev.* **2021**, *29*, 670–679. [CrossRef]
31. Mueller, S.M.; Immoos, M.; Anliker, E.; Drobnjak, S.; Boutellier, U.; Toigo, M. Reduced Bone Strength and Muscle Force in Women 27 Years After Anorexia Nervosa. *J. Clin. Endocrinol. Metab.* **2015**, *100*, 2927–2933. [CrossRef] [PubMed]
32. Germain, N.; Genteuil, C.D.; Belleton, G.; Da Silva, T.L.; Exbrayat, C.; Degas, F.; Hammour, A.; Gay, A.; Ravey, B.; Massoubre, C.; et al. Continuous Glucose Monitoring Assessment in Patients Suffering from Anorexia Nervosa Reveals Chronic Prolonged Mild Hypoglycemia All over the Nycthemeron. *Eur. Eat. Disord. Rev.* **2023**, *31*, 402–412. [CrossRef] [PubMed]
33. Uotani, N.; Noma, S.; Akamine, M.; Miyawaki, T. Continuous Glucose Monitoring for Detection of Glycemic Variability, Hypoglycemia, and Hyperglycemia in Women with Eating Disorders. *BioPsychoSocial Med.* **2022**, *16*, 22. [CrossRef] [PubMed]
34. Lee, J.L.; Oh, E.S.; Lee, R.W.; Finucane, T.E. Serum Albumin and Prealbumin in Calorically Restricted, Nondiseased Individuals: A Systematic Review. *Am. J. Med.* **2015**, *128*, 1023.e1–1023.e22. [CrossRef] [PubMed]
35. Hussain, A.A.; Hübel, C.; Hindborg, M.; Lindkvist, E.; Kastrup, A.M.; Yilmaz, Z.; Støving, R.K.; Bulik, C.M.; Sjögren, J.M. Increased Lipid and Lipoprotein Concentrations in Anorexia Nervosa: A Systematic Review and Meta-Analysis. *Int. J. Eat. Disord.* **2019**, *52*, 611–629. [CrossRef] [PubMed]
36. Sproston, N.R.; Ashworth, J.J. Role of C-Reactive Protein at Sites of Inflammation and Infection. *Front. Immunol.* **2018**, *9*, 754. [CrossRef] [PubMed]
37. Dolezalova, R.; Lacinova, Z.; Dolinkova, M.; Kleiblova, P.; Haluzikova, D.; Housa, D.; Papezova, H.; Haluzik, M. Changes of Endocrine Function of Adipose Tissue in Anorexia Nervosa: Comparison of Circulating Levels versus Subcutaneous MRNA Expression. *Clin. Endocrinol.* **2007**, *67*, 674–678. [CrossRef] [PubMed]
38. Lawson, E.A.; Miller, K.K.; Mathur, V.A.; Misra, M.; Meenaghan, E.; Herzog, D.B.; Klibanski, A. Hormonal and Nutritional Effects on Cardiovascular Risk Markers in Young Women. *J. Clin. Endocrinol. Metab.* **2007**, *92*, 3089–3094. [CrossRef]
39. Mariani, S.; di Giorgio, M.R.; Barbaro, G.; Contini, S.; Lubrano, C.; Donini, L.M.; Lenzi, A.; Gnessi, L. Inverse Association of Circulating SIRT1 and Adiposity: A Study on Underweight, Normal Weight, and Obese Patients. *Front. Endocrinol.* **2018**, *9*, 449. [CrossRef] [PubMed]
40. Haluzíková, D.; Dostálová, I.; Kaválková, P.; Roubíček, T.; Mráz, M.; Papežová, H.; Haluzík, M. Serum Concentrations of Adipocyte Fatty Acid Binding Protein in Patients with Anorexia Nervosa. *Physiol. Res.* **2009**, *58*, 577–581. [CrossRef] [PubMed]
41. Misra, M.; Miller, K.K.; Tsai, P.; Stewart, V.; End, A.; Freed, N.; Herzog, D.B.; Goldstein, M.; Riggs, S.; Klibanski, A. Uncoupling of Cardiovascular Risk Markers in Adolescent Girls with Anorexia Nervosa. *J. Pediatr.* **2006**, *149*, 763–769.e1. [CrossRef] [PubMed]
42. Caso, J.R.; MacDowell, K.S.; Soto, M.; Ruiz-Guerrero, F.; Carrasco-Díaz, Á.; Leza, J.C.; Carrasco, J.L.; Díaz-Marsá, M. Dysfunction of Inflammatory Pathways and Their Relationship with Psychological Factors in Adult Female Patients with Eating Disorders. *Front. Pharmacol.* **2022**, *13*, 846172. [CrossRef] [PubMed]
43. Kells, M.R.; Roske, C.; Watters, A.; Puckett, L.; Wildes, J.E.; Crow, S.J.; Mehler, P.S. Vitamin D and Hypophosphatemia in Patients with Anorexia Nervosa and Avoidant/Restrictive Food Intake Disorder: A Case Control Study. *J. Eat. Disord.* **2023**, *11*, 195. [CrossRef] [PubMed]
44. Casper, R.C. Might Starvation-Induced Adaptations in Muscle Mass, Muscle Morphology and Muscle Function Contribute to the Increased Urge for Movement and to Spontaneous Physical Activity in Anorexia Nervosa? *Nutrients* **2020**, *12*, 2060. [CrossRef] [PubMed]
45. Achamrah, N.; Coëffier, M.; Jésus, P.; Charles, J.; Rimbert, A.; Déchelotte, P.; Grigioni, S. Bone Mineral Density after Weight Gain in 160 Patients with Anorexia Nervosa. *Front. Nutr.* **2017**, *4*, 46. [CrossRef] [PubMed]
46. Lopes, M.P.; Robinson, L.; Stubbs, B.; dos Santos Alvarenga, M.; Araújo Martini, L.; Campbell, I.C.; Schmidt, U. Associations between Bone Mineral Density, Body Composition and Amenorrhoea in Females with Eating Disorders: A Systematic Review and Meta-Analysis. *J. Eat. Disord.* **2022**, *10*, 173. [CrossRef] [PubMed]
47. Lee, L.C.; Liong, C.-Y.; Jemain, A.A. Partial Least Squares-Discriminant Analysis (PLS-DA) for Classification of High-Dimensional (HD) Data: A Review of Contemporary Practice Strategies and Knowledge Gaps. *Analyst* **2018**, *143*, 3526–3539. [CrossRef] [PubMed]

nutrients

Article

Ultrasound Cut-Off Values for Rectus Femoris for Detecting Sarcopenia in Patients with Nutritional Risk

Daniel de Luis Roman [1,2,*,†], José Manuel García Almeida [3], Diego Bellido Guerrero [4,*,‡], Germán Guzmán Rolo [5], Andrea Martín [5], David Primo Martín [1,2], Yaiza García-Delgado [6], Patricia Guirado-Peláez [3,7], Fiorella Palmas [8], Cristina Tejera Pérez [4,9], María García Olivares [7,10,11], María Maíz Jiménez [12], Irene Bretón Lesmes [13], Carlos Manuel Alzás Teomiro [14], Juan Manuel Guardia Baena [15], Laura A. Calles Romero [16], Inmaculada Prior-Sánchez [17], Pedro Pablo García-Luna [18], María González Pacheco [19,20], Miguel Ángel Martínez-Olmos [21,22,23], Blanca Alabadí [24,25], Valeria Alcántara-Aragón [26], Samara Palma Milla [27], Tomás Martín Folgueras [28], Andrea Micó García [29], Begoña Molina-Baena [30], Henry Rendón Barragán [31], Pablo Rodríguez de Vera Gómez [32], María Riestra Fernández [33,34], Ana Jiménez Portilla [35], Juan J. López-Gómez [1,2], Nuria Pérez Martín [6], Natalia Montero Madrid [3,7,36], Alba Zabalegui Eguinoa [8], Cristina Porca Fernández [4,9,37], María José Tapia Guerrero [7,10], Marta Ruiz Aguado [12,38], Cristina Velasco Gimeno [13], Aura D Herrera Martínez [14,39], María Novo Rodríguez [15], Natalia C. Iglesias Hernández [16], María de Damas Medina [17], Irene González Navarro [18], Francisco Javier Vílchez López [19,20], Antía Fernández-Pombo [21] and Gabriel Olveira [7,10,36,40]

1 Endocrinology and Nutrition Department, Clinical Universitary Hospital of Valladolid, 47003 Valladolid, Spain; dprimoma@saludcastillayleon.es (D.P.M.); jlopezgo@saludcastillayleon.es (J.J.L.-G.)
2 Investigation Centre Endocrinology and Nutrition, Faculty of Medicine, University of Valladolid, 47003 Valladolid, Spain
3 Department of Endocrinology and Nutrition, Hospital Universitario Virgen de la Victoria, 29010 Málaga, Spain; jgarciaalmeida@gmail.com (J.M.G.A.); pguirado1991@gmail.com (P.G.-P.); nataly_montero@hotmail.com (N.M.M.)
4 Department of Endocrinology and Nutrition, Complejo Hospitalario Universitario de Ferrol (CHUF), 15405 Ferrol, A Coruña, Spain; cristina.tejera.perez@sergas.es (C.T.P.); cris88_pf@hotmail.com (C.P.F.)
5 Medical Department, Abbott Laboratories, 28050 Madrid, Spain; german.guzman1@abbott.com (G.G.R.); andrea.martin@abbott.com (A.M.)
6 Department of Endocrinology and Nutrition, Complejo Hospitalario Universitario Insular-Materno Infantil, 35016 Gran Canaria, Spain; ygarciadelgado@gmail.com (Y.G.-D.); nuriapm@hotmail.com (N.P.M.)
7 Institute of Biomedical Research in Malaga (IBIMA)-Bionand Platform, University of Malaga, 29590 Málaga, Spain; mery.garcia.96@gmail.com (M.G.O.); mjtapiague@gmail.com (M.J.T.G.); gabrielm.olveira.sspa@juntadeandalucia.es (G.O.)
8 Endocrinology and Nutrition Department, Hospital Universitari Vall D'Hebron, 08036 Barcelona, Spain; fiorellaximena.palmas@vallhebron.cat (F.P.); alba.zabalegui@vallhebron.cat (A.Z.E.)
9 Epigenomics in Endocrinology and Nutrition Group, Santiago Health Research Institute (IDIS), 34113 Santiago de Compostela, Spain
10 Endocrinology and Nutrition Department, Hospital Regional Universitario de Málaga, 29010 Málaga, Spain
11 Department of Medicine and Surgery, Malaga University, 29010 Malaga, Spain
12 Department of Endocrinology and Nutrition, University Hospital 12 de Octubre, 28041 Madrid, Spain; mariamaizj@gmail.com (M.M.J.); marta.ruiz84@gmail.com (M.R.A.)
13 Endocrinology and Nutrition Unit, Hospital General Universitario Gregorio Marañón, 28007 Madrid, Spain; irenebreton@gmail.com (I.B.L.); cvelascog@salud.madrid.org (C.V.G.)
14 Reina Sofía University Hospital, 14004 Córdoba, Spain; alzas94@hotmail.com (C.M.A.T.); aurita.dhm@gmail.com (A.D.H.M.)
15 Service of Endocrinology and Nutrition, University Hospital Virgen de las Nieves, 41013 Granada, Spain; guardiabaena@gmail.com (J.M.G.B.); marianovor@hotmail.com (M.N.R.)
16 Endocrinology and Nutrition Service, Basurto University Hospital, 48903 Bilbao, Spain; lauraaraceli.callesromero@osakidetza.eus (L.A.C.R.); nataliacovadonga.iglesiashernandez@osakidetza.eus (N.C.I.H.)
17 Endocrinology Service, Complejo Hospitalario de Jaén, 23007 Jaén, Spain; priorsanchez@hotmail.com (I.P.-S.); mdedamasm@gmail.com (M.d.D.M.)
18 Endocrinology and Nutrition Clinical Management Unit, Institute of Biomedicine of Seville (IBiS), Hospital Universitario Virgen del Rocío/CSIC/University of Seville, 41013 Seville, Spain; garcialunapp@yahoo.es (P.P.G.-L.); irenegonzalez1@gmail.com (I.G.N.)
19 Endocrinology and Nutrition Department, Hospital Universitario Puerta del Mar, 11009 Cádiz, Spain; mariagonzaleznutricion@gmail.com (M.G.P.); franvilchez1977@gmail.com (F.J.V.L.)

[20] Biomedical Research and Innovation Institute of Cádiz (INiBICA), 11009 Cádiz, Spain
[21] Division of Endocrinology and Nutrition, University Clinical Hospital of Santiago de Compostela, 15706 Santiago de Compostela, Spain; miguel.angel.martinez.olmos@sergas.es (M.Á.M.-O.); antiafpombo@gmail.com (A.F.-P.)
[22] Molecular Endocrinology Research Group, Health Research Institute of Santiago de Compostela-IDIS, 15706 Santiago de Compostela, Spain
[23] CIBERObn, National Health Institute Carlos III, 28031 Madrid, Spain
[24] Service of Endocrinology and Nutrition, Hospital Clínico Universitario of Valencia, 46010 Valencia, Spain; blanca.alabadi@gmail.com
[25] INCLIVA Biomedical Research Institute, 46010 Valencia, Spain
[26] Endocrinology and Nutrition Department, Marqués de Valdecilla University Hospital, 39008 Santander, Spain; v.alcantara.aragon@gmail.com
[27] Clinical Nutrition and Dietetics Unit, Endocrinology and Nutrition Service, University Hospital of La Paz, 28046 Madrid, Spain; palmamillasamara@gmail.com
[28] Endocrinology and Nutrition Service, Hospital Universitario de Canarias, 38320 Tenerife, Spain; tmf7312@hotmail.com
[29] Endocrinology and Nutrition Service, La Fe University and Polytechnic Hospital, 46026 Valencia, Spain; andrea.mico@hotmail.com
[30] Deparment of Endocrinology and Nutrition, Hospital Universitario de la Princesa, Instituto de Investigación Sanitaria Princesa (IIS-IP), 28006 Madrid, Spain; bmolinabaena@hotmail.com
[31] Endocrinology and Nutrition, FEA Endocrinology and Nutrition, Navarra University Hospital, 31008 Pamplona, Spain; hereba17@gmail.com
[32] Endocrinology and Nutrition Service, Virgen Macarena University Hospital, 41009 Seville, Spain; pablordevera@gmail.com
[33] Endocrinology Service, Cabueñes University Hospital, 33394 Gijón, Spain; mriestra.fernandez@gmail.com
[34] Health Research Institute of the Principality of Asturias (ISPA), 33011 Oviedo, Spain
[35] Endocrinology and Nutrition Service, Consorci Hospital General Universitari de València, 46014 Valencia, Spain; anajipor@gmail.com
[36] Department of Medicine and Dermatology, Faculty of Medicine, University of Malaga, 29010 Málaga, Spain
[37] Professor Novoa Santos Foundation, 15405 A Coruña, Spain
[38] i+12 Research Institute, 28041 Madrid, Spain
[39] Maimonides Institute for Biomedical Research of Cordoba (IMIBIC), 14004 Córdoba, Spain
[40] CIBER of Diabetes and Associated Metabolic Diseases, Carlos III Health Institute, 28029 Madrid, Spain
* Correspondence: dadluis@yahoo.es (D.d.L.R.); diegobellido@gmail.com (D.B.G.)
† Current address: Department of Endocrinology and Nutrition, Hospital Clínico Universitario de Valladolid (HCUV), Av. Ramón y Cajal 3, 47003 Valladolid, Spain.
‡ Current address: Department of Endocrinology and Nutrition, Complejo Hospitalario de Ferrol, Av. da Residencia, S/N, 15405 Ferrol, A Coruña, Spain.

Abstract: Background: A nationwide, prospective, multicenter, cohort study (the Disease-Related caloric-protein malnutrition EChOgraphy (DRECO) study) was designed to assess the usefulness of ultrasound of the rectus femoris for detecting sarcopenia in hospitalized patients at risk of malnutrition and to define cut-off values of ultrasound measures. Methods: Patients at risk of malnutrition according to the Malnutrition Universal Screening Tool (MUST) underwent handgrip dynamometry, bioelectrical impedance analysis (BIA), a Timed Up and Go (TUG) test, and rectus femoris ultrasound studies. European Working Group on Sarcopenia in Older People (EWGSOP2) criteria were used to define categories of sarcopenia (at risk, probable, confirmed, severe). Receiver operating characteristic (ROC) and area under the curve (AUC) analyses were used to determine the optimal diagnostic sensitivity, specificity, and predictive values of cut-off points of the ultrasound measures for the detection of risk of sarcopenia and probable, confirmed, and severe sarcopenia. Results: A total of 1000 subjects were included and 991 of them (58.9% men, mean age 58.5 years) were evaluated. Risk of sarcopenia was detected in 9.6% patients, probable sarcopenia in 14%, confirmed sarcopenia in 9.7%, and severe sarcopenia in 3.9%, with significant differences in the distribution of groups between men and women ($p < 0.0001$). The cross-sectional area (CSA) of the rectus femoris showed a significantly positive correlation with body cell mass of BIA and handgrip strength, and a significant negative correlation with TUG. Cut-off values were similar within each category of sarcopenia, ranging between 2.40 cm^2 and 3.66 cm^2 for CSA, 32.57 mm and 40.21 mm for the X-axis, and 7.85 mm and 10.4 mm for the Y-axis. In general, these cut-off values showed high sensitivities, particularly for the categories of confirmed and severe sarcopenia, with male patients also showing better sensitivities than women.

Conclusions: Sarcopenia in hospitalized patients at risk of malnutrition was high. Cut-off values for the better sensitivities and specificities of ultrasound measures of the rectus femoris are established. The use of ultrasound of the rectus femoris could be used for the prediction of sarcopenia and be useful to integrate nutritional study into real clinical practice.

Keywords: sarcopenia; nutritional ultrasound; ultrasound cut-off values; rectus femoris; malnutrition; nutritional risk

1. Introduction

Sarcopenia has been classically defined as an age-related decline in skeletal muscle mass and function with adverse effects on quality of life and survival [1], but the European Working Group on Sarcopenia in Older People (EWGSOP2) has recently published an updated consensus definition that uses low muscle strength as the key characteristic for the condition rather than low muscle mass [2]. When low muscle strength, low muscle quantity/quality, and low physical performance are all detected, sarcopenia is considered severe [2].

A wide variety of tests and tools are available for the assessment of muscle in clinical practice, the selection of which may depend upon the availability of resources in the healthcare setting. The SARC-F questionnaire is a five-item simple clinical symptom index that is self-reported by patients as a screen for sarcopenia risk [3]. Measuring handgrip strength is also simple and inexpensive, but accurate measurement requires the use of a calibrated handheld dynamometer under well-defined test conditions with interpretive data from appropriate reference populations [4]. Based on data of two studies [5,6], normal reference values for the Spanish population have been reported.

On the other hand, measuring the quantity and quality of muscle mass has been positioned as a crucial aspect for the diagnosis of disease-related malnutrition (DRM). In this context, nutritional ultrasound that evaluates fat-free mass is an emerging cheap, portable, and non-invasive technique that quantifies muscle in malnutrition [7–9], with advantages over computed tomography (CT), magnetic resonance imaging (MRI), or dual photon X-ray absorptiometry (DXA) techniques that may be less accessible in clinical practice and involve a high healthcare cost, especially CT and MRI [8]. Bioelectrical impedance analysis (BIA) of muscle mass may be preferable to DXA, but validated prediction equations for specific populations are necessary [2]. In addition, DXA and BIA do have cut-off values for muscle quantity, but these methods do not provide indexes for muscle quality, whereas CT and MRI can measure both muscle quantity and quality, but clear cut-off points are still undefined [10].

Muscle ultrasound evaluates muscle volume and area, the length of the fascicles, and the angle of the muscle pennation in transverse and longitudinal positions, as well as subcutaneous fat [9]. However, standardization of methods and measures is still needed. In 2018, the SARCUS (SARCopenia through UltraSound) Working Group [10] reported a consensus proposition for anatomical landmarks of ultrasonographic muscle assessment, with recommendations for patient positioning, system settings, and components to be measured. The application of ultrasound to measure sarcopenia has been recently updated by the SARCUS group, including a detailed description of measuring points and muscle parameters for 39 muscles/muscle groups [11]. In a previous study of our group, standardization of the ultrasound measurement of quadriceps rectus femoris for use in clinical practice was described [9].

However, data on ultrasound cut-off values for predicting low muscle mass status are scarce. Sari et al. [12] reported cut-off values for the gastrocnemius medialis and rectus abdominis in patients with systemic sclerosis. Barotsis et al. [13] predicted sarcopenia from ultrasonographically measured muscle thickness of the vastus intermedius, rectus femoris, medial head of the gastrocnemius, and geniohyoid based on receiver operating characteristic (ROC) analysis. Fukumoto et al. [14] estimated cut-off values of the rectus femoris, vastus intermedius, gastrocnemius, and soleus muscles to detect low muscle mass for sarcopenia. Finally, Eşme et al. [15] reported cut-off values for the gastrocnemius, rectus femoris cross-sectional area, and external and internal oblique for predicting sarcopenia in patients with sarcoidosis.

This prospective multicenter cohort study was designed to assess the usefulness in clinical practice of nutritional ultrasound for the diagnosis of sarcopenia in patients at nutritional risk and to establish cut-off values of different ultrasound measures in patients at risk of sarcopenia and in those with probable, confirmed, and severe sarcopenia.

2. Materials and Methods

2.1. Design and Study Population

This was a nationwide, prospective, multicenter, cohort study (the DRECO study, "Disease-Related caloric-protein malnutrition EChOgraphy") carried out at the Services of Endocrinology and Nutrition of public hospitals throughout Spain. The objectives of the study were to assess the contribution of ultrasound of the rectus femoris for diagnosing sarcopenia in hospitalized patients at risk of malnutrition, and to define cut-off values of ultrasound parameters for the identification of risk of sarcopenia and probable, confirmed, and severe sarcopenia.

Between March and December 2022, consecutive patients aged 18 to 85 years admitted to medical–surgical departments of the participating hospitals (excluding intensive care units [ICUs]) who were diagnosed of being at risk of malnutrition during the first week of hospital stay were eligible if informed consent had been obtained. Exclusion criteria were the presence of liver dysfunction (aminotransferase levels > 3 times the upper reference limit); chronic renal failure (glomerular filtration rate < 45 mL/min/1.73 m^2); previous ICU stays during the index hospital admission; cancer patients with Eastern Cooperative Oncology Group (ECOG) performance status $\geq$ 3 points [16]; eating disorders; any musculoskeletal disease preventing unassisted walking ability; dementia, cognitive impairment, or any neurological/psychiatric condition that may interfere with the study procedures; a life expectancy of less than 6 months; and refusal to sign the informed consent form.

The study protocol was approved by the Ethics Committee for Clinical Research (CEIC) of the Health Council of the Andalusian Health Service (protocol code ALM-DRECO-2021-01, approval date 1 February 2022) and the individual Institutional Review Boards of the participating hospitals. Written informed consent was obtained from all patients. The study was conducted in accordance with the principles of the Declaration of Helsinki and registered in ClinicalTrials.gov (NCT05433831) https://clinicaltrials.gov/study/NCT05433831 (accessed on 14 May 2024).

2.2. Assessment of Malnutrition and the Risk of Sarcopenia

Screening for the risk of sarcopenia was assessed using the SARC-F questionnaire [17,18] and the malnutrition risk was assessed by the Malnutrition Universal Screening Tool (MUST) [19].

Risk of sarcopenia was defined in the presence of an SARC-F score $\geq$ 4.

2.3. Ultrasound Measurements

Ultrasound measurements of the unilateral (right side) rectus femoris were performed at each participating center by an experienced medical sonographer blinded to the clinical data and other results of nutritional assessment using a commercially available portable ultrasound system with a 4–10 cm linear tube (UProbe L6C Ultrasound Scanner, Guangzhou Sonostar Technologies Co., Ltd., Guangzhou, China). Abdominal and anterior thigh muscle measurements were performed with the patient lying supine with their knees extended and relaxed. A linear 7.5–10 kHz ultrasound probe was used. The acquisition site was located two-thirds of the way along the femur length, measured between the anterior superior iliac spine and the upper edge of the patella. The transducer was placed perpendicular to the long axis of the thigh with excessive use of contact gel and minimal pressure to avoid compression of the muscle. All parameters were taken as an average of three consecutive measurements in the dominant leg. We measured the transversal axis of the cross-sectional area (CSA) in cm^2; the X-axis and Y-axis in mm, which corresponded to the linear measurement of the distance between the muscular limits of the rectus femoris (lateral and anteroposterior); the X-axis/Y-axis ratio; and the total fat tissue in mm. All US parameters were also normalized and divided by height squared (in cm^2 for rectus femoris).

2.4. Study Variables

Other data recorded included sociodemographic and anthropometric characteristics, handgrip strength, bioimpedance analysis (BIA), the Timed Up and Go (TUG) test, and biochemical data. Handgrip strength was determined using the Jamar dynamometer (J A Preston Corporation, New York, NY, USA). The dominant hand was tested. Three measurements were taken, and the average was reported and compared with the published population reference data that were used as cut-off points [5]. Total body BIA (50 kHz frequency) (Akern EFG BIA 101 Anniversary) was used to determine phase angle (degrees), total body water (%), fat mass (kg), lean mass (kg), body cell mass (kg), and appendicular skeletal muscle mass (ASMM) (kg). The TUG test was used to assess functionality. A colored tape was marked 3 m away from an armless chair in which participants were sitting. Participants were asked to walk 3 m, turn around the marked tape, and return to the chair as fast as they could. A timer was set as soon as the patient stood up from the chair and was stopped when the patient was seated again. At least one practice trial was performed before the test. A TUG-score of $\geq$20 s was identified as a cut-off point for sarcopenia [2]. Biochemical variables included serum levels of albumin (g/dL), prealbumin (g/dL), C-reactive protein (CRP) (mg/L), and the CRP/prealbumin ratio.

2.5. Categories of Sarcopenia

The presence of risk of sarcopenia was defined by the identification of an SARC-F score $\geq$ 4; probable sarcopenia was defined by an SARC-F score $\geq$ 4 and low handgrip strength based on cut-off reference values (10th percentile) for the Spanish population [5]. In all patients, sarcopenia assessment was carried out according to EWGSOP2 criteria to detect confirmed sarcopenia as criteria of probable sarcopenia plus abnormal ASMM on BIA (<7.0 kg/m^2 for men and <5.5 kg/m^2 for women) [2] and severe sarcopenia as criteria of confirmed sarcopenia plus TUG $\geq$ 20 s [2].

2.6. Outcomes

The primary outcome of this study was to assess the usefulness of ultrasound of the rectus femoris for detecting sarcopenia in hospitalized patients at risk of malnutrition. The secondary outcome was to define cut-off values of the different ultrasound measures for the diagnosis of risk of sarcopenia, probable sarcopenia, confirmed sarcopenia, and severe sarcopenia.

2.7. Statistical Analysis

For the purpose of this study, the sample was distributed by quotas to cover 50% men and 50% women and stratified by 10-year age ranges. It was estimated that a large sample of 1000 patients would be adequate to assess the outcomes of the study. The inclusion of at least 40 patients per center was expected from about 20–25 hospitals. Patients were admitted to the Services of Endocrinology and Nutrition, in which screening for disease-related malnutrition is routinely performed, and referred to a nutritional support team to complete the nutritional assessment and treatment.

Categorical variables are expressed as frequencies and percentage, and continuous variables as mean and standard deviation ($\pm$SD). The chi-square test or Fisher's exact test were used for the comparison of qualitative variables, and Student's t test, two-way analysis of variance (ANOVA), the Mann–Whitney U test, or the Kruskal–Wallis test for the comparison of quantitative variables according to conditions of application. Bonferroni correction was applied as a multiple comparison procedure. The correlation between ultrasound variables (CSA, *X*-axis, *Y*-axis) and mean handgrip strength, BIA (body cell mass), and TUG was assessed with the Spearman rank-order correlation coefficient (rho). Correlations of 0–0.19 were regarded as very weak, 0.2–0.39 as weak, 0.40–0.59 as moderate, 0.6–0.79 as strong, and 0.8–1 as very strong. Receiver operating characteristic (ROC) and area under the curve (AUC) analyses were used to determine the optimal diagnostic sensitivity, specificity, and predictive values of cut-off points of the ultrasound measures for the detection of risk of sarcopenia and probable, confirmed, and severe sarcopenia. The cut-off points were determined by the AUC method that showed the best specificity and sensitivity values for the test in question, as well as the Youden index (sensitivity + specificity − 1). Analyses were performed for the overall study population as well as separately for men and women. Statistical significance was set at $p < 0.05$. Statistical Analysis System (SAS) version 9.4 was used for data analysis.

3. Results

3.1. General Characteristics of Patients

During the study period, a total of 1000 hospitalized patients were screened for risk of malnutrition; 9 of them refused to participate in the study after inclusion, so 991 patients were finally included in the study (58.9% men and 41.1% women). The mean age was 58.5 ± 16.5 years, mean weight 63.6 ± 14.8 kg, and mean body mass index (BMI) 22.9 ± 4.8 kg/m^2. Sociodemographic and anthropometric characteristics, risk of malnutrition, and results of dynamometry, BIA, TUG, and biochemical variables in all patients as well as in men and women are shown in Table 1.

Table 1. General characteristics of patients and distribution of study variables by sex.

Variables	All Patients	Men	Women	Difference	*p*
	(*n* = 991)	(*n* = 585)	(*n* = 406)	(*n* = 991)	
Age, years, mean ± SD	58.5 ± 16.5	58.9 ± 16.5	57.8 ± 16.3	−1.1 ± 1.1	0.33
Weight, kg, mean ± SD	63.7 ± 14.8	68.5 ± 14.2	56.7 ± 12.9	−11.8 ± 0.9	<0.0001
BMI, kg/m^2, mean ± SD	22.9 ± 4.8	23.4 ± 4.7	22.3 ± 4.9	−1.1 ± 0.3	0.0004
Handgrip strength, kg, mean ± SD (*n* = 963)	25.0 ± 10.8	30.0 ± 10.2	17.8 ± 6.8	−12.2 ± 0.5	<0.0001
EWGSOP2 cut-off (men 27 kg, women 16 kg) (*n* = 963)					
Normal, *n* (%)	321 (33.3)	188 (33.1)	133 (33.7)	−55 (0.60)	0.889
Abnormal, *n* (%)	642 (66.7)	380 (66.9)	262 (66.3)	−118 (0.60)	
BIA, mean ± SD					
Phase angle, degrees, (*n* = 907)	5.02 ± 1.11	5.20 ± 1.17	4.76 ± 0.96	−0.44 ± 0.1	<0.0001
Total body water, % (*n* = 939)	73.53 ± 6.14	74.05 ± 5.85	72.75 ± 6.48	−1.3 ± 0.4	0.001
Fat mass, kg (*n* = 958)	15.13 ± 8.40	14.63 ± 8.17	15.85 ± 8.67	1.22 ± 0.5	0.027
Lean mass, kg (*n* = 968)	48.06 ± 10.09	53.36 ± 8.90	40.52 ± 6.10	−12.84 ± 0.5	<0.0001
Body cell mass, kg (*n* = 934)	23.46 ± 6.40	26.25 ± 6.14	19.46 ± 4.28	−6.79 ± 0.3	<0.0001
Appendicular skeletal muscle mass, kg/m^2 (*n* = 937)	6.33 ± 1.63	6.75 ± 1.71	5.72 ± 1.27	−1.03 ± 0.1	<0.0001
EWGSOP2 cut-off (men 7 kg/m^2, women 5.5 kg/m^2) (*n* = 937)					
Normal, *n* (%)	474 (50.6)	265 (47.4)	209 (55.3)	−56 (7.9)	0.019
Abnormal, *n* (%)	463 (49.4)	294 (52.6)	169 (44.7)	−125 (−7.9)	

Table 1. *Cont.*

Variables	All Patients	Men	Women	Difference	p
	(n = 991)	(n = 585)	(n = 406)	(n = 991)	
Ultrasound rectus femoris, mean ± SD					
Cross-sectional area, cm^2 (n = 869)	3.80 ± 1.37	4.09 ± 1.42	3.33 ± 1.13	−0.76 ± 0.1	<0.0001
X-axis, mm, (n = 979)	37.16 ± 5.87	38.65 ± 5.73	34.99 ± 5.39	−3.66 ± 0.4	<0.0001
Y-axis, mm (n = 981)	10.45 ± 3.54	11.10 ± 3.80	9.51 ± 2.89	−1.59 ± 0.2	<0.0001
X-axis/Y-axis ratio, mm (n = 979)	3.93 ± 1.35	3.88 ± 1.42	4.0 ± 1.26	0.12 ± 0.1	0.18
Total fat tissue, mm (n = 940)	7.09 ± 4.73	5.44 ± 3.38	9.41 ± 5.35	3.97 ± 0.3	<0.0001
TUG, s, mean ± SD (n = 829)	13.65 ± 7.70	12.53 ± 6.64	15.21 ± 8.73	2.68 ± 0.5	<0.0001
EWGSOP2 cut-off ≥ 20 s in men and women, (n = 829)					
Normal, n (%)	696 (84.0)	426 (88.4)	270 (77.8)	−156 (−10.6)	0.0005
Abnormal, n (%)	133 (16.0)	56 (11.6)	77 (22.2)	21 (10.6)	
Biochemical data, mean ± SD					
Albumin, g/dL (n = 925)	3.45 ± 0.76	3.45 ± 0.73	3.45 ± 0.81	0 ± 0.1	0.977
Prealbumin, mg/dL (n = 677)	17.89 ± 8.22	17.77 ± 8.47	18.07 ± 7.86	0.30 ± 0.5	0.638
C-reactive protein (CRP), mg/L (n = 905)	45.56 ± 65.97	48.0 ± 63.8	42.1 ± 68.9	−5.9 ± 4.3	0.185
CPR/prealbumin ratio (n = 659)	5.15 ± 12.62	5.90 ± 13.14	4.09 ± 11.78	−1.81 ± 0.8	0.07

BMI: body mass index. CRP: C-reactive protein. SD: standard deviation; GLIM. Global Leadership Initiative on Malnutrition; SGA: Subjective Global Assessment; BIA: bioimpedance analysis; EWGSOP2: European Working Group on Sarcopenia in Older People; TUG: Timed Up and Go; low handgrip strength based on cut-off reference values (10th percentile) for the Spanish population [5].

There were statistically significant differences between men and women in most study variables, except for the risk of malnutrition, biochemical variables, and the percentages of patients with normal or abnormal handgrip strength and ASMM when the corresponding cut-off points recommended by the EWGSOP2 [2] were applied. Women compared with men showed significantly lower values of BMI, mean handgrip strength, all BIA parameters except for fat mass, and all ultrasound measures except for total fat tissue and preperitoneal and total fat on abdominal ultrasound examination. The percentage of women with an abnormal TUG test was significantly higher than that of men (Table 1).

3.2. Prevalence of Sarcopenia

As shown in Table 2, most patients (62.8%) were not at risk of sarcopenia and did not fulfill the criteria for sarcopenia. Risk of sarcopenia was identified in 9.6% of patients and probable sarcopenia in 14.0%. Confirmed sarcopenia was found in 9.7% of patients and severe sarcopenia in 3.9%. There were statistically significant differences ($p < 0.0001$) in the distribution of categories of sarcopenia between men and women, with higher percentages of absence of sarcopenia and confirmed and severe sarcopenia among men, whereas the risk of sarcopenia and probable sarcopenia was more common among women (Figure 1).

3.3. Correlation between Ultrasound Variables, Handgrip Strength, BIA, and TUG

The CSA of the rectus femoris showed a significantly positive correlation the X-axis, Y-axis, body cell mass of BIA, and handgrip strength, and a significant negative correlation with TUG. The X-axis and Y-axis showed the same pattern than the CSA, with significant positive correlations with body cell mass of BIA and handgrip strength, and negative correlations with TUG. Body cell mass of BIA and handgrip strength correlated significantly with ultrasound variables but showed a negative correlation with TUG. In general, correlations ranged between moderate and strong, but in the case of TUG, correlations were mostly weak (Table 3).

Table 2. Categories of sarcopenia and distribution by sex.

Categories	All Patients (n = 990)	Men (n = 584)	Women (n = 406)	Difference (n = 990)
Sarcopenia, n (%)				
Absence	621 (62.8)	399 (68.3)	222 (54.7)	−177 (−13.6)
At risk	95 (9.6)	46 (7.9)	49 (12.1)	3 (4.2)
Probable	139 (14.0)	55 (9.4)	84 (20.7)	29 (11.3)
Confirmed	96 (9.7)	58 (9.9)	38 (9.4)	−20 (−0.5)
Severe	39 (3.9)	26 (4.5)	13 (3.2)	−13 (−1.3)

Risk for sarcopenia: in all patients, sarcopenia assessment was carried out according to EWGSOP2 criteria to detect confirmed sarcopenia as criteria of probable sarcopenia plus abnormal ASMM on BIA (<7.0 kg/m^2 for men and <5.5 kg/m^2 for women) and severe sarcopenia as criteria of confirmed sarcopenia plus TUG $\geq$ 20 s.

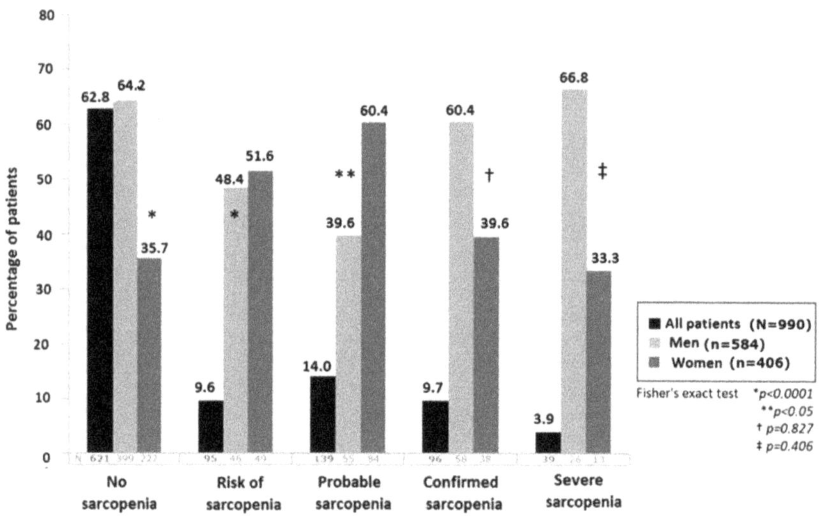

Figure 1. Percentage of patients in the different categories of sarcopenia for the overall study population and distributed by sex.

Table 3. Correlations between the study variables.

Variables	CSA cm^2	X-Axis mm	Y-Axis mm	Handgrip Strength, kg	BIA, Body Cell Mass, kg	TUG, s
CSA, cm^2	-	n = 867 rho = 0.624 p < 0.001	n = 869 rho = 0.788 p < 0.001	n = 850 rho = 0.426 p < 0.001	n = 822 rho = 0.519 p < 0.001	n = 738 rho = −0.290 p < 0.001
X-axis, mm	n = 867 rho = 0.624 p < 0.001	-	n = 979 rho = 0.393 p < 0.001	n = 955 rho = 0.411 p < 0.001	n = 924 rho = 0.368 p < 0.001	n = 822 rho = −0.246 p < 0.001
Y-axis, mm	n = 869 rho = 0.788 p < 0.001	n = 979 rho = 0.393 p < 0.001	-	n = 957 rho = 0.391 p < 0.001	n = 926 rho = 0.548 p < 0.001	n = 823 rho = −0.340 p < 0.001
Handgrip strength, kg	n = 850 rho = 0.425 p < 0.001	n = 955 rho = 0.411 p < 0.001	n = 957 rho = 0.391 p < 0.001	-	n = 912 rho = 0.633 p < 0.001	n = 815 rho = −0.466 p < 0.001

Table 3. *Cont.*

Variables	CSA cm^2	X-Axis mm	Y-Axis mm	Handgrip Strength, kg	BIA, Body Cell Mass, kg	TUG, s
BIA, body cell mass, kg	$n = 822$ rho = 0.519 $p < 0.001$	$n = 924$ rho = 0.368 $p < 0.001$	$n = 926$ rho = 0.548 $p < 0.001$	$n = 912$ rho = 0.633 $p < 0.001$	-	$n = 786$ rho = −0.300 $p < 0.001$
TUG, s	$n = 738$ rho = −0.290 $p < 0.001$	$n = 822$ rho = −0.242 $p < 0.001$	$n = 823$ rho = −0.340 $p < 0.001$	$n = 815$ rho = −0.466 $p < 0.001$	$n = 786$ rho = −0.300 $p < 0.001$	-

CSA: cross-sectional area by ultrasound of rectus femoris; BIA: bioimpedance analysis; TUG: Timed Up and Go; *X* axis by ultrasound of rectus femoris; *Y*-axis by ultrasound of rectus femoris; *X*/*Y* axis ratio by ultrasound of rectus femoris; rho: Spearman's correlation coefficient; *n* = number of patients.

3.4. Ultrasound Cut-Off Points for Detecting Sarcopenia

Cut-off values of the main ultrasound measures in the groups of patients categorized by risk of sarcopenia, probable sarcopenia, confirmed sarcopenia, and severe sarcopenia as well as according to sex are shown in Table 4. In general, the cut-off values were similar within each category of sarcopenia, ranging from 2.40 cm^2 to 3.66 cm^2 for CSA, 32.57 mm to 40.21 mm for the X-axis, and 7.85 mm to 10.4 mm for the *Y*-axis. In general, these cut-off values were associated with high sensitivities for all ultrasound measures, particularly for the categories of confirmed and severe sarcopenia, with male patients also showing better sensitivities compared with females. However, specificities and positive predictive values were low, but negative predictive values were consistently high. The most favorable cut-off value was 8.65 mm for the *Y*-axis for men with severe sarcopenia, with an AUC of 0.801, sensitivity of 80.8%, and specificity of 77.3%, followed by 3.48 cm^2 for the CSA in men with confirmed sarcopenia, with an AUC of 0.777, sensitivity of 81.4%, and specificity of 66.9%.

Table 4. Cut-off points of ultrasound variables of the rectus femoris for detecting sarcopenia in all study patients and distributed by sex.

Variables	Sarcopenia Category	Study Patients	Cut-Off Value	AUC	Sensitivity %	Specificity %	Predictive Values	
							Positive %	Negative %
Cross-sectional area (CSA), cm^2	Risk of sarcopenia	All patients	3.37	0.629	58.5	61.5	45.8	72.7
		Men	3.48	0.647	56.4	66.6	42.4	77.8
		Women	2.97	0.556	50.0	62.5	51.7	60.8
	Probable sarcopenia	All patients	3.37	0.634	64.4	59.1	28.7	86.6
		Men	3.48	0.700	66.7	66.9	35.9	87.8
		Women	3.37	0.548	70.0	41.5	20.9	86.2
	Confirmed sarcopenia	All patients	3.66	0.680	81.0	49.5	20.0	94.3
		Men	3.48	0.777	81.4	66.4	26.9	85.9
		Women	2.4	0.483	89.1	16.3	14.8	90.2
	Severe sarcopenia	All patients	3.41	0.669	78.1	55.3	6.4	98.5
		Men	3.41	0.818	95.2	66.6	10.8	99.7
		Women	3.12	0.597	72.7	49.7	4.8	98.1

Table 4. *Cont.*

Variables	Sarcopenia Category	Study Patients	Cut-Off Value	AUC	Sensitivity %	Specificity %	Predictive Values Positive %	Predictive Values Negative %
X-axis, mm	Risk of sarcopenia	All patients	37.37	0.583	58.3	56.0	44.3	69.1
		Men	40.1	0.579	68.6	45.8	37.2	75.7
		Women	37.41	0.534	72.5	35.0	48.3	60.3
	Probable sarcopenia	All patients	33.55	0.610	37.6	79.3	34.5	80.4
		Men	40.21	0.634	77.4	46.0	30.7	86.8
		Women	32.57	0.620	51.2	73.7	34.1	84.9
	Confirmed sarcopenia	All patients	38.3	0.579	73.3	46.7	18.3	91.5
		Men	38.3	0.687	76.2	59.8	24.6	93.6
		Women	34.41	0.584	74.5	43.4	16.4	91.9
	Severe sarcopenia	All patients	38.3	0.613	76.9	45.4	5.7	97.8
		Men	37.82	0.725	76.9	62.4	9.2	98.2
		Women	37.69	0.579	53.8	67.9	5.8	97.8
Y-axis, mm	Risk of sarcopenia	All patients	9.59	0.628	56.9	63.5	48.3	71.2
		Men	9.66	0.652	55.7	70.2	46.6	77.2
		Women	8.57	0.563	48.9	65.1	53.9	60.4
	Probable sarcopenia	All patients	9.59	0.645	62.4	61.2	31.8	84.7
		Men	9.66	0.691	64.2	70.0	39.8	86.4
		Women	7.85	0.583	44.0	73.7	30.8	83.2
	Confirmed sarcopenia	All patients	9.66	0.686	71.9	59.4	22.3	92.8
		Men	9.66	0.775	78.6	69.7	30.8	94.9
		Women	10.4	0.534	74.5	35.4	14.7	90.3
	Severe sarcopenia	All patients	8.77	0.716	74.4	67.6	9.0	98.4
		Men	8.65	0.801	80.8	77.3	14.9	98.8
		Women	8.77	0.558	61.5	56.0	4.6	97.7
X/*Y* axis ratio	Risk of sarcopenia	All patients	5.19	0.598	89.9	25.3	60.0	66.7
		Men	4.63	0.624	35.7	83.8	50.7	73.5
		Women	4.95	0.552	24.7	86.6	60.81	57.8
	Probable sarcopenia	All patients	4.63	0.598	37.1	79.9	35.0	81.3
		Men	4.64	0.638	40.1	83.1	42.3	81.7
		Women	4.95	0.533	27.4	83.8	31.1	81.2
	Confirmed sarcopenia	All patients	4.19	0.661	60.0	68.3	23.5	91.2
		Men	4.66	0.708	52.4	84.0	36.1	91.1
		Women	4.16	0.582	62.7	61.0	19.4	91.6
	Severe sarcopenia	All patients	4.19	0.666	66.7	66.7	79.5	97.9
		Men	4.67	0.577	57.7	82.2	13.8	97.5
		Women	4.26	0.602	69.2	63.0	6.08	98.3

Risk for sarcopenia: in all patients, sarcopenia assessment was carried out according to EWGSOP2 criteria to detect confirmed sarcopenia as criteria of probable sarcopenia plus abnormal ASMM on BIA (<7.0 kg/m^2 for men and <5.5 kg/m^2 for women) and severe sarcopenia as criteria of confirmed sarcopenia plus TUG $\geq$ 20 s.

4. Discussion

It is well known that sarcopenia is one of the most important health problems in elderly people with a high rate of adverse outcomes. Data of a systematic review and meta-analysis of 35 articles with a total of 58,404 individuals revealed an overall prevalence of 10% in both men and women, with a substantial proportion of old people having sarcopenia, even in healthy populations [20]. Sarcopenia has been associated with an increased risk of mortality, falls, fractures, and poor quality of life [21], so timely detection can be effective in reducing the burden of disease. In this respect, ultrasound provides a safe, cost-effective, and rapid means of assessing the musculoskeletal system [22] and is very promising in geriatric practice in the context of sarcopenia [23]. The present real clinical practice study in shows that in a large population of inpatients undergoing routine screening for the risk of malnutrition, ultrasound examination of the rectus femoris was a feasible technique for detecting sarcopenia, particularly in cases of confirmed and severe sarcopenia defined by a combination of SARC-F score, handgrip strength, ASMM on BIA, and results of TUG. It should be noted that definitions of these variables were based on standard interpretation of the SARC-F questionnaire ($\geq$4 points) and the use of reference values for handgrip strength using a Jamar dynamometer already reported in a Spanish population by gender and age groups [5] and cut-points of ASMM and TUG proposed by the EWGSOP2 group for the diagnosis of sarcopenia [2]. In fact, the strict definitions of the categories of sarcopenia (at risk, probable, confirmed, and severe) for which ultrasound cut-off values of the rectus femoris have been estimated are a strength of this study and an important contribution of the present findings.

There are few studies on thigh muscle evaluation by ultrasound of the rectus femoris in the diagnosis of sarcopenia [13–15], but a direct comparison with our findings cannot be established due to methodological differences in acquisition points and the ultrasound parameters considered. Ultrasound measurements of abdominal and calf muscle thickness was found to be a useful screening method in predicting low-muscle-mass status in patients with systemic sclerosis, with a high sensitivity (92.3%) for both the gastrocnemius medialis and rectus abdominis and negative predictive value (97.9% and 97.6%, respectively) [12]. In this study, however, ultrasound assessment of the rectus femoris was not performed. In another prospective study of 94 individuals with a mean age of 75.6 years referred for sarcopenia screening to a rehabilitation department of a university hospital in Patras, Greece [13], thickness of the rectus femoris was measured between its deep and superficial fascia. It was found that the likelihood of sarcopenia was 11.9 and 6.9 times greater for transverse and longitudinal section thickness lower than the cut-off points of 1.54 cm and 1.59 cm, respectively, for which sensitivities of 68.8% and 81.3% and specificities of 65.4% and 51.3% were reported [13]. These data, however, are difficult to compare with our study as the acquisition points were not described. In a cross-sectional study of 204 community-dwelling older adults (mean age 75.4 years) and 59 younger adults (mean age 22.3 years), lower limb muscle thickness was evaluated to assess sarcopenia [14]. The cut-off point of rectus femoris muscular thickness based on 2 SD below the young adults was 1.85 cm for males and 1.42 cm for females, corresponding to a prevalence of low muscular mass of 69.4% and 36.7%, respectively. In this study, the muscular thickness of the rectus femoris was defined as the distance between the superficial and deep fascia of the muscle. Finally, in a study of 40 patients with a mean age of 53.2 years, a cut-off value of the rectus femoris cross-sectional area of 5.65 mm^2 showed a sensitivity of 76% and a specificity of 69% for predicting sarcopenia [15]. In our study, CSA showed cut-off points ranging between 3.37 and 3.66 cm^2, with sensitivities of 58.5% for predicting the risk of sarcopenia and 64.4%, 81%, and 78.1% for probable, confirmed, and severe sarcopenia, respectively.

An interesting aspect of our study was the analysis of the distribution of the study variables by sex, with values in general being higher in male patients than in female patients. The assessment of differences in nutritional-related variables between men and women provides valuable information at the time of targeting nutritional interventions. In a systematic review and meta-analysis of 107 RCTs, a greater proportion of gender-targeted interventions than gender-neutral studies were effective in improving nutrition [24]. In relation to ultrasound cut-off values for the evaluation of sarcopenia, men show higher cut-off points than women in practically all categories of sarcopenia, a fact that should be taken into consideration in practice. However, differences in cut-off values of patients stratified by age were not evaluated. On the other hand, as may be expected, there were statistically significant correlations between ultrasound variables and handgrip strength, BIA, and TUG, which is consistent with data reported in previous studies [14,15].

The field of US muscle assessment is clearly growing, with more research groups using this technique to give more hands-on information on the muscles described. However, a clear standardization remains absent. A large number of variables can influence the use of US for the determination of sarcopenia. The first factor is the location of the muscle that we can measure; a multitude of areas, up to 39 upper extremity muscles (upper arm, lower arm, and hand), lower extremity muscles (upper leg, lower leg, foot), and head and neck muscles, have been evaluated in the literature [11]. We decided to measure the rectus femoris [25–29] as a well-known muscle with previous clinical studies. It is one of the most evaluated muscles in the literature and very accessible to an untrained observer, and therefore, each one must have sarcopenia cut-off points and different parameters (x-axis, y-axis, circumference, area, fascicle length, echo-intensity pennation angle and so on). In our present study, we report the cut-off points for sarcopenia in this specific muscle. Second, whereas a resting period of a minimum of 30 min was previously proposed, new data show that when changing from a standing to a supine position, after 5 min, a normalization of measurements can occur. In our protocol, the US image was captured in the supine position. Finally, some muscles can easily be delineated through the use of specific anatomical landmarks, but others will still require an ultrasonographic visualization before exact measuring points can be identified, for example, suprahyoid musculature of the neck or the flexor hallucis brevis in the foot [11]. A recent revision of Niels et al. [30] indicated that ultrasound of the rectus femoris muscle to diagnose sarcopenia has been shown to be a promising method in multiple clinical populations and it is necessary to implement protocols in clinical practice [31], like our present study.

Several limitations should be noted when interpreting this study. The results may not be generalizable to other muscle groups, as only the rectus femoris was assessed. However, this location of muscle is easily accessible for ultrasound in the supine position and has an excellent association with whole body muscle mass [31]. Although there are different muscle structures that can be evaluated, many studies focus on the rectus femoris or combinations of various muscle groups involving large muscle bundles with functional importance to patients in terms of gait. Measurement of the rectus femoris of the quadriceps is one of the most referenced measurements due to its correlation with strength and tests of execution or functional performance [25–29,32]. The data from our work can be extrapolated only to patients at potential risk of malnutrition when hospitalized and older than 18 years. Our data cannot be generalized to ICU patients, considering the design and inclusion criteria of our protocol. The data may vary depending on the image acquisition equipment as well as the protocol used for the acquisition of these ultrasound images; thus, the DRECO study protocol has been recently published [33]. Inter- and intra-observer variability may be a confounding factor in our results that should be considered in future studies. Finally, the absence of recording physical activity may be a limitation in the interpretation of the results.

However, the large sample size and the assessment of global cut-off values of ultrasound measures of the rectus femoris, as well as those for men and women, are important strengths and differential features of this study. Also, estimates of cut-off values according to the categories of sarcopenia are relevant scientific contributions of this study.

5. Conclusions

In a large population of patients admitted to the medical–surgical departments of public hospitals throughout Spain who were routinely screened for risk of malnutrition using validated instruments, 9.6% were at risk of sarcopenia, 14% had probable sarcopenia, and 9.7% had confirmed sarcopenia. Severe sarcopenia was detected in almost 4%. Based on these categories of sarcopenia, cut-off values for the better sensitivities and specificities of different ultrasound measures of the rectus femoris are established for the global study population as well as for male and female patients. Ultrasound of the rectus femoris can be used for the prediction of sarcopenia. The findings of the present clinical study are useful to integrate nutritional ultrasound in real clinical practice.

Author Contributions: D.d.L.R., J.M.G.A., D.B.G., G.G.R. and G.O. contributed to the conception of the study and investigation and the acquisition, validation, and supervision of data. D.d.L.R. and G.O. contributed to the data curation and interpretation of results. D.d.L.R. wrote the original draft. D.d.L.R., J.M.G.A., D.B.G., G.G.R., A.M., D.P.M., Y.G.-D., P.G.-P., F.P., C.T.P., M.G.O., M.M.J., I.B.L., C.M.A.T., J.M.G.B., L.A.C.R., I.P.-S., P.P.G.-L., M.G.P., M.Á.M.-O., B.A., V.A.-A., S.P.M., T.M.F., A.M.G., B.M.-B., H.R.B., P.R.d.V.G., M.R.F., A.J.P., J.J.L.-G., N.P.M., N.M.M., A.Z.E., C.P.F., M.J.T.G., M.R.A., C.V.G., A.D.H.M., M.N.R., N.C.I.H., M.d.D.M., I.G.N., F.J.V.L., A.F.-P. and G.O contributed to the design of the study, revised the manuscript critically for important intellectual content, and approved the final version of the manuscript. G.G.R. and A.M. contributed to the funding acquisition. The authors decline the use of artificial intelligence, language models, machine learning, or similar technologies to create content or assist with writing or editing of the manuscript. All authors have read and agreed to the published version of the manuscript.

Funding: This research was funded in part by Abbott Laboratories, but the founding source has no role in the design of the study, analysis, interpretation of data, or decisions regarding the publication of results.

Institutional Review Board Statement: The study protocol was approved by the Ethics Committee for Clinical Research (CEIC) of the Health Council of the Andalusian Health Service (protocol code ALM-DRECO-2021-01, approval date 1 February 2022) and the individual Institutional Review Boards of the participating hospitals.

Informed Consent Statement: Informed consent was obtained from all subjects involved in this study.

Data Availability Statement: The original contributions presented in the study are included in the article, further inquiries can be directed to the corresponding author due to privacy reasons.

Conflicts of Interest: G.G.R. and A.M are full employees of Abbott Laboratories. None of the remaining authors have any conflicts of interest. The authors declare that the project was conducted in the absence of any commercial or financial relationships that could be construed as a potential conflict of interest.

References

1. Rosenberg, I.H. Sarcopenia: Origins and clinical relevance. *J. Nutr.* **1997**, *127* (Suppl. S5), 990S–991S. [CrossRef] [PubMed]
2. Cruz-Jentoft, A.J.; Bahat, G.; Bauer, J.; Boirie, Y.; Bruyère, O.; Cederholm, T.; Cooper, C.; Landi, F.; Rolland, Y.; Sayer, A.A.; et al. Sarcopenia: Revised European consensus on definition and diagnosis. *Age Ageing* **2019**, *48*, 601. [CrossRef] [PubMed]
3. Malmstrom, T.K.; Miller, D.K.; Simonsick, E.M.; Ferrucci, L.; Morley, J.E. SARC-F: A symptom score to predict persons with sarcopenia at risk for poor functional outcomes. *J. Cachexia Sarcopenia Muscle* **2016**, *7*, 28–36. [CrossRef] [PubMed]
4. Roberts, H.C.; Denison, H.J.; Martin, H.J.; Patel, H.P.; Syddall, H.; Cooper, C.; Sayer, A.A. A review of the measurement of grip strength in clinical and epidemiological studies: Towards a standardised approach. *Age Ageing* **2011**, *40*, 423–429. [CrossRef] [PubMed]
5. Sánchez Torralvo, F.J.; Porras, N.; Abuín Fernández, J.; García Torres, F.; Tapia, M.J.; Lima, F.; Soriguer, F.; Gonzalo, M.; Rojo Martínez, G.; Olveira, G. Normative reference values for hand grip dynamometry in Spain. Association with lean mass. *Nutr. Hosp.* **2018**, *35*, 98–103. [CrossRef] [PubMed]
6. Mateo Lázaro, M.L.; Penacho Lázaro, M.A.; Berisa Losantos, F.; Plaza Bayo, A. New tables on hand strength in the adult population from Teruel. *Nutr. Hosp.* **2008**, *23*, 35–40. [PubMed]
7. Mateos-Angulo, A.; Galán-Mercant, A.; Cuesta-Vargas, A.I. Ultrasound muscle assessment and nutritional status in institutionalized older adults: A pilot study. *Nutrients* **2019**, *11*, 1247. [CrossRef]

8. García Almeida, J.M.; García García, C.; Bellido Castañeda, V.; Bellido Guerrero, B. A new nutritional approach. Assessment of the patient nutritional status: Function and body composition. *Nutr. Hosp.* **2018**, *35*, 1–4.
9. García-Almeida, J.M.; García-García, C.; Vegas-Aguilar, I.M.; Ballesteros Pomar, M.D.; Cornejo-Pareja, I.M.; Fernández Medina, B.; de Luis Román, D.A.; Bellido Guerrero, D.; Bretón Lesmes, I.; Tinahones Madueño, F.J. Nutritional ultrasound®: Conceptualisation, technical considerations and standardisation. *Endocrinol. Diabetes Nutr.* **2023**, *70* (Suppl. 1), 74–84. [CrossRef]
10. Perkisas, S.; Baudry, S.; Bauer, J.; Beckwee, D.; De Cock, A.-M.; Hobbelen, H.; Jager-Wittenaar, H.; Kasiukiewicz, A.; Landi, F.; Marco, E.; et al. Application of ultrasound for muscle assessment in sarcopenia: Towards standardized measurements. *Eur. Geriatr. Med.* **2018**, *9*, 739–757. [CrossRef]
11. Perkisas, S.; Bastijns, S.; Baudry, S.; Bauer, J.; Beaudart, C.; Beckwée, D.; Cruz-Jentoft, A.; Gasowski, J.; Hobbelen, H.; Jager-Wittenaar, H.; et al. Application of ultrasound for muscle assessment in sarcopenia: 2020 SARCUS update. *Eur. Geriatr. Med.* **2021**, *12*, 45–59. [CrossRef] [PubMed]
12. Sari, A.; Esme, M.; Aycicek, G.S.; Armagan, B.; Kilic, L.; Ertenli, A.I.; Halil, M.G.; Akdogan, A. Evaluating skeletal muscle mass with ultrasound in patients with systemic sclerosis. *Nutrition* **2020**, *84*, 110999. [CrossRef] [PubMed]
13. Barotsis, N.; Galata, A.; Hadjiconstanti, A.; Panayiotakis, G. The ultrasonographic measurement of muscle thickness in sarcopenia. A prediction study. *Eur. J. Phys. Rehabil. Med.* **2020**, *56*, 427–437. [CrossRef] [PubMed]
14. Fukumoto, Y.; Ikezoe, T.; Taniguchi, M.; Yamada, Y.; Sawano, S.; Minani, S.; Asai, T.; Kimura, M.; Ichihashi, N. Cut-off values for lower limb muscle thickness to detect low muscle mass for sarcopenia in older adults. *Clin. Interv. Aging* **2021**, *16*, 1215–1222. [CrossRef] [PubMed]
15. Eşme, M.; Karcıoğlu, O.; Öncel, A.; Ayçiçek, G.; Deniz, O.; Ulaşlı, S.S.; Köksal, D.; Doğu, B.B.; Cankurtaran, M.; Halil, M. Ultrasound assessment of sarcopenia in patients with sarcoidosis. *J. Ultrasound Med.* **2021**, *41*, 951–959. [CrossRef] [PubMed]
16. Oken, M.M.; Creech, R.H.; Tormey, D.C.; Horton, J.; Davis, T.E.; McFadden, E.T.; Carbone, P.P. Toxicity and response criteria of the Eastern Cooperative Oncology Group. *Am. J. Clin. Oncol.* **1982**, *5*, 649–655. [CrossRef] [PubMed]
17. Malmstrom, T.K.; Morley, J.E. SARC-F: A simple questionnaire to rapidly diagnose sarcopenia. *J. Am. Med. Dir. Assoc.* **2013**, *14*, 531–532. [CrossRef] [PubMed]
18. Sanchez-Rodriguez, D.; Marco, E.; Davalos-Yerovi, V.; Lopez-Escobar, J.; Messaggi-Sartor, M.; Barrera, C.; Ronquillo-Moreno, N.; Vazquez-Ibar, O.; Calle, A.; Inzitari, M.; et al. Translation and validation of the spanish version of the SARC-F questionnaire to assess sarcopenia in older people. *J. Nutr. Health Aging* **2019**, *23*, 518–524. [CrossRef] [PubMed]
19. Stratton, R.J.; Hackston, A.; Longmore, D.; Dixon, R.; Price, S.; Stroud, M.; King, C.; Elia, M. Malnutrition in hospital outpatients and inpatients: Prevalence, concurrent validity and ease of use of the 'malnutrition universal screening tool' ('MUST') for adults. *Br. J. Nutr.* **2004**, *92*, 799–808. [CrossRef]
20. Shafiee, G.; Keshtkar, A.; Soltani, A.; Ahadi, Z.; Larijani, B.; Heshmat, R. Prevalence of sarcopenia in the world: A systematic review and meta- analysis of general population studies. *J. Diabetes Metab. Disord.* **2017**, *16*, 21. [CrossRef]
21. Xia, L.; Zhao, R.; Wan, Q.; Wu, Y.; Zhou, Y.; Wang, Y.; Cui, Y.; Shen, X.; Wu, X. Sarcopenia and adverse health-related outcomes: An umbrella review of meta-analyses of observational studies. *Cancer Med.* **2020**, *9*, 7964–7978. [CrossRef] [PubMed]
22. Patil, P.; Dasgupta, B. Role of diagnostic ultrasound in the assessment of musculoskeletal diseases. *Ther. Adv. Musculoskelet. Dis.* **2012**, *4*, 341–355. [CrossRef] [PubMed]
23. Ticinesi, A.; Meschi, T.; Narici, M.V.; Lauretani, F.; Maggio, M. Muscle Ultrasound and sarcopenia in older individuals: A clinical perspective. *J. Am. Med. Dir. Assoc.* **2017**, *18*, 290–300. [CrossRef] [PubMed]
24. Sharkey, T.; Whatnall, M.C.; Hutchesson, M.J.; Haslam, R.L.; Bezzina, A.; Collins, C.E.; Ashton, L.M. Effectiveness of gender-targeted versus gender-neutral interventions aimed at improving dietary intake, physical activity and/or overweight/obesity in young adults (aged 17–35 years): A systematic review and meta-analysis. *Nutr. J.* **2020**, *19*, 78. [CrossRef] [PubMed]
25. Primo, D.; Izaola, O.; Gómez, J.J.L.; de Luis, D. Correlation of the Phase Angle with Muscle Ultrasound and Quality of Life in Obese Females. *Dis. Markers* **2022**, *2022*, 7165126. [CrossRef] [PubMed]
26. López-Gómez, J.J.; Izaola-Jauregui, O.; Almansa-Ruiz, L.; Jiménez-Sahagún, R.; Primo-Martín, D.; Pedraza-Hueso, M.; Ramos-Bachiller, B.; González-Gutiérrez, J.; De Luis-Román, D. Use of Muscle Ultrasonography in Morphofunctional Assessment of Amyotrophic Lateral Sclerosis (ALS). *Nutrients* **2024**, *16*, 1021. [CrossRef] [PubMed]
27. de Luis, D.A.; Lopez Gomez, J.J. Morphofunctional Nutritional assessment in clinical Practice: A new approach to assessing Nutritional Status. *Nutrients* **2023**, *5*, 4300. [CrossRef] [PubMed]
28. López-Gómez, J.J.; García-Beneitez, D.; Jiménez-Sahagún, R.; Izaola-Jauregui, O.; Primo-Martín, D.; Ramos-Bachiller, B.; Gómez-Hoyos, E.; Delgado-García, E.; Pérez-López, P.; De Luis-Román, D.A. Nutritional Ultrasonography, a Method to Evaluate Muscle Mass and Quality in Morphofunctional Assessment of Disease Related Malnutrition. *Nutrients* **2023**, *15*, 3923. [CrossRef] [PubMed]
29. Lopez, J.J.; Gutierrez, C.; Izaola, O.; Primo, D.; Gomez, E.; Jimenez, R.; de Luis, D. Real World practice study of the effect of a specific oral nutritional supplement for diabetes mellitus on the morphofuncitional assessment and proteinenergy requirements. *Nutrients* **2022**, *14*, 4802. [CrossRef]
30. Nies, I.; Ackermans, L.L.G.C.; Poeze, M.; Blokhuis, T.J.; Bosch, J.A.T. The Diagnostic Value of Ultrasound of the Rectus Femoris for the diagnosis of Sarcopenia in adults: A systematic review. *Injury* **2022**, *53*, S23–S29. [CrossRef]
31. Lee, S.J.; Janssen, I.; Heymsfield, S.B.; Ross, R. Relation between whole-body and regional measures of human skeletal muscle. *Am. J. Clin. Nutr.* **2004**, *80*, 1215–1221. [CrossRef] [PubMed]

32. Ticinesi, A.; Meschi, T.; Maggio, M.; Narici, M.V. Application of ultrasound for muscle assessment in sarcopenia: The challenge of implementing protocols for clinical practice. *Eur. Geriatr. Med.* **2018**, *10*, 155–156. [CrossRef] [PubMed]
33. Almeida, J.M.G.; Bellido, D.; De Luis, D.; Rolo, G.G.; Olveira, G. Protocol for a prospective cohort study on the feasibility of application of nutritional ultrasound in the diagnosis and follow-up of patients with nutritional risk at hospital discharge: Study on body composition and function (DRECO). *BMJ Open* **2023**, *13*, e074945. [CrossRef] [PubMed]

nutrients

MDPI

Article

Validation of an Artificial Intelligence-Based Ultrasound Imaging System for Quantifying Muscle Architecture Parameters of the Rectus Femoris in Disease-Related Malnutrition (DRM)

Sergio García-Herreros [1], Juan Jose López Gómez [2,3], Angela Cebria [1], Olatz Izaola [2,3], Pablo Salvador Coloma [1], Sara Nozal [1], Jesús Cano [1], David Primo [2], Eduardo Jorge Godoy [1,*] and Daniel de Luis [2,3,*]

[1] DAWAKO Medtech S.L., Parc Cientific de la Universitat de Valencia, Calle del Catedratic Agustín Escardino Benlloch, 9, 46980 Paterna, Spain; sgarcia@dawako.es (S.G.-H.); acebria@dawako.es (A.C.); psalvador@dawako.es (P.S.C.); snozal@dawako.es (S.N.); jcano@dawako.es (J.C.)

[2] Investigation Centre Endocrinology and Nutrition, Faculty of Medicine, University of Valladolid, 47003 Valladolid, Spain; jlopezgo@saludcastillayleon.es (J.J.L.G.); oizaolaj@saludcastillayleon.es (O.I.); dprimoma@saludcastillayleon.es (D.P.)

[3] Endocrinology and Nutrition Department, Clinical Universitary Hospital of Valladolid, 47003 Valladolid, Spain

* Correspondence: egodoy@dawako.es (E.J.G.); dluisro@saludcastillayleon.es (D.d.L.)

Abstract: (1) Background: The aim was to validate an AI-based system compared to the classic method of reading ultrasound images of the rectus femur (RF) muscle in a real cohort of patients with disease-related malnutrition. (2) Methods: One hundred adult patients with DRM aged 18 to 85 years were enrolled. The risk of DRM was assessed by the Global Leadership Initiative on Malnutrition (GLIM). The variation, reproducibility, and reliability of measurements for the RF subcutaneous fat thickness (SFT), muscle thickness (MT), and cross-sectional area (CSA), were measured conventionally with the incorporated tools of a portable ultrasound imaging device (method A) and compared with the automated quantification of the ultrasound imaging system (method B). (3) Results: Measurements obtained using method A (i.e., conventionally) and method B (i.e., raw images analyzed by AI), showed similar values with no significant differences in absolute values and coefficients of variation, 58.39–57.68% for SFT, 30.50–28.36% for MT, and 36.50–36.91% for CSA, respectively. The Intraclass Correlation Coefficient (ICC) for reliability and consistency analysis between methods A and B showed correlations of 0.912 and 95% CI [0.872–0.940] for SFT, 0.960 and 95% CI [0.941–0.973] for MT, and 0.995 and 95% CI [0.993–0.997] for CSA; the Bland–Altman Analysis shows that the spread of points is quite uniform around the bias lines with no evidence of strong bias for any variable. (4) Conclusions: The study demonstrated the consistency and reliability of this new automatic system based on machine learning and AI for the quantification of ultrasound imaging of the muscle architecture parameters of the rectus femoris muscle compared with the conventional method of measurement.

Keywords: artificial intelligence; disease-related malnutrition; muscle architecture parameters; reproducibility; reliability; ultrasound imaging

1. Introduction

Disease-related malnutrition (DRM) [1] is a prevalent health issue that poses a significant challenge in our healthcare system, affecting 20% to 50% of hospitalized patients [2,3]. Its presence can lead to increased complications and mortality risk. The Effect of Early Nutritional Support on Frailty, Functional Outcomes, and Recovery of Malnourished Medical Inpatients Trial EFFORT study demonstrated that patients diagnosed with malnutrition according to Global Leadership Initiative on Malnutrition (GLIM) criteria were at higher risk for adverse clinical outcomes [4]. This condition also raises hospitalization costs [5]. Malnutrition may be linked with other conditions such as sarcopenia, characterized by muscle mass and function loss, which was traditionally associated with aging and frailty, but in 2019, the European Working Group on Sarcopenia in Older People (EWGSOP2) raised secondary sarcopenia associated with several diseases [6]. Sarcopenia might affect up to 15% of malnourished patients and 32% of cachexic older adults, increasing the risk of complications in different patient groups [7,8]. Scientific nutritional societies advise early medical nutrition treatment for at-risk medical and surgical patients to provide appropriate Medical Nutrition Therapy and prevent potential complications. In this context, measuring muscle mass is crucial for diagnosing DRM and loss of muscle mass. Muscle ultrasound, which evaluates fat-free mass and fat mass, is an emerging technique that quantifies muscle in malnutrition [8]. It has advantages over computed tomography (CT), magnetic resonance imaging (MRI), or dual photon X-ray absorptiometry (DXA) techniques due to being cheap, portable, and non-invasive [9]. Additionally, bioelectrical impedance analysis (BIA) of muscle mass may be preferable to DXA; however, specific populations require validated prediction equations [6]. Furthermore, while DXA and BIA have cut-off values for assessing muscle quantity but not quality indexes; CT and MRI can measure both quantity and quality, although clear cut-off points are still undefined [10]. Ultrasound assessment of muscle volume, area, fascicle length, and muscle pennation angle in both transverse and longitudinal positions is a valuable clinical technique [10].

However, there remains a need for the standardization of methods and measures. The SARCopenia through Ultrasound (SARCUS) Working Group proposed anatomical landmarks for ultrasonographic muscle assessment in 2018 with guidelines on patient positioning, system settings, and components to be measured [10]. Recently updated by the SARCUS group, ultrasound's application to measuring sarcopenia includes detailed descriptions of measurement points and muscle parameters for various muscles and muscle groups [11]. Previously, we described the standardization of ultrasound measurement of rectus femoris specifically tailored for clinical practice [9]. The main problem of muscle ultrasound is the great interobserver variability that exists. Therefore, automatic analyzing systems based on AI and machine learning algorithms can help homogenize the results obtained with muscle ultrasound. In this context, the objective of this study was to validate the use of a novel software tool for medical conventional ultrasound B-mode Ultrasound Imaging System. This automatic system is a cloud-based web application software (i.e., software as a medical device) for the visualization, quantification, and analysis of medical ultrasound images with the capability to be used with any computer and compatibility with the DICOM®-Digital Imaging and Communications in Medicine, the international standard for medical images and related information [12]. AI is developing fast. It is right now changing our lives by improving healthcare (e.g., making diagnosis more precise, enabling better prevention of diseases). AI is a collection of technologies that combine data, algorithms, and computing power. Advances in computing and the increasing availability of data are therefore key drivers of the current upsurge of AI [13].

As ultrasound instruments have become smaller, less expensive, and easier to use, diagnostic ultrasound has become increasingly popular among a wide variety of physicians. The ultrasound imaging technique has replaced or complemented many radiographic and nuclear medicine procedures and has opened new areas of diagnostic investigation, especially in the evaluation of patients with DRM through the study of the quality and quantity of muscle.

Considering the importance that muscle ultrasound, and especially RF, has in nutritional assessment and the possible interobserver variability in this technique, it is important to develop automatic assessment systems that allow obtaining reliable parameters from the ultrasound images captured in real-world practice. Without a doubt, these AI analysis systems are still unknown outside of research areas, however, they will be implemented in many areas of clinical image analysis. Clinical studies are scarce, so our work attempts to validate the new system in real clinical practice.

The aim was to validate an AI-based system compared to the classic method of reading ultrasound images of the rectus femur (RF) muscle in a real cohort of patients with disease-related malnutrition.

2. Materials and Methods

2.1. Subjects

A total of one hundred consecutive adult patients with disease-related malnutrition (DRM) aged 18 to 85 years were considered eligible if they had been diagnosed (with DRM) during the visit to our Nutritional Unit and provided informed consent.

Malnutrition was assessed by the Global Leadership Initiative on Malnutrition (GLIM) criteria [14].

The constructed dataset consisted of two sets of measurements, one corresponding to the measurements realized by a conventional method for rater 1 (i.e., method A) and the other one is the set of measurements performed by PIIXMED^{TM}, rater 2 (i.e., method B). The raters were kept blinded to the initial findings, (i.e., measurements for each muscle, for each MAP parameter, and the same variable for each rater).

2.2. Inclusion/Exclusion Criteria

Exclusion criteria included liver dysfunction (aminotransferase levels > 3 times the upper reference limit); chronic renal failure (glomerular filtration rate < 45 mL/min/1.73 m^2); previous Intensive Care Unit (ICU) stay during the last hospital admission; cancer patients with an Eastern Cooperative Oncology Group performance status $\geq$ 3 points; eating disorders; any musculoskeletal disease preventing unassisted walking ability; dementia, cognitive impairment, or any neurological/psychiatric condition that may interfere with study procedures; life expectancy of less than six months; and refusal to sign the informed consent form.

2.3. Ethics Committee

The study protocol received approval from the Ethics Committee for Clinical Research of the Health Council of HCUVA (protocol code PIP23341, approval date November 2023), as well as from the individual Institutional Review Boards of the participating hospitals. Written informed consent was acquired from all patients involved in the study.

2.4. Screening Process

In all patients, a conventional ultrasound determination of the rectus femoris (RF) was performed by the same investigator, capturing the ultrasound images and subsequently analyzing them with the automatic system PIIXMED^{TM}, (Dawako Medtech S.L., Valencia, Spain). This cloud-based web system is a convolutional neural network (CNN), with a U-net architecture, see Figure 1.

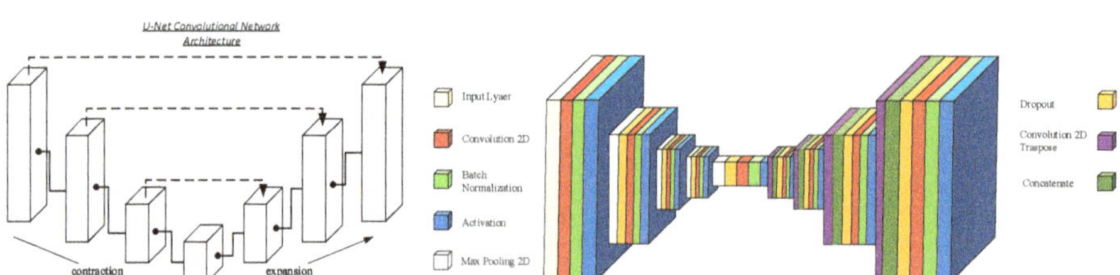

(**a**) (**b**)

Figure 1. The U-net is a convolutional network architecture for fast and precise segmentation of images. Up to now, it has outperformed the prior best method (a sliding-window convolutional network). (**a**) Generic U-Net architecture; (**b**) specifically developed U-Net architecture for automatic musculoskeletal system segmentation depicting the constitutive layers in the contraction and expansion phases.

Ultrasound assessments of the unilateral (right) RF were conducted in all patients at risk of malnutrition by a skilled medical sonographer who was unaware of the clinical data and the other results of the nutritional assessment. A portable ultrasound system with a 4–10 cm linear probe (UProbe L6C Ultrasound Scanner, Guangzhou Sonostar Technologies Co., Ltd., Guangzhou, China) was utilized for anterior thigh muscle measurements while the patient lay supine with extended and relaxed knees.

The acquisition site was located two-thirds along the length of the femur, between the anterior superior iliac spine and the upper edge of the patella. The transducer was positioned perpendicularly to minimize pressure on the muscle during measurement using excessive contact gel.

All parameters were measured manually using the incorporated tools of the ultrasound device averaged over three consecutive measurements in the dominant leg, including the cross-sectional area (CSA) in cm^2, the Y-axis (Transverse muscle thickness (MT)) in millimeters (mm) of the quadriceps rectus femoris muscles, and subcutaneous fat thickness (SFT) in mm. The Image JR program version 1.54 f (National Institutes of Health NIH, Bethesda, MD, USA) was used to determine echogenicity; this program is a method to treat radiological images developed by the National Health Institute (NIH). After the acquisition of the ultrasound images and the subsequent processing of these images by the PIXMED™ system, the following analysis methodology was conducted.

1. Compare the measurements of the unilateral (right) RF of the patients performed by the expert evaluator (rater 1) using the standard tools included in the ultrasound image device (i.e., method A), see Figure 2, with those obtained by applying the PIIXMED™ Ultrasound Imaging System (Dawako Medtech S.L., Valencia, Spain) (rater 2) (i.e., method B) [15–19] on the same acquired raw images, see Figures 3 and 4.
2. Calculate and evaluate the inter-rater reliability of quantitative muscle architecture parameters (MAP) of the unilateral (right) RF measurements performed by the expert evaluator (rater 1) (i.e., method A) against the measurements using the automated PIIXMED™ Ultrasound Imaging System (rater 2) (Dawako Medtech S.L., Valencia, Spain) (i.e., method B) on the same acquired raw images.

The MAP variables measured and analyzed by PIIXMED™ in this study were the RF thickness and cross-sectional area in the transverse plane (MT, and CSA) and the subcutaneous fat thickness (SFT) in its longitudinal plane.

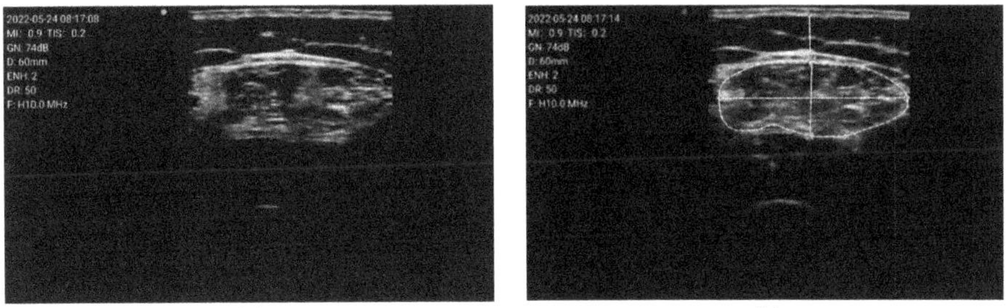

(a) (b)

Figure 2. (**a**) Acquired raw ultrasound image of the unilateral (right) quadriceps rectus femoris muscle in the transverse plane measure by rater 1 (i.e., method A); (**b**) Measurement of the variables by the conventional method using the ultrasound imaging device tools, by rater 1 (i.e., method A), for the parameters of the cross-sectional area, the Y-axis, i.e., transverse muscle thickness (MT), and the subcutaneous fat thickness (SFT).

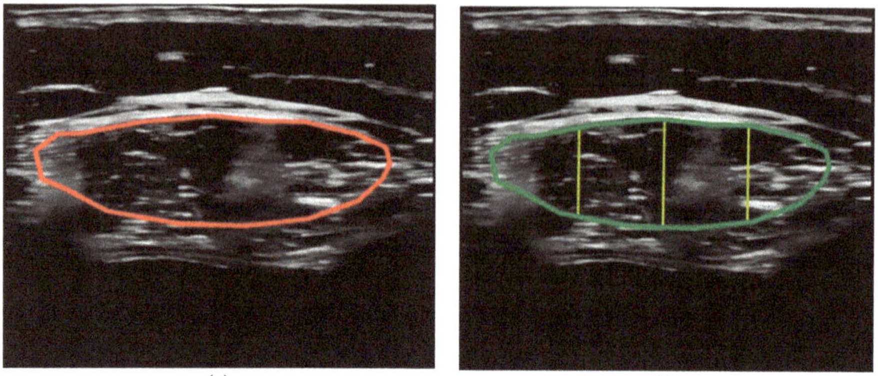

(a) (b)

Figure 3. (**a**) Acquired raw ultrasound image of the unilateral (right) quadriceps rectus femoris muscle in the transverse plane obtained by rater 1, scaled and automatically segmented (red color line) by PIIXMEDTM (rater 2—method B); (**b**) PIIXMEDTM processing (i.e., rater 2—method B) of the segmented transverse ultrasound image to obtain the results of CSA (green color), and MT (three yellow lines and their mean value) parameters.

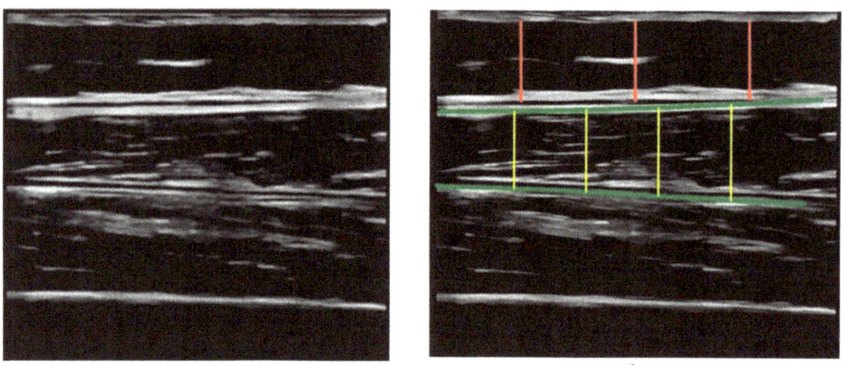

(a) (b)

Figure 4. (**a**) Acquired raw ultrasound image of the unilateral (right) quadriceps rectus femoris muscle in the longitudinal plane obtained by rater 1 and scaled by PIIXMEDTM (rater 2—method B); (**b**) PIIXMEDTM processing (i.e., rater 2—method B) of the automatically segmented longitudinal ultrasound image, upper and deep aponeurosis (green color), to obtain the results of the SFT (three red lines and their mean value) parameter and the longitudinal thickness (four yellow lines and their mean value), MT, not used in this study.

2.5. Statistical Analysis

Previous statistical analysis and power and sample size determination were performed to ensure the study was adequately powered to detect meaningful effects and achieve specific statistical goals. The level of statistical power was set to 80% and a curve of sensitivity was obtained with a result of 84 subjects as the sample size. The factors for calculating the sample size were the level of 95% confidence interval, a significance level (α) of 5%, and the variability (standard deviation) of the data.

It is important to assess the number of measurement errors by evaluating the reproducibility and reliability of measurements [20]. In the context of a study, it is important to consider other statistical measures in conjunction with assessing reproducibility (i.e., the variation in the same measurement made on a subject under changing circumstances or by different operators).

To evaluate the magnitude of error between repeated measurements, the Coefficient of Variation (CV) was used, which is a standardized measure of the dispersion of a probability distribution [21]. The CV is a statistical measure used to assess the relative variability of a set of data points, expressed as a percentage and calculated by dividing the standard deviation by the mean and then multiplying by 100. The Coefficient of Variation is particularly useful when comparing the variability of datasets with different units or scales. It provides a standardized measure, allowing for a more meaningful comparison of the relative variability between datasets.

After the normality of the data was assessed using Kolmogorov–Smirnov test statistics for normally distributed variables, such as MT, the correlation between method A and method B was estimated using Pearson's (i.e., r) linear relationship. For non-normally distributed variables like SFT and CSA, the correlation between method A and method B was estimated using Spearman's rank correlation test for association between the two variables, (i.e., ρ).

Also, Linear Regression analysis was applied to evaluate reproducibility by obtaining the percentage of the explained variation (i.e., r^2), which represents the proportion of the variance in the dependent variable that can be explained by the independent variable in a linear model, being a measure of the goodness of fit.

Then, the Intraclass Correlation Coefficient (ICC) was used to evaluate reliability to assess the consistency or agreement under changing conditions or different raters. There are three versions of the ICC introduced in the literature depending on the experimental design and goals of the study [22–24]. The commonly used models of ICC are as follows: one-way random effects, two-way random effects, and two-way mixed effects. The one-way random effect was selected for the objective of this study, (i.e., assessing the reliability and consistency of measurements made by different raters or instruments on the same subjects). The classification of Intraclass Correlation Coefficient (ICC) scores varies from 0 to 1. Higher ICC values indicate greater agreement or consistency between measurements. ICC values above 0.75 are considered excellent, between 0.60 and 0.74 good, between 0.40 and 0.59 fair to moderate, and below 0.40 poor.

Together with ICC, the Bland–Altman analysis method was used [25] to assess the agreement between two measurement techniques or observers. It is a scatter plot of the differences between the two methods against their average. The analysis provides insights into the agreement, bias, and limits of agreement between the two methods. The Bland–Altman plot is widely used to visualize the difference in two continuous measurements from the same individual, graphed according to the average value of the two measures. In terms of the musculoskeletal system, this is highly valuable to assess measurements taken on the same patient by two different operators. This method can also be used for assessing two measurements made by the same operator or two measurements using different techniques or in different environments [20].

The software package used for statistical analysis and calculations was RStudio 2023.06.0 Build 421—(Posit Software, PBC formerly RStudio, PBC. The open-source data science company, 250 Northern Ave, Suite 420, Boston, MA, USA 02210 844-448-1212). RStudio is a complete, integrated software package that provides all the data manipulation, visualization, statistics, and automated reporting.

3. Results

3.1. Dataset

The database of samples in the study was made up of 100 patients (40% male and 60% female), see Table 1. All patients had nutritional DRM, with one phenotypic and one etiological criteria [15].

Table 1. Parameters of patients with DRM.

Parameters	
Age (years)	56.9 ± 16
Weight (kg)	55.6 ± 14.7
BMI (kg/m^2)	20.9 ± 4.3
Sex (male/female)	40/60

3.2. *Summary and Descriptive Analysis*

The calculation of the univariate summary statistics for all the variables in the dataset. The number of observations, mean value, standard deviation, standard error, minimum and maximum values, skewness, and kurtosis of the distributions for SFT and MT are shown in Table 2.

Table 2. Summary and descriptive statistical analysis of the dataset.

	Subcutaneous Fat Thickness (SFT)		Muscle Thickness (MT)		Cross-Sectional Area (CSA)	
	Method A	**Method B**	**Method A**	**Method B**	**Method A**	**Method B**
N	100	100	100	100	100	100
Mean	0.70	0.74	1.10	1.04	3.47	3.52
SD	0.41	0.42	0.34	0.29	1.27	1.30
Min	0.00	0.03	0.50	0.53	1.06	1.10
Max	2.30	2.20	2.25	2.04	9.30	9.46
Skewness	1.21	0.93	0.54	0.42	1.00	0.97
Kurtosis	1.94	0.78	0.27	0.11	3.08	2.96
SE	0.04	0.04	0.03	0.03	0.13	0.13

3.3. *Coefficient of Variation (CV)*

The CV measurements obtained using the two methods showed similar values with no significant differences in absolute values and coefficients of variation: 58.39–57.68% for SFT, 30.50–28.36% for MT, and 36.50–36.91% for CSA using method A and method B, respectively. The results are shown in Table 3.

Table 3. The table shows the CV for the distributions of method A and method B for each of the MAP variables.

	Coefficient of Variation (%) Method A and Method B		
Method	Subcutaneous Fat Thickness (SFT)	Muscle Thickness (MT)	Cross-Sectional Area (CSA)
A	58.39	30.50	36.50
B	57.68	28.36	36.91

3.4. *Pearson and Spearman Correlation Coefficients*

Table 4 shows the results of correlations between methods A and B, showing significantly higher values for very strong correlations, with 0.864 Spearman's monotonic positive correlation and p (value) = 5.2×10^{-32} for SFT (a); 0.969 for Pearson's linear relationship correlation and p (value) = 4.8×10^{-61} for MT (b); 0.991 Sperman's correlation, and p (value) = 1.9×10^{-86} for CSA (c).

Table 4. Correlations between methods.

Correlation between Method A and Method B		
Variables	Correlation	*p*_value
Subcutaneous Fat Thickness (SFT)	0.864 +	5.2×10^{-32}
Muscle Thickness (MT)	0.969 *	4.82×10^{-61}
Cross-Sectional Area (CSA)	0.991 +	1.92×10^{-86}

* Pearson's Correlation; + Spearman's Correlation.

3.5. Linear Regression Analysis

In the context of Linear Regression analysis, the R-squared (r^2) value represents the proportion of the variance in the dependent variable (i.e., method B) that can be explained by the independent variable (i.e., method A) in the model. It is a measure of the goodness of fit of the regression model and describes how well one variable can be used to predict the value of the other or the strength of their relationship. Figure 5 also shows (in set) the results obtained for R-squared (r^2) with values of 0.83 and *p* (value) = 4.8×10^{-40} for SFT (a); 0.94 and *p* (value) = 4.8×10^{-61} for MT (b); and 0.99 and *p* (value) = 6.4×10^{-102} for CSA (c).

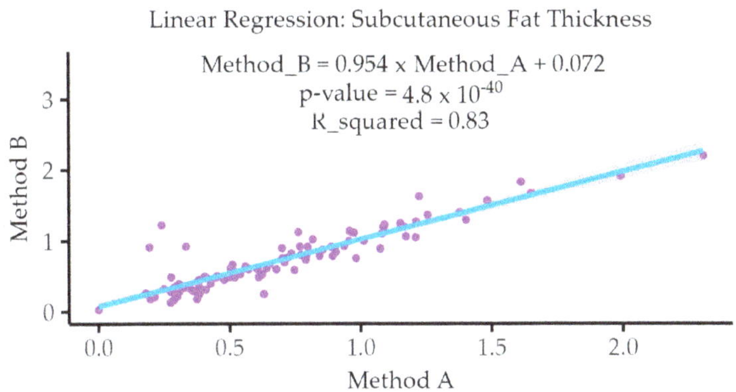

(**a**)

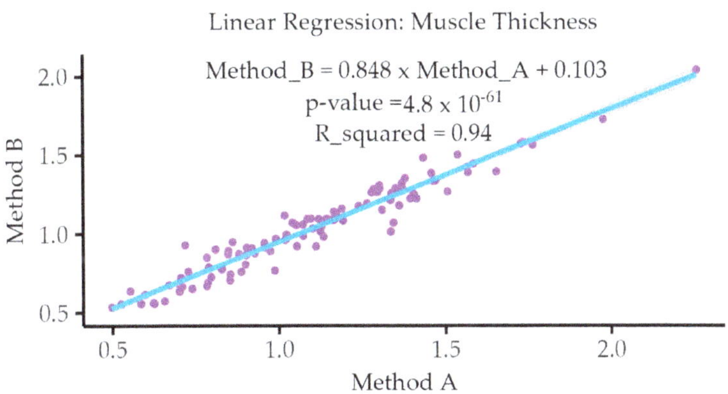

(**b**)

Figure 5. *Cont.*

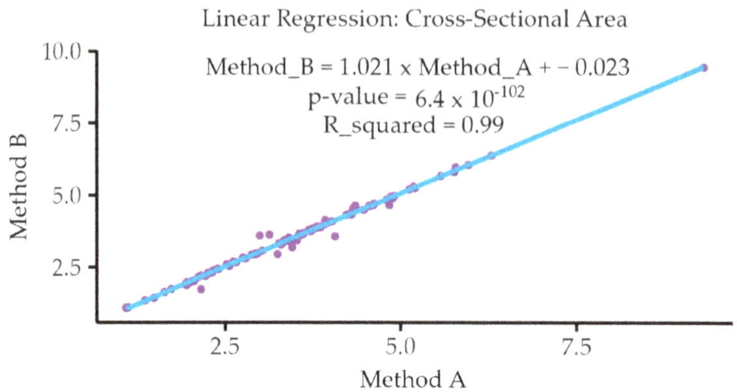

(c)

Figure 5. Results of the Linear Regression (r^2) for SFT (**a**); MT (**b**); and CSA (**c**).

3.6. Intraclass Correlation Coefficient (ICC)

The Intraclass Correlation Coefficient (ICC) results are detailed in Table 5. where the ICC coefficients are shown for the three variables (i.e., SFT (a), MT (b), and CSA (c)) under the three first columns of the table, with Excellent Reliability (ICC $\geq$ 0.9) indicating almost perfect agreement for the Single Fixed Raters and Average Fixed Raters.

Table 5. Complete detail of the statistical results for the ICC and Bland–Altman analysis of the MAP variables: (a) subcutaneous fat thickness (SFT); (b) muscle thickness (MT); (c) cross-sectional area (CSA).

Subcutaneous Fat Thickness (SFT)							
ICC			**Bland Altman Test**				
Raters	**ICC Coeff.**	**CI 95%**	**Mean Diff.**	**SE Diff.**	**CI 95% Diff.**	**SD Diff.**	**Lim. 95% Agreement**
Single fixed raters Average fixed raters	0.912 0.954	[0.872, 0.940] [0.931, 0.969]	−0.04	0.017	[−0.07, −0.005]	0.174	[−0.38, 0.30]

(a)

Muscle Thickness							
ICC			**Bland Altman Test**				
Raters	**ICC Coeff.**	**CI 95%**	**Mean Diff.**	**SE Diff.**	**CI 95% Diff.**	**SD Diff.**	**Lim. 95% Agreement**
Single fixed raters Average fixed raters	0.960 0.980	[0.941, 0.973] [0.970, 0.986]	0.065	0.009	[0.047, 0.082]	0.089	[−0.11, 0.24]

(b)

Cross-Sectional Area (CSA)							
ICC			**Bland Altman Test**				
Raters	**ICC Coeff.**	**CI 95%**	**Mean Diff.**	**SE Diff.**	**CI 95% Diff.**	**SD Diff.**	**Lim. 95% Agreement**
Single fixed raters Average fixed raters	0.995 0.998	[0.993, 0.997] [0.996, 0.998]	−0.051	0.013	[−0.076, −0.026]	0.127	[−0.3, 0.20]

(c)

3.7. Bland–Altman Analysis and Plots

It involves creating a scatter plot of the differences between the two methods against their average. The analysis provides insights into the agreement, bias, and limits of agreement between the two methods.

As can be seen in the plots in Figure 6, there is a consistent spread of points for the three variables (i.e., SFT (a), MT (b), and CSA (c)), with a few outliers falling outside of the LoA. These limits of agreement indicate where the true mean (and future measurements) is likely to lie. Also, the spread of points is quite uniform around the bias lines with no evidence of strong bias in any variable. In the case of the SFT (a)—bias = −0.04, and LoA = [−0.38, 0.30]; for MT (b)—bias = 0.065, and LoA = [−0.11, 0.24]; and for CSA (c)—bias = −0.051, and LoA = [−0.3, 0.20]. Table 5 describes all the quantitative results of the Bland–Altman analysis.

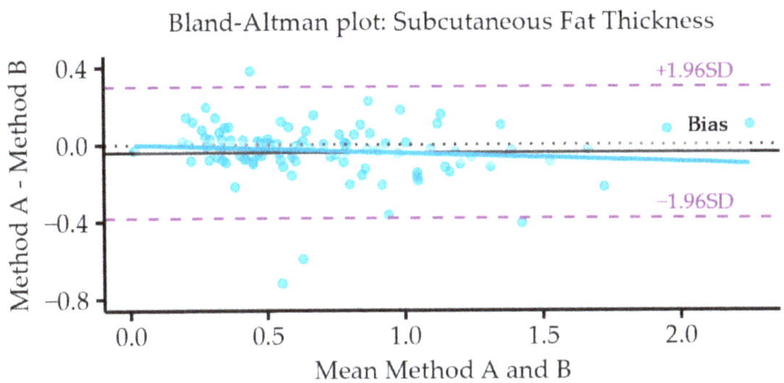

(a)

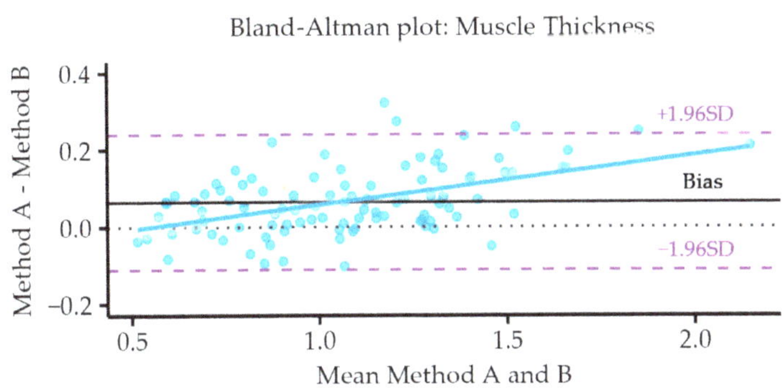

(b)

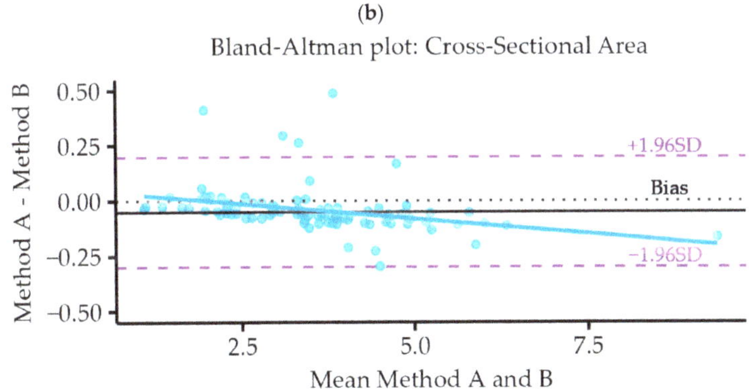

(c)

Figure 6. Bland–Altman analysis and plots to assess the agreement between the measurements performed by the two methods and between different measurements for each method for (**a**) subcutaneous fat thickness (SFT); (**b**) muscle thickness (MT); (**c**) cross-sectional area (CSA).

4. Discussion

Our study shows how the automatic ultrasound image analyzing system based on machine learning and AI can analyze ultrasound images of the rectus femoris (RF) with the same consistency and reliability as a trained sonographer.

There is an increasing focus in the research on assessing muscle mass using ultrasound. New studies indicate that measuring the area of the QRF muscle can be correlated with other factors such as fat-free mass, handgrip strength, and exercise capacity [26,27]. The clinical significance of ultrasound lies in its ability to assess muscle mass involvement in diagnosing malnutrition [26,28].

One of the significant challenges related to the effectiveness of ultrasound is in diagnosing malnutrition in various clinical scenarios. While specific cut-off points have not been determined yet, there are already publications attempting to identify the RF area with suitable sensitivity and specificity as a criterion for malnutrition. For instance, a multicenter study has established that a muscle area at the midpoint of the femur below 6 cm^2 for men or 4.47 cm^2 for females demonstrates adequate sensitivity and specificity in diagnosing malnutrition associated with PEW (protein-energy wasting) hemodialysis syndrome, a condition characterized by malnutrition, inflammation, and muscle wasting syndrome [27].

Despite the previously mentioned data, conventional analysis of ultrasound images of the muscle by an observer can have great variability and is also time-consuming during clinical consultation. If there is doubt, the arrival of automatic systems for analyzing ultrasound images could improve these limitations.

Our automatic system based on machine learning for the visualization and automatic analysis of medical ultrasound images is a cloud-based diagnostic aid tool referred to herein as a biomarker identification system for the generation, processing, and reporting of biosignal biomarkers and quantitative ultrasound image biomarkers. The cloud-based web system is a convolutional neural network (CNN) with a U-net architecture designed for the automatic segmentation of regions of interest (ROI). The U-Net receives images as input and returns segmentation maps as output. This architecture has been developed by the department of computer science at the University of Freiburg [29].

The network architecture for this study was designed to work with fewer training images and produce more accurate segmentations than previous proposals. The processing algorithms are based on the open-source Python package for the extraction of features and image biomarkers from medical imaging (i.e., Radiomics) [30]. Radiomics is a rapidly developing field of research focused on the extraction of quantitative features from medical images, thus converting these digital images into minable, high-dimensional data, which offer unique biological information that can enhance our understanding of disease processes and provide clinical decision support [31,32].

Our automatic system supports feature extraction in 2D for conventional B-Mode ultrasound imaging and can be used to calculate single values per feature for a region of interest (i.e., segment-based). From the features identified in the images and the application of the different algorithms, diverse biomarkers are extracted and processed to analyze, among others, the anatomical measures, the mean echogenicity of the region of interest (ROI), the muscle quality based on histogram analysis of echogenicity, the texture, and other non-linear algorithms like fractality (i.e., fractal dimension).

These biomarkers are automatically integrated into a structured report together with the results of the analysis to assist the physician in the diagnosis and assessment of a patient. Other automatic analyzing systems in ultrasound, based on machine learning and AI, are developed for pathologies such as breast cancer [33,34] or thyroid nodule characterization [35], generating in these pathologies an improvement in the speed of diagnosis and the accuracy of the prognoses compared with traditional methods. An example in nutrition is the evaluation of sarcopenia in patients with hepatocellular carcinoma [36].

To date, there is no automatic machine learning system that has evaluated muscle mass in patients with malnutrition related to disease, this being the first work to demonstrate its consistency and reliability in a pathology such as DRM with a high prevalence in our area [37].

Our study has some limitations. Firstly, it has only been conducted in patients with malnutrition related to disease, therefore it can only be generalized to patients with this pathology. Secondly, it was conducted in a single center, and there may be some selection bias. Thirdly, although the use of US is not a widespread technique in the determination of muscle mass in patients with DRM, clinical guidelines recommend its use [14] and a recent study has shown a good correlation with CT as a gold standard technique [38]. Fourthly, only one muscle has been evaluated, the RF. Finally, this automated method should be also replicated (and cross-validated) with another cohort and against MRI/CT [39,40] However, it also has strengths: the determination of the RF ultrasound image was perfectly standardized and only one researcher performed the ultrasounds on all patients.

5. Conclusions

Our study demonstrated the consistency and reliability of our new automatic system based on machine learning and AI for visualization and an automatic analysis system for the quantification of ultrasound imaging of the rectus femoris muscle compared with a conventional analysis by ultrasound in patients with disease-related malnutrition. These findings should be reproduced in future studies with a larger sample size and using other muscle groups. Without a doubt, this automated ultrasound image analysis system based on machine learning can help in the assessment of muscle mass in patients at risk of malnutrition and in patients with other entities.

Author Contributions: Conceptualization, D.d.L., J.J.L.C., S.N. and E.J.G.; methodology, D.d.L. and E.J.G.; software, A.C., S.N. and J.C.; validation, D.d.L. and E.J.G.; formal analysis, D.d.L.; investigation, E.J.G. and S.G.-H.; resources, D.d.L. and E.J.G.; data curation, A.C. and S.N.; writing—original draft preparation, D.d.L. and E.J.G.; writing—review and editing, S.G.-H., A.C., J.C., D.P., O.I., S.N. and P.S.C.; supervision, D.d.L. and E.J.G.; project administration, D.d.L. and E.J.G. All authors have read and agreed to the published version of the manuscript.

Funding: This research received no external funding.

Institutional Review Board Statement: The study was conducted in accordance with the Declaration of Helsinki of 1975 (https://www.wma.net/what-we-do/medical-ethics/declaration-of-helsinki/, accessed on 4 June 2024), revised in 2013, and the study protocol received approval from the Ethics Committee for Clinical Research of the Health Council of HCUVA (protocol code PIP23341, approval date November 2023), as well as from the individual Institutional Review Boards of the participating hospitals.

Informed Consent Statement: Informed consent was obtained from all subjects involved in the study before they participated in the study.

Data Availability Statement: Data are unavailable due to privacy and ethical restrictions.

Acknowledgments: We thank Agustín Maciá Barber and DAWAKO Medtech S.L. for providing administrative and technical support, for assistance in the use of the DAWAKO's Clinical spaces and equipment, and for comments on the manuscript.

Conflicts of Interest: Authors Sergio García-Herreros, Angela Cebria, Pablo Salvador Coloma, Sara Nozal, Jesús Cano and Eduardo Jorge Godoy were employed by the company DAWAKO Medtech S.L. The remaining authors declare that the research was conducted in the absence of any commercial or financial relationships that could be construed as a potential conflict of interest.

References

1. López-Gómez, J.J.; Bachiller, B.R.; de Luis Roman, D. Management of disease-related malnutrition: A real-world experience with a novel concentrated high-protein energy-dense oral nutritional supplement. *Postgrad. Med.* **2024**, *136*, 52–59. [CrossRef]
2. Álvarez-Hernández, J. Prevalencia y costes de la malnutrición en pacientes hospitalizados: Estudio PREDyCES®. *Nutr. Hosp.* **2012**, *27*, 1049–1059.
3. Merker, M. Association of baseline inflammation with effectiveness of nutritional support among patients with disease-related malnutrition: A secondary analysis of a randomized clinical trial. *JAMA Netw. Open* **2020**, *3*, e200663. [CrossRef] [PubMed]

4. Kaegi-Braun, N. Validation of modified GLIM criteria to predict adverse clinical outcome and response to nutritional treatment: A secondary analysis of a randomized clinical trial. *Clin. Nutr.* **2022**, *41*, 795–804. [CrossRef]
5. León-Sanz, M.; Brosa, M.; Planas, M.; García-de-Lorenzo, M.; Celaya-Pérez, S.; Alvarez, J. PREDyCES study: The cost of hospital malnutrition in Spain. *Nutrition* **2015**, *31*, 1096–1102. [CrossRef] [PubMed]
6. Cruz-Jentoft, A.J. Sarcopenia: Revised European consensus on definition and diagnosis. *Age Ageing* **2019**, *48*, 16–31. [CrossRef]
7. Gingrich, A. Prevalence and overlap of sarcopenia, frailty, cachexia and malnutrition in older medical inpatients. *BMC Geriatr.* **2019**, *19*, 120. [CrossRef]
8. Park, B. Consensus-defined sarcopenia predicts adverse outcomes after elective abdominal surgery: Meta-analysis. *BJS Open* **2023**, *7*, 065. [CrossRef] [PubMed]
9. Garcia-Almeida, J.M. Nutritional ultrasound®: Conceptualisation, technical considerations and standardisation. *Endocrinol. Diabetes Nutr.* **2023**, *70*, 74–84. [CrossRef]
10. Perkisas, S. Application of ultrasound for muscle assessment in sarcopenia: Towards standardized measurements. *Eur. Geriatr. Med.* **2018**, *9*, 739–757. [CrossRef]
11. Perkisas, S.; Bastijns, S.; Sanchez-Rodriguez, D.; Piotrowicz, K.; De Cock, A.M.; Full SARCUS Working Group. Application of ultrasound for muscle assessment in sarcopenia: 2020 SARCUS update: Reply to the letter to the editor: SARCUS working group on behalf of the Sarcopenia Special Interest Group of the European Geriatric Medicine Society. *Eur. Geriatr. Med.* **2021**, *12*, 427–428. [CrossRef] [PubMed]
12. Standard, D. Digital Imaging and Communication in Medicine. Strateg. Doc. Available online: https://www.dicomstandard.org/ (accessed on 25 March 2024).
13. Cath, S.; Wachter, B.; Mittelstadt, M.; Floridi, L. Artificial intelligence and the 'good society': The US, EU, and UK approach. *Sci. Eng. Ethics* **2018**, *24*, 505–528. [PubMed]
14. Cederholm, T. GLIM criteria for the diagnosis of malnutrition—A consensus report from the global clinical nutrition community. *J. Cachexia. Sarcopenia Muscle* **2019**, *10*, 207–217. [CrossRef] [PubMed]
15. Haralick, R.M.; Shanmugam, K.; Dinstein, I.H. Textural features for image classification. *IEEE Trans. Syst. Man. Cybern.* **1973**, *6*, 610–621. [CrossRef]
16. Galloway, M.M. Texture analysis using gray level run lengths. *Comput. Graph. Image Process.* **1975**, *4*, 172–179. [CrossRef]
17. Penn, A.I.; Loew, M.H. Estimating fractal dimension with fractal interpolation function models. *IEEE Trans. Med. Imaging* **1997**, *16*, 930–937. [CrossRef] [PubMed]
18. Yu, S.; Lakshminarayanan, V. Fractal dimension and retinal pathology: A meta-analysis. *Appl. Sci.* **2021**, *11*, 2376. [CrossRef]
19. Romero, F.; Alonso, F.J. A comparison among different Hill-type contraction dynamics formulations for muscle force estimation. *Mech. Sci.* **2016**, *7*, 19–29. [CrossRef]
20. Bunting, K.V.; Steeds, R.P.; Slater, L.T.; Rogers, J.K.; Gkoutos, G.V.; Kotecha, D. A Practical Guide to Assess the Reproducibility of Echocardiographic Measurements. *J. Am. Soc. Echocardiogr.* **2019**, *32*, 1505–1515. [CrossRef]
21. Reed, G.F.; Lynn, F.; Meade, B.D. Use of coefficient of variation in assessing variability of quantitative assays. *Clin. Vaccine Immunol.* **2002**, *9*, 1235–1239. [CrossRef]
22. Shrout, P.E.; Fleiss, J.L. Intraclass Correlations: Uses in Assessing Rater Reliability. *Psychol. Bull.* **1979**, *86*, 420–428. [CrossRef] [PubMed]
23. Rankin, G.; Stokes, M. Reliability of assessment tools in rehabilitation: An illustration of appropriate statistical analyses. *Clin. Rehabil.* **1998**, *12*, 187–199. [CrossRef] [PubMed]
24. Liljequist, D.; Elfving, B.; Skavberg Roaldsen, K. Intraclass correlation—A discussion and demonstration of basic features. *PLoS ONE* **2019**, *14*, e0219854. [CrossRef] [PubMed]
25. Bland, J.M.; Altman, D.G. Statistical methods for assessing agreement between two methods of clinical measurement. *Lancet* **1986**, *327*, 307–310. [CrossRef]
26. López-Gómez, J.J. Nutritional Ultrasonography, a method to evaluate Muscle Mass and Quality in Morphofunctional Assessment of Disease Related Malnutrition. *Nutrients* **2023**, *15*, 3923. [CrossRef] [PubMed]
27. Sahathevan, S. Association of ultrasound-derived metrics of the quadriceps muscle with protein energy wasting in hemodialysis patients: A multicenter cross-sectional study. *Nutrients* **2020**, *12*, 3597. [CrossRef] [PubMed]
28. de Luis Roman, D.A.; Lopez Gomez, J.J. Morphofunctional Nutritional Assessment in Clinical Practice: A New Approach to Assessing Nutritional Status. *Nutrients* **2023**, *15*, 4300. [CrossRef] [PubMed]
29. Ronneberger, O.; Fischer, P.; Brox, T. U-net: Convolutional networks for biomedical image segmentation. In Proceedings of the Medical Image Computing and Computer-Assisted Intervention—MICCAI 2015: 18th International Conference, Munich, Germany, 5–9 October 2015; Proceedings, Part III 18. pp. 234–241.
30. Van Griethuysen, J.J.M. Computational radiomics system to decode the radiographic phenotype. *Cancer Res.* **2017**, *77*, e104–e107. [CrossRef]
31. McCague, C. Introduction to radiomics for a clinical audience. *Clin. Radiol.* **2023**, *78*, 83–98. [CrossRef]
32. Abramson, R.G.; Burton, K.R.; Yu, J.P.; Scalzetti, E.M.; Yankeelov, T.E.; Rosenkrantz, A.B.; Mendiratta-Lala, M.; Bartholmai, B.J.; Ganeshan, D.; Lenchik, L.; et al. Methods, and challenges in quantitative imaging biomarker development. *Acad. Radiol.* **2015**, *22*, 25–32. [CrossRef]

33. Raza, A.; Ullah, N.; Khan, J.A.; Assam, M.; Guzzo, A.; Aljuaid, H. Deep Breast Cancer Net: A Novel Deep Learning Model for Breast Cancer Detection Using Ultrasound Images. *Appl. Sci.* **2023**, *13*, 2082. [CrossRef]
34. Rabiei, R.; Ayyoubzadeh, S.M.; Sohrabei, S.; Esmaeili, M.; Atashi, A. Prediction of Breast Cancer using Machine Learning Approaches. *J. Biomed. Phys. Eng.* **2022**, *12*, 297–308. [CrossRef] [PubMed]
35. Anari, S.; Tataei Sarshar, N.; Mahjoori, N.; Dorosti, S.; Rezaie, A. Review of deep learning approaches for thyroid cancer diagnosis. *Math. Probl. Eng.* **2022**, *20*, 5052435. [CrossRef]
36. Liu, Z. Deep learning-based radiomics allows for a more accurate assessment of sarcopenia as a prognostic factor in hepatocellular carcinoma. *J. Zhejiang Univ. B* **2024**, *25*, 83–90. [CrossRef] [PubMed]
37. Jiménez, C.B.; Ovalle, H.F.; Moreno, M.F.; Aller de la Fuente, R.; de Luis Román, D. Undernutrition measured by the Mini Nutritional Assessment (MNA) test and related risk factors in older adults under hospital emergency care. *Nutrition* **2019**, *66*, 142–146. [CrossRef] [PubMed]
38. Palmas, F.; Mucarzel, F.; Ricart, M.; Lluch, A.; Burgos, R. Body composition assessment with ultrasound muscle measurement: Optimization through the use of semi-automated tools in colorectal cancer. *Front. Nutr.* **2024**, *11*, 1372816. [CrossRef] [PubMed]
39. Naruse, M.; Trappe, S.; Trappe, T.A. Human skeletal muscle size with ultrasound imaging: A comprehensive review. *J. Appl. Physiol.* **2022**, *132*, 1267–1279. [CrossRef]
40. Ahtiainen, J.P.; Hoffren, M.; Hulmi, J.J.; Pietikäinen, M.; Mero, A.A.; Avela, J.; Häkkinen, K. Panoramic ultrasonography is a valid method to measure changes in skeletal muscle cross-sectional area. *Eur. J. Appl. Physiol.* **2010**, *108*, 273–279. [CrossRef]

nutrients MDPI

Systematic Review

Morphofunctional Assessment beyond Malnutrition: Fat Mass Assessment in Adult Patients with Phenylketonuria—Systematic Review

Luis M. Luengo-Pérez [1,2,*], Mercedes Fernández-Bueso [2], Carlos Guzmán-Carmona [3], Ana López-Navia [3] and Claudia García-Lobato [2]

1 Medical Sciences Department, Faculty of Medicine and Health Sciences, University of Extremadura, 06006 Badajoz, Spain
2 Clinical Nutrition and Dietetics Unit, Endocrinology and Nutrition Section, Badajoz University Hospital, 06008 Badajoz, Spain; mmercedes.fernandez@salud-juntaex.es (M.F.-B.); claudia.garcial@salud-juntaex.es (C.G.-L.)
3 Endocrinology and Nutrition, Don Benito-Villanueva de la Serena Hospital Complex, 06400 Don Benito, Spain; carlos.guzman@salud-juntaex.es (C.G.-C.); ana.lopezn@salud-juntaex.es (A.L.-N.)
* Correspondence: luismluengo@unex.es

Abstract: Morphofunctional assessment was developed to evaluate disease-related malnutrition. However, it can also be used to assess cardiometabolic risk, as excess adiposity increases this risk. Phenylketonuria (PKU) is the most prevalent inherited metabolic disease among adults, and obesity in PKU has recently gained interest, although fat mass correlates better with cardiometabolic risk than body mass index. In this systematic review, the objective was to assess whether adult patients with PKU have higher fat mass than healthy controls. Studies of adult PKU patients undergoing dietary treatment in a metabolic clinic reporting fat mass were included. The PubMed and EMBASE databases were searched. Relevance of articles, data collection, and risk of bias were evaluated by two independent reviewers. Ten articles were evaluated, six with a control group, including 310 subjects with PKU, 62 with mild hyperphenylalaninemia, and 157 controls. One study reported a significant and four a tendency towards an increased fat mass in all patients or only females with PKU. Limitations included not having a healthy control group, not reporting sex-specific results and using different techniques to assess fat mass. Evaluation of fat mass should be included in the morphofunctional assessment of cardiometabolic risk in adult patients with PKU.

Keywords: phenylketonuria; body composition; body fat; morphofunctional assessment; cardiovascular risk; metabolic diseases

1. Introduction

Morphofunctional assessment of patients' nutritional status was first developed for disease-related malnutrition [1,2]. Malnutrition is an issue of concern in patients with inherited metabolic diseases (IMDs), some of whom have neurological manifestations, and most of whom are on restrictive dietary treatment.

Nevertheless, there are IMDs with a known increased cardiometabolic risk, such as homocystinuria and glycogen storage disease type III, while most patients with IMDs in adult metabolic clinics are patients with phenylketonuria (PKU), in whom a possible increased risk and prevalence of obesity have recently been discussed [3–5].

Newborn screening programs, together with dietary treatment, have led to an increase in the life expectancy of patients with PKU, with a growing number of patients aged 50 or older, in whom prevention of acquired cardiovascular and metabolic diseases should be considered, although it is not known whether the risk of cardiometabolic disease is similar or different to that of the general population.

Obesity, as an excess of total body adiposity, could increase the risk of acquired cardiometabolic disease. Adipose tissue has different biological endocrine, autocrine, and paracrine functions [6], and may increase the risk of cardiometabolic disease depending on its type and location [7,8].

In a global morphofunctional assessment of a patient's nutritional status, fat mass should be evaluated as a morphological assessment of cardiometabolic risk. Excess adiposity and visceral fat are not well evaluated by body mass index (BMI) or other anthropometric methods. The Global Leadership Initiative on Malnutrition recommends anthropometry, only when technical approaches to assess muscle mass are not available [9]. Most available clinical fat assessment techniques are bioelectrical impedance analysis (BIA), and nutritional ultrasound, while others such as dual X-ray absorptiometry (DXA), computed tomography (CT), or magnetic resonance imaging (MRI) are less available or only opportunistic [10].

The objective of this systematic review was to evaluate whether patients with PKU have a higher cardiometabolic risk due to excess fat mass than people without hyperphenylalaninemia (hPA).

2. Materials and Methods

2.1. Protocol and Selection Criteria

This study was developed according to the Grading of Recommendations Assessment, Development and Evaluation (GRADE) systematic approach for evidence synthesis [11,12].

The inclusion and exclusion criteria for articles were defined following the PECO (Population, Exposure, Comparator, and Outcome) format [13].

Inclusion criteria were: Adult patients with PKU (population, exposure) undergoing dietary treatment at a metabolic diseases clinic (exposure); although published studies including a control group (comparator) were preferred, those without a control group were not excluded provided they were randomized controlled trials (RCTs), as well as non-randomized controlled trials (non-RCTs), or observational studies (case series, cohort, case-control, and cross-sectional), providing information about fat mass (outcome). Exclusion criteria: Pediatric population, patients with diseases other than PKU, lack of data on fat mass. The project has been registered at Open Science Framework (OSF): https://osf.io/f2xvn, accessed on 3 may 2024.

2.2. Search Strategy, Study Selection, and Data Collecction

A scientific literature search was performed on PubMed, and Embase databases on 21 September 2023 and updated on April 1st, 2024. Medical Subject Headings (MeSH) and text terms related to fat mass and PKU were used. Limits to "adult" patients and to the English, German, French, Portuguese, and Spanish languages were introduced. As the result in PubMed was only 9 articles, the "adult" limit was ignored at this stage of the review to obtain 33 articles (see Section 3.1).

All articles identified in the previous search were included in the screening process, but those with animals, seven more with pediatric populations only, two different studies with other inherited metabolic diseases and unrelated diseases, as well as duplicates, were subsequently excluded.

Two independent reviewers (L.M.L.-P. and C.G.-L.) assessed the relevance of the titles and abstracts of the articles. Full-text articles were reviewed when titles and abstracts did not provide enough information and were selected for their interest to assess eligibility according to the criteria in Section 2.1. As a secondary search strategy, the references included in the selected articles were screened to avoid missing relevant studies. There were some articles without a control group, with differences between reviewers, and it was decided to include them to avoid missing data, as the number of articles was low.

Data items from each study were extracted by two authors (L.M.L.-P. and M.F.-B.). Data included were: first author, country, year, study design, method, sample characteristics, including comparison with control group, and fat mass (outcome).

2.3. Assessment of Risk of Bias in Individual Studies

Two reviewers (L.M.L.-P. and M.F.-B.) independently evaluated the risk of bias of selected studies using the National Institutes of Health (NIH) Quality Assessment Tool for Observational Cohort and Cross-Sectional Studies [14], including the items related to: Statement of the research question or objective, definition of the study population, rate of eligible persons, inclusion and exclusion criteria, sample size justification, when and how exposure and outcome were measured, blinding of outcome assessors, rate of follow-up, and adjustment of confounding variables. Disagreements between reviewers were resolved by consensus, with the highest risk of bias identified when there were differences.

3. Results

3.1. Study Selection

A total of 149 articles were identified in EMBASE and 33 in PubMed (without "Adult" limit). Figure 1 shows the flow diagram of the review process following the PRISMA model [15].

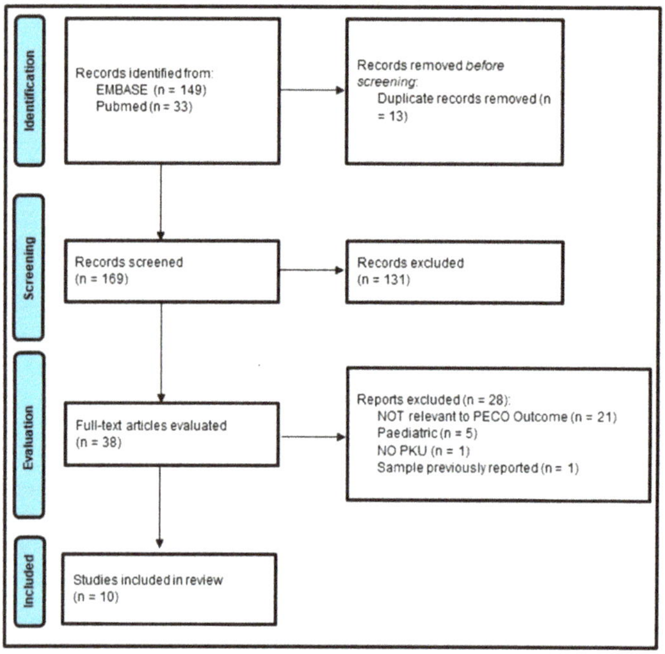

Figure 1. Study flow diagram following PRISMA model.

After removing 13 duplicates, the titles and abstracts of the remaining 169 articles were assessed for relevance, and a total of 38 full-text articles were selected for evaluation.

Among these 38 articles, 22 did not provide information about body composition, 5 included an exclusively or predominantly pediatric sample, and another one did not include patients with PKU but healthy volunteers. (See Supplementary Material). The remaining 10 articles fulfilled all inclusion criteria (Section 2.1) and were included for quantitative analysis [16–25].

3.2. Study Characteristics

A summary of the 10 articles reviewed is shown in Table 1.

There was only one longitudinal study [20], with a follow-up of six months. The remaining 9 studies were cross-sectional, although one of them [23] was a cross-sectional study of a subset of 15 participants from a previously published randomized, crossover trial [26], and another one included baseline data from a longitudinal study [18].

Table 1. Summary of the studies included in the systematic review.

Reference (Country)	Study Design (Duration of Follow-Up)	Sample Size (Age)	Controls (Age)	Sex (F/M)	Other	Risk of Bias [1]
Alghamdi et al. 2021 (UK) [16]	Cross-sectional	10 (33.9 ± 5.0)	9 (28.8 ± 5.9)	P: 6/4 C: 6/3	Mixed pediatric and adult sample	High
Barta et al. 2022 (Hungary) [17]	Cross-sectional	50 (F 31 ± 7.8, M 26.6 ± 7.6)	40 (F 26.5, M 24)	P: 27/23 C: 20/20	-	High
Jani et al. 2017 (USA) [18]	Cross-sectional	27 (28.8, [19.5–54.6])	NO	18/9	Mixed pediatric and adult sample, compared with reference US population	High
Mezzomo et al. 2023 (Brazil) [19]	Cross-sectional	36 (25.36 ± 5.14)	33 (28.27 ± 6.15)	P: 16/20 C: 21/12	-	Moderate
Montanari et al. 2022 (Italy) [20]	Longitudinal (6 months)	4 (n.a.)	NO	n.a.	Mixed pediatric and adult sample	High
Rocha et al. 2012 (Portugal) [21]	Cross-sectional	26 (22.8 ± 3.0)	29 (23.6 ± 4.7)	n.a.	Mixed pediatric and adult sample	Moderate
Rojas Agurto et al. 2023 (Chile) [22]	Cross-sectional	24 (39.3)	24 (38.4)	P: 10/14 C: 10/14		High
Stroup et al. 2018 (USA) [23]	Cross-sectional	15 (15–50)	NO	9/6	Included 3 adolescents (15–17 y)	High
Weng et al. 2020 (Taiwan) [24]	Cross-sectional	22 (15.23 ± 5.23 [8–27])	22 (19.73 ± 10.6 [8–39])	P: 12/10 C: 12/10	Correlates inversely with protein intake Adult subjects number not shown	High
Zerjav Tansek et al. 2020 (Slovenia) [25]	Cross-sectional	96 (48 adults) (22.2 ± 11.4)	NO/62 mild HPA (14.4 ± 6.8)	P: 50/46 HPA: 22/40	Compared with mild HPA, not healthy controls	High

[1] Assessed using the National Institutes of Health (NIH) Quality Assessment Tool for Observational Cohort and Cross-Sectional Studies [14]. Abbreviations: AFM: abdominal fat mass, C: control group, F: female, FM: fat mass, FMI: fat mass index, HPA: hyperphenylalaninemia, M: male, n.a.: not available, P: PKU patients group, UK: United Kingdom; USA: United States of America. n.b.: When samples were with mixed pediatric and adult populations, only adult (or older than 15/16) results are shown.

Five studies were developed in Europe [16,17,20,21,25], four in America [18,19,22,23], and one in Asia [24]. All of them, but Rocha et al. (2012) [21], were published between 2017 and 2023.

Three studies did not include a control group [18,20,23], and Jani et al. [18] compared patients with PKU with the USA reference population. These three studies included 46 patients with PKU. The other six articles included 168 patients with PKU and 157 non-HPA-matched controls [16,17,19,21,22,24], and the last study, by Zerjav Tansek et al. [25], compared outcomes in 96 patients with PKU and 62 patients with mild HPA. Considering all the articles, outcomes in 310 subjects with PKU, 62 with mild HPA, and 157 with non-HPA were communicated.

All studies included both female and male participants (patients with PKU and controls), but two of them did not report the number of each [20,22], and the other four did not report female and male results separately (Table 2) [16,21,24,25].

Most articles included a mixed sample of pediatric and adult patients (and controls). Whenever adult data were presented separately [16,18,20,21], only these data were taken into consideration. Rocha et al. [21] included as adult patients those aged 16 or older.

Two other studies with mixed pediatric-adult samples, reported the proportion of adult patients [25] or did not report [24], but neither of them reported adult data separately. The remaining 3 studies included only [17,19] or mainly [23] adult patients, as Stroup et al. included 3 patients aged 15 to 17 among their sample of 15 patients.

All the included studies assessed body composition, as fat mass was the PECO outcome inclusion criteria of this review (Section 2.1). Body composition was assessed by BIA [17,19,21,24] and DXA [18,22,23,25] in four articles each, and plethysmography [20] and deuterium [16] were the methods used in the remaining two studies.

Table 2. Fat mass outcome from references that do NOT report adult female and male fat mass separately.

Reference (Country)	Parameter, Technique	PKU	Control	Difference	*p*
Alghamdi et al. 2021 (UK) [16]	FM (%) FMI Deuterium	39.4 ± 8.2 12.9 ± 4.6	34.3 ± 11.1 11.0 ± 5.8	+5.1 +1.8	n.a. n.a.
Rocha et al. 2012 (Portugal) [21]	FM (%), BIA	23.8 (13.9, 35.5)	23.8 (17.9, 34.3)	0	0.964
Rojas Agurto et al. 2023 (Chile) [22]	FM (kg), DXA	23.15	24.56	−1.41	n.a.
Weng et al. 2020 (Taiwan) [24]	FM (%), BIA	20.74 ± 8.9	18.67 ± 7.52	+2.07	0.4635
Zerjav Tansek et al. 2020 (Slovenia) [25]	FM (%) AFM (%) DXA	25.8 ± 6.8 22.7 ± 7.8	25.4 ± 6.7 21.1 ± 7.2 (HPA)	+0.4 +1.6	0.758 0.204

Data reported as mean ± standard deviation or mean (P25, P75). Abbreviations: AFM: abdominal fat mass, BIA: bioelectrical impedance analysis, DXA: dual X-ray absorptiometry, FM: fat mass, FMI: fat mass index, HPA: hyperphenylalaninemia, n.a.: not available, UK: United Kingdom. n.b.: When samples were with mixed pediatric and adult populations, only adult (or older than 15/16) results are shown.

Two studies [20,23] did not compare fat mass in patients with PKU with any other group. Among the six articles that included patients with PKU and non-HPA-matched controls [16,17,19,21,22,24], only Barta et al. [17] found that adult female patients with PKU had significantly more fat mass than non-HPA matched controls. Jani et al. [18] found a similar outcome comparing patients with PKU to the US reference population, but significance was not provided. Zerjav Tansek et al. [25] found that only patients with classic PKU had significantly lower fat mass than patients with non-classic PKU, but they included data from the pediatric population, with no other differences in whole-body or abdominal fat mass.

Fat mass from cross-sectional studies is shown in Table 2 (data reported without differences by sex)and Table 3 (male and female data separately).

Table 3. Fat mass outcome from references that report adult female and male fat mass separately.

Reference (Country)	Parameter, Technique	Female PKU	Female Control	Difference	Male PKU	Male Control	Difference
Barta et al. 2022 (Hungary) [17]	FM (%), BIA	36.7 (30.6, 40.2)	24.7 (22.2, 30.8)	+12.0 *	18.7 (14.3, 29.8)	19.4 (15.07, 24.5)	−0.7
Jani et al. 2017 (USA) [18]	FMI, DXA	38.9 *** (30.8, 64.3)	40.7 **	−1.8	23.4 *** (13.8, 81.4)	28.7 **	+5.3
Mezzomo et al. 2023 (Brazil) [19]	FM (%), BIA	36.2 (20.1, 49.0)	28.4 (15.9, 46.4)	+7.2	17.4 (10.1, 29.5)	23.3 (12.1, 27.2)	−5.9
Stroup et al. 2018 (USA) [23]	FM (%), DXA	36.5 ± 2.5	-	-	24.5 ± 4.8	-	-

* $p = 0.078$; all the rest, $p > 0.05$. ** USA reference population as control group. Data reported as mean ± standard deviation or mean (P25, P75) or *** mean (max, min). Abbreviations: BIA: bioelectrical impedance analysis, DXA: dual X-ray absorptiometry, FM: fat mass, FMI: fat mass index, USA: United States of America. n.b.: When samples were with mixed pediatric and adult populations, only adult (or older than 15/16) results are shown.

3.3. *Risk of Bias Assessment*

Two of the studies [19,21] were fair, with a moderate risk of bias, and the remaining eight [16–18,20,22–25] were poor, with high risk of bias. Figure 2 shows the degree of compliance with the selected items (see Section 2.3) from the NIH Quality Assessment Tool for Observational Cohort and Cross-Sectional Studies [14]. Risk of bias analysis from every individual study is available in the Supplementary Material, Section S3—Figure S1.

3.4. *Synthesis of Results*

3.4.1. Patients with PKU vs. Controls

Six of the studies [16,17,19,21,22,24] compared fat mass in patients with PKU with non-HPA controls, and only one of them, by Barta et al. [17], found significantly higher fat mass in adult female patients with PKU compared with matched healthy controls (35.8% vs. 24.7%, $p = 0.028$). No other significant differences in fat mass were found.

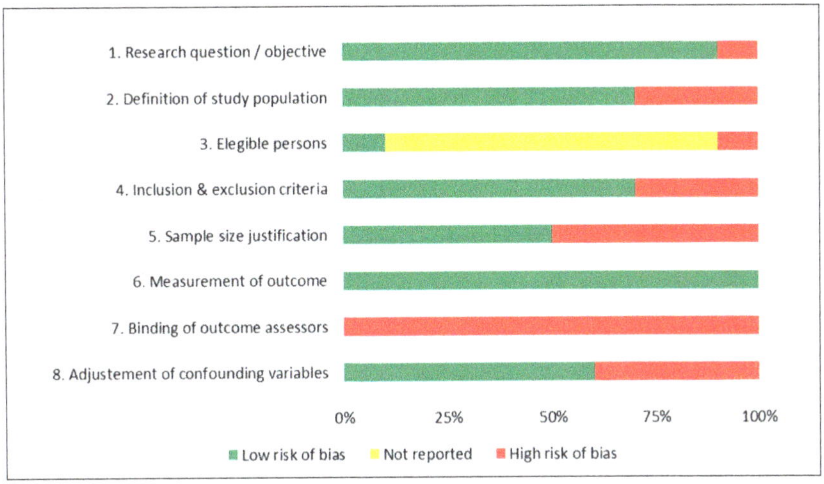

Figure 2. Risk of bias: judgments about each risk of bias item presented as percentages across all included studies.

Zerjav Tansek et al. [25] found that the proportion of whole-body fat by DXA was significantly (p = 0.04) lower in patients with classic PKU (24.3% ± 6.4) compared to non-classic PKU (27.6% ± 6.9), but they did not compare with healthy volunteers.

3.4.2. Patients with PKU without Control Group

Three studies did not include a control group [18,20,23].

Jani et al. [18] only showed that the median fat mass index by DXA in 26 adult patients with PKU (mainly females) was 9.1 (range: 5.3–29.5) and the median fat mass in males was 30.9 kg (17.1–51.4) and 23.4 kg (13.8–81.4) in females, and compared these results with the median fat mass in the US reference population, 23.7 and 28.7 kg, respectively.

Stroup et al. [23] found fat mass by DXA in 6 males with PKU was 24.5% ± 4.8, and, in 9 females, 36.5% ± 2.5, but included 20% of subjects aged less than 18.

Montanari et al. [20] found a median basal fat mass of 15.2% by plethysmography, which increased significantly after 6 months of study to 19.6%, and which increased from the 25th to the 50th percentile in females but did not change in males.

3.4.3. Metabolic Control

In the study by Alghamdi et al. [16], all adults with PKU had poor metabolic control, as 100% of phenylalanine measurements were above age-specific targets.

In the sample of Barta et al. [17], poor metabolic control of PKU, defined as mean Phe level > 600 µmol/L over the course of 10 years, was observed in 35% and 67% of male and female patients with PKU, respectively, and there was no significant inverse correlation between amino acid supplementation intake and fat mass.

Mezzomo et al. [19] observed good metabolic control of PKU in 41.67% (15/36) of the sample, being 65% (13/20) in males and 12.5% (2/16) in females, but they did not present the results of fat mass related to metabolic control, although the authors said, "The individuals with PKU evaluated here are young adults with inadequate metabolic control of the disease, with males being eutrophic and females being overweight and excess BF".

Montanari et al. [20] found that metabolic control of PKU was worse (not significantly) at the end of the study.

Rocha et al. [21] observed that 40.5% of their patients older than 16 years had good metabolic control of PKU. The authors found that the prevalence of overweight was higher in patients with poor metabolic control, but they did not report fat mass with respect to metabolic control.

Rojas Agurto et al. [22] compared a group of patients with PKU under strict follow-up with another group of patients who stopped attending metabolic control visits, but they found no significant differences in their body fat mass.

The remaining articles [18,23–25] did not provide information regarding metabolic control of PKU.

As information on metabolic control in PKU is scarce and heterogeneous, it was not possible to explore the association between metabolic control and fat mass.

3.4.4. Sex

Five of the studies did not show differentiated adult fat mass in females and males [16,21,22,24,25], although Rocha et al. found a non-significantly higher fat mass in females with PKU, including children (27.5%) than in healthy controls (26.1%, $p = 0.192$).

Among the five ones that did show these data, Barta et al. [17] found that adult female patients with PKU had significantly more fat mass than control females. Mezzomo et al. [19] found no significant differences. Jani et al. [18] did not compare with a control group but with a US reference population. Montanari et al. [20] found that female patients with PKU increased their fat mass at the end of the study. Stroup et al. [23] did not compare fat mass in PKU patients with a control group.

3.4.5. Body Fat Mass

Fat mass was assessed by DXA in 4 studies [18,22,23,25], BIA in another 4 [17,19,21,24], and by plethysmography [20] or deuterium [16] in one study each. This heterogeneity made it unfeasible to compare the body fat mass outcome.

3.4.6. Moderate vs. Poor Risk of Bias Studies

Only two of the studies [19,21] were considered fair, with a moderate risk of bias, and these found no significant differences in fat mass between patients with PKU and healthy controls. Among the studies with a high risk of bias [16–18,22–25], Barta et al. [17] found a significantly higher fat mass in female patients with PKU compared to healthy controls.

4. Discussion

Morphofunctional assessment of patients' nutritional status was first developed for disease-related malnutrition [1,2]. Malnutrition is an issue of concern in patients with IMDs with severe neurological complications, but there are IMDs with known increased cardiometabolic risk, and most patients with IMDs in adult metabolic clinics are patients with PKU, in whom a possible risk and prevalence of obesity has recently been discussed [3–5], as obesity could increase acquired cardiometabolic risk.

4.1. Inherited Metabolic Diseases with Known Higher Cardiovascular Risk

Homocystinuria is an IMD with a well-characterized acquired increased cardiometabolic risk. Although McCully and Wilson proposed the "Homocysteine Theory of Atherosclerosis" [27] in 1975, it was not until the 1990s that increased serum levels of total homocysteine were recognized as a new independent risk factor for cardiovascular disease [28].

A direct association has been found between increased plasma total homocysteine levels and cardiovascular disease [29]. Hyperhomocysteinemia leads to:

- vascular endothelial injury and dysfunction, with less release of nitric oxide, thus favoring endothelial dysfunction and the atherothrombotic process [30];
- proliferation of vascular wall smooth muscle cells [31]; lipid peroxidation, with oxidation of LDL-C through the generation of the superoxide radical [32];
- a prothrombotic state favored by an increase in the activity of coagulation factors V and XII and a higher production of thromboxane A2 (a potent platelet aggregator), favoring the genesis of vascular disease [33];

- intraluminal venous thrombi formation [34].

Cardiovascular risk in homocystinuria is expounded in the result of two meta-analyses of case-control and prospective studies, indicating that for every 5 υmol/L of increased homocysteine, the risk of ischemic heart disease increases by 56.8%, and the risk of stroke by 61.3% [35,36].

Another IMD with a known increased cardiometabolic risk is glycogen storage disease type 1, which induces hyperlactacidemia, hyperlipidemia, and hyperuricemia [37]. The marked hyperlipidemia may be due to increased de novo lipidogenesis and release of lipids into the blood compartment [38], and decreased clearance and uptake, on account of reduced activity of lipoprotein lipase and hepatic lipase [39]. Arterial dysfunction is also present, leading to an increased cardiovascular risk due to hyperlipemia [40].

Most IMDs do not lead per se to a higher cardiometabolic risk than in the general population, but this risk could be increased in patients with excess adiposity.

4.2. Adipose Tissue and Cardiometabolic Risk

Adipose tissue (AT) is a complex and dynamic endocrine organ. Its biological variability, depending on its location and metabolic state, affects individuals and their cardiometabolic risk [7,8].

There are two major types of adipose tissue in the body (classified by phenotype and functional role): White adipose tissue (WAT) and brown adipose tissue (BAT). WAT can be found in two main anatomical depots: Ectopic or visceral adipose tissue (VAT), which is strongly associated with cardiometabolic risk, and subcutaneous adipose tissue (SAT) [7,8]. VAT has higher levels of macrophages, regulatory T cells, natural killer T cells, and eosinophils than SAT [7], and both display differences in angiogenesis and sympathetic inervation [41].

ATs are known to have endocrine, autocrine, and paracrine functions [6].

In obesity, the secretion of hormones and adipokines is different compared to normal weight individuals [42–45]. This results in an increased risk of coronary artery calcification, carotid artery intimal media thickening, and left ventricular hypertrophy [44–46].

Adyponectin is reduced in obesity, increasing the risk of hypertension, myocardial hypertrophy, and endothelial dysfunction; omentin, SPARC, and nefastin-1 levels, which are inversely correlated with cardiovascular disease, are also reduced in obesity. Hyperleptinemia is associated with cardiovascular remodeling, prothrombotic effects, and endothelial dysfunction; resistin, angiotensinogen, and visfatin are also expressed in VAT, increased in obesity, and related to high blood pressure; chemerin is associated with inflammatory markers in metabolic syndrome; other adipokines such as lipocalin-2 (LCN2), vaspin, FSTL1, SFRP5, CTRPs, FAM19A5, WISP1,PGRN, apelin, RBP4, PAI-1 are also secreted by AT, and their levels have a correlation with major risk of CV disease [7,43].

Cardiovascular disease (CVD) is a leading cause of morbidity and mortality worldwide. Obesity, or more precisely, increased ectopic adiposity, is associated with cardiometabolic abnormalities such as hypertension, dyslipidemia, and insulin resistance [7,8]. Fat mass distribution should be considered the main indicator of CV risk, and therefore fat mass must be evaluated in the morphofunctional assessment of cardiometabolic risk.

4.3. Morphofunctional Assessment of Cardiometabolic Risk

Visceral fat can be assessed by means of anthropometric measurements. The most commonly used marker [47], body mass index (BMI), should not be useful [42,47], as its main limitation is the inability to discern the composition and distribution of fat mass from muscle mass. Therefore, other anthropometric markers focused on the measurement of central fat mass, which are more closely related to cardiometabolic risk, are also employed [48].

Waist circumference (WC) is the anthropometric marker that best predicts intra-abdominal fat mass [49,50]. A waist circumference > 102 cm in men and >88 cm in women is considered a marker of cardiometabolic risk [51]. Other anthropometric measurements that can estimate visceral fat are waist-to-height ratio [52], waist-to-hip ratio [52], and relative fat mass, which considers WC, height, and sex to express total body fat as a percentage and shows a stronger correlation between total body fat and BMI [53,54].

Visceral adipose index is a mixed morphological and functional parameter. It is based on WC and BMI, as well as triglycerides and HDL cholesterol, and shows a strong association with visceral adipose tissue composition measured by MRI. It also indirectly expresses visceral adipose tissue function and insulin sensitivity by using different formulae according to sex and ethnicity [55,56].

Anthropometric techniques are imprecise for evaluating visceral/ectopic fat mass, and more specific evaluation methods are available [1,10,57].

Bioelectrical impedance analysis (BIA) performs an estimation of body composition, including fat mass, by measuring the resistance of body tissues to electrical currents. These currents are of low intensity and high frequency [58]. The main limitation of BIA when assessing adipose tissue, in addition to the limitations of its own estimation, is the hydration variation, as BIA estimates FFM assuming that FFM is constantly hydrated to 73.2% [59]. FFM hydration status is also higher in individuals with obesity; therefore, total body composition estimates are affected [59,60].

Nutritional Ultrasound® (NU) is a tool capable of evaluating adipose tissue (visceral and muscular ectopic adipose tissues). The distribution of ectopic adipose tissue is represented by preperitoneal visceral fat (PVF), which is related to other adipose tissue deposits as intrahepatic fat. There are limitations in PVF measurement in persons with obesity due to the impossibility of covering the layer depth with nutritional ultrasound [61]. Ectopic adipose infiltration of muscle is a type of ectopic adipose tissue that is known as myosteatosis. NU evaluates muscular ectopic adipose tissue by measuring echointensity, as fat is usually more echolucent and superficially distributed [62,63]. Echointensity can be assessed from two points of view. Qualitatively, according to hypo, iso, or hyperintensity; quantitatively, using grayscale analysis on ultrasound with different available software [64]. Furthermore, color Doppler ultrasound can be used to observe quadricep rectus femoris vascularization. Muscle fat infiltration involves decreased vascular flow [65].

Due to radiation exposure, **computed tomography** (CT) is generally not used as a first choice for body composition measurement, but rather to evaluate the body composition of CTs previously performed for another purpose. Tissue is measured using a quantitative scale in Hounsfield units (HU), a measure of body tissue attenuation compared to water [16]. Muscle mass, visceral, subcutaneous, pericardial, intermuscular, and intramuscular adipose tissue can be identified based on predetermined HU values [58,66]. For muscle adipose tissue assessment, either intermuscular adipose tissue (IMAT) or muscle attenuation can be measured [67]. Low muscle attenuation is associated with increased muscle fat content as well as decreased specific strength [68]. The area of the different tissues can be determined manually or through software, with a typical range attributed to fat, from −195 to −45 HU [58,66,69].

Magnetic resonance imaging (MRI), compared to CT, provides a better definition of soft tissues, especially fat [70]. MRI is a useful tool for measuring muscle mass and subcutaneous, visceral, and ectopic adipose tissue [71] and shows a high correlation with CT [72]. However, MRI is not a first-choice technique for body composition assessment due to its higher cost and lower availability.

Dual-energy X-ray absorptiometry (DXA) performs a full-body scan using low doses of radiation in a short period of time, with high precision and accuracy. DXA indirectly measures lean mass and fat mass. DXA has a good correlation with BIA, CT, and MRI, although CT and MRI are more accurate in the assessment of visceral fat and ectopic adipose tissue, and DXA cannot measure intramuscular fat mass [58].

CT, MRI, and DXA are usually less available in clinics than BIA and NU. Other techniques to evaluate ectopic fat are more experimental, such as plethysmography and deuterium dilution, but they have also been included in the systematic review.

In the **functional assessment** of cardiometabolic risk, it should be taken into account that adipokines produced in the adipose tissue are key to insulin resistance, inflammation, and tissue dysfunction [73]. Ectopic/visceral adipose tissue is characterized by tissue infiltration by macrophages and leukocytes and the secretion of inflammatory cytokines, including C-reactive protein, IL-6, plasminogen activator inhibitor-1 (PAI-1) and TNF-α [74,75]. Ectopic adipose tissue also modifies the plasma lipid profile through increased lipolysis and the release of free fatty acids, decreased expression of lipoprotein lipase (LPL), and increased expression of cholesterol ester transfer protein (CETP). This leads to a lipid profile characterized by hypertriglyceridemia, increased LDL and low-density lipoproteins, and low HDL cholesterol levels [75].

For the consequences of ectopic fat deposition, the functional assessment of cardiometabolic risk should include blood pressure, glucose (HOMA-IR), lipid metabolism (HDL-cholesterol, triglycerides, and their ratio), and inflammatory markers (PCR).

This systematic review focuses on morphological fat assessment in patients with PKU, the most prevalent IMD in adult metabolic clinics [76].

4.4. Summary of Evidence

The association between PKU and obesity had been previously explored in three systematic reviews, one of which included a meta-analysis. The first one, in children and adolescents only, found that overweight was a common outcome in this population [77], the second one, with adults and pediatric populations with PKU, found no differences in BMI between patients with PKU and healthy controls, but patients with classical PKU had a significantly higher BMI than healthy controls [4], and the last one, only in adults, found patients with PKU had a higher BMI but also a higher prevalence of obesity than healthy controls, but with inconsistent results when compared with the general population [5].

Nevertheless, no published systematic review was found on the assessment of fat mass in patients with PKU, despite the fact that fat mass (namely ectopic fat mass) correlated better with cardiometabolic risk than BMI.

One six-month longitudinal follow-up study [20] and nine observational studies [16–19,21–25] were reviewed, including a cross-sectional analysis of two other studies [18], and a cross-sectional study [23] of a subset of 15 participants from a previously published randomized crossover trial [26].

Only six of the studies compared results with a non-hPA control group [16,17,19,21,22,24], while the longitudinal study [20] and the remaining three observational studies did not [18,23,25]. Only Barta et al. [17] found a significantly higher fat mass in female patients with PKU, although Alghamdi et al. [16], and Weng et al. (including children) [24] found a non-significantly higher fat mass in patients with PKU versus non-hPA controls, while Mezzomo et al. [19], and Rocha et al. [21] reported a higher non-significant fat mass in female patients with PKU vs. non-hPA females.

In the only longitudinal study included [20], there was a significant increase in fat mass percentile in female patients with PKU, but not in males, although all of them were in a 6-month follow-up interventional study with a GMP formula. This may reflect how fast fat mass can fluctuate over time, at least in women, and it is related to the results from cross-sectional studies, which reflect a tendency towards higher fat mass in female PKU patients than in females in the general population.

As body composition changes with age, it is necessary that outcomes are only studied in adult samples or, at least, reported separately for pediatric patients and controls. Four of the selected articles [16,18,20,21] included both pediatric and adult patients, but they were included because they reported outcome data separately for adults [16,18,20] or patients older than 16 years [21] without increasing the risk of bias. Stroup et al. [23] included three patients (20%) aged 15 or older. The study with the highest risk of bias due to the inclusion of data from pediatric patients is that of Weng et al. [24], as they did not report the number of adults in the PKU or control groups, nor did they report outcome data for adults separately.

Among these six studies that compared results in patients with PKU with a control group, the ones from Mezzomo et al. [19] and Rocha et al. [21] were evaluated with moderate risk of bias, according to the NIH Quality Assessment Tool for Observational

Cohort and Cross-Sectional Studies [14], and reported a tendency towards higher fat mass among female patients with PKU (Rocha et al., including pediatric patients). The remaining 4 studies, assessed as high risk of bias, reported no tendency [22], tendency towards [16,24] or significantly higher [17] fat mass in patients with PKU.

Exposure was defined as PKU under treatment, but different levels of exposure (compliance, BH4 treatment, etc.) were not reported in most cases. Good metabolic control in patients with PKU was defined as the Phe concentration in a single sample [18], the median [21] or average [22] concentration in the previous year or the preceding 10 years [17], attendance at follow-up appointments [22], and regular intake of protein substitutes without Phe were also considered [17,22].

Barta et al. did not find any significant correlation between metabolic control and body composition [17]. Rojas Agurto et al. [22] reported that patients with PKU and poor metabolic control had a fat mass of 24.4 (18.1–32.4) kg compared to 21.1 (16–30.2) kg in patients with good metabolic control, but did not show statistical analysis. Rocha et al. found that patients with poor metabolic control had a prevalence of overweight and obesity of 42.9%, compared with 27.9% in patients with good metabolic control, but they did not report the relationship between fat mass and metabolic control [21].

Fat mass was not adjusted for other variables related to fat mass deposition, such as energy intake, physical activity, sociocultural status, or family history.

The quality of the evidence was very low due to the risk of bias in the studies reviewed, but it may be enough to raise the possibility of higher fat mass, and subsequently, an increased cardiometabolic risk in people with PKU.

In the context of morphofunctional assessment of patients with PKU, body fat mass and, when available, ectopic fat mass should be included in the morphological evaluation as biomarkers for the early detection of cardiometabolic risk, followed by functional evaluation including HOMA-IR, triglycerides, HDL-cholesterol, LDL-cholesterol, and PCR. Protein substitutes need to be designed in order to avoid insulin resistance, dyslipidemia, and systemic inflammation.

4.5. Strengths and Limitations of This Study

There are some limitations to this systematic review. Just 10 studies were evaluated, after rejecting 28 (see Supplementary Material) [4,26,78–103], and only six of which included a matched control group, and all these six studies were observational, which have a higher risk of bias due to confounding variables than randomized clinical trials.

The populations included in the studies were diverse in terms of age, disease severity, type of treatment and adherence, and metabolic control. Zerjav Tansek et al. [25] compared fat mass in patients with PKU with HPA as controls and in patients with classic PKU compared to non-classic PKU. In this study, 50% of the patients with PKU but only 13% of benign HPA patients were adults, and the proportion of females was similar in both groups (51–52%), but outcomes from adults vs. non-adults and females vs. males were not differentiated, despite the fact that the fat mass in females is higher and changes with age, both physiologically.

Five of the studies did not report separately fat mass in adult females and males [16,21,22,24,25], although fat mass is physiologically different according to sex and should be reported properly. There are five studies from Europe [16,17,20,21,25], two from the USA, two from South America, and one from Asia. As there are differences in body composition according to ethnicity, it is difficult to compare the results.

There are also differences in the metabolic control of patients with PKU, with the proportion of patients in good metabolic control ranging from 65% in males in Mezzomo et al. [19] to 0% in the study by Alghamdi et al. [16], as all phenylalanine measurements were above age-specific targets.

The methods employed for fat mass assessment were also different: DXA in four [18,22,23,25] and BIA in another four [17,19,21,24]. Alghamdi et al. [16] assessed fat mass by deuterium but did not report sex-specific results. Montanari et al. [20] measured fat mass with plethysmography in 4 adults (45% of subjects); fat mass was not a primary objective in this study, and they do not show adult data separately.

There were also different ways of presenting the fat mass outcome. Jani et al. [18] presented fat mass outcome as a fat mass index and distinguished between adult and pediatric populations, but not between females and males. They also presented median fat mass in kilograms, as Rojas Agurto et al. [22], which can be influenced by height, and so fat mass index or percentage could be better alternatives. The only study reporting ectopic fat mass (abdominal fat mass), which correlates better with cardiometabolic risk, is the one from Zerjav Tansek et al. [25], but they did not report female abdominal fat mass results apart from male results.

The strength of the evidence was very low because only two of the trials had a moderate risk of bias and the other eight had a high risk, resulting in a limited quality of evidence for the body fat-mass percentage. Furthermore, differences from the technique employed to evaluate fat mass, absence of control group in four articles [18,20,23,25], absence of separated data from females and males [16,18,21–24], and age of patients and controls included, were not adjusted for and it not possible to conduct a meta-analysis.

To our knowledge, this is the first systematic review regarding fat mass assessment in patients with PKU. The following methodology was used in this systematic review:

- Followed the PRISMA guidelines
- Clearly defined the objective of this review
- Defined inclusion and exclusion criteria according to the PECO format
- Included both PubMed and EMBASE databases in the search strategy
- Presented the full search strategies for both databases, including any filters and limits used
- Searched the reference lists of the included studies
- Described the study selection process using the PRISMA-model flow diagram
- Provided the list of excluded studies and the reasons for their exclusion in the Supplementary Material
- Provided a table with the main characteristics of the included studies
- Study selection, data search, and assessment of risk of bias and quality of evidence were performed by two independent authors
- Described the rationale for the review in the context of existing knowledge
- Provided an interpretation of the results in the context of the evidence
- Discussed the limitations of the evidence included in the review and the limitations of the review process itself.

This systematic review provides an updated overview of the evidence on fat mass in patients with PKU and may be useful to assess body and ectopic fat mass as a part of morphofunctional assessment and to include cardiometabolic disease assessment, prevention, and follow-up programs for patients with PKU in adult IMD clinics.

Morphofunctional assessment of cardiometabolic risk should be complemented by a functional evaluation, which is proposed to include not only known major cardiovascular risk factors (dyslipidemia, high blood pressure, diabetes mellitus, and smoking) but also known markers of these conditions (HOMA-IR) or systemic inflammation (PCR).

5. Conclusions

Fat mass (namely ectopic fat mass) correlates with cardiometabolic risk better than BMI, and therefore fat mass should be assessed preferentially, as a global morphofunctional assessment of nutritional state should include not only disease-related malnutrition but also cardiometabolic risk.

There were no significant differences in fat mass between adult patients with PKU and healthy controls, although a tendency towards higher fat mass in patients, particularly among women, was shown.

The quality of the evidence was very low due to the risk of bias in the studies reviewed, but it may be enough to raise the possibility of an increased cardiometabolic risk in people with PKU.

As a second part of morphofunctional assessment, after morphological fat mass assessment, functional evaluation of dyslipidemia, insulin resistance, and systemic inflammation should be performed.

More evidence is needed on body composition, body and ectopic fat mass, and cardiometabolic risk in patients with PKU.

Supplementary Materials: The following supporting information can be downloaded at: https://www.mdpi.com/article/10.3390/nu16121833/s1, S1: Search details. S2: List of excluded studies and their reasons. S3: Figure S1: Summary of the risk of bias of every reviewed study including every selected item from the "Guidance for assessing the quality of cohort and cross-sectional studies".

Author Contributions: Conceptualization, L.M.L.-P.; methodology, L.M.L.-P.; validation, L.M.L.-P., C.G.-L. and M.F.-B.; formal analysis, L.M.L.-P., C.G.-L. and M.F.-B.; investigation, L.M.L.-P., C.G.-L. and M.F.-B.; data curation, L.M.L.-P., C.G.-L. and M.F.-B.; writing—original draft preparation, all authors; writing—review and editing, all authors; visualization, all authors; supervision, L.M.L.-P.; project administration, L.M.L.-P.; funding acquisition, L.M.L.-P. All authors have read and agreed to the published version of the manuscript.

Funding: This research received no external funding. Article processing charge has been paid by Sociedad Extremeña de Diabetes, Endocrinología y Nutrición (SEDiEN), Spain.

Informed Consent Statement: Informed consent was obtained in every study included in the meta-analysis.

Data Availability Statement: Data available at: Review fat mass PKU.

Acknowledgments: Authors like to thank SEDiEN for their support for this publication.

Conflicts of Interest: The authors declare no conflicts of interest.

References

1. Almeida, J.M.G.; García, C.G.; Castañeda, V.B.; Guerrero, D.B. Nuevo enfoque de la nutrición. Valoración del estado nutricional del paciente: Función y composición corporal. *Nutr. Hosp.* **2018**, *35*, 1–14. [CrossRef]
2. García, C.G.; Almeida, J.M.G.; Aguilar, I.M.V.; Castañeda, V.B.; Guerrero, D.B. Morphofunctional assessment of patient nutritional status: A global approach. *Nutr. Hosp.* **2021**, *38*, 592–600. [CrossRef]
3. Rocha, J.C.; MacDonald, A.; Trefz, F. Is overweight an issue in phenylketonuria? *Mol. Genet. Metab.* **2013**, *110*, S18–S24. [CrossRef] [PubMed]
4. Rodrigues, C.; Pinto, A.; Faria, A.; Teixeira, D.; van Wegberg, A.M.J.; Ahring, K.; Feillet, F.; Calhau, C.; MacDonald, A.; Moreira-Rosário, A.; et al. Is the Phenylalanine-Restricted Diet a Risk Factor for Overweight or Obesity in Patients with Phenylketonuria (PKU)? A Systematic Review and Meta-Analysis. *Nutrients* **2021**, *13*, 3443. [CrossRef]
5. Tankeu, A.T.; Pavlidou, D.C.; Superti-Furga, A.; Gariani, K.; Tran, C. Overweight and obesity in adult patients with phenylketonuria: A systematic review. *Orphanet J. Rare Dis.* **2023**, *18*, 37. [CrossRef] [PubMed]
6. Coelho, M.; Oliveira, T.; Fernandes, R. Biochemistry of adipose tissue: An endocrine organ. *Arch. Med. Sci.* **2013**, *9*, 191–200. [CrossRef]
7. Koenen, M.; Hill, M.A.; Cohen, P.; Sowers, J.R. Obesity, Adipose Tissue and Vascular Dysfunction. *Circ. Res.* **2021**, *128*, 951–968. [CrossRef]
8. Oikonomou, E.K.; Antoniades, C. The role of adipose tissue in cardiovascular health and disease. *Nat. Rev. Cardiol.* **2018**, *16*, 83–99. [CrossRef]
9. Compher, C.; Cederholm, T.; Correia, M.I.T.D.; Gonzalez, M.C.; Higashiguch, T.; Shi, H.P.; Bischoff, S.C.; Boirie, Y.; Carrasco, F.; Cruz-Jentoft, A.; et al. Guidance for assessment of the muscle mass phenotypic criterion for the Global Leadership Initiative on Malnutrition diagnosis of malnutrition. *J. Parenter. Enter. Nutr.* **2022**, *46*, 1232–1242. [CrossRef]
10. Luengo-Pérez, L.M.; Fernández-Bueso, M.; Ambrojo, A.; Guijarro, M.; Ferreira, A.C.; Pereira-Da-Silva, L.; Moreira-Rosário, A.; Faria, A.; Calhau, C.; Daly, A.; et al. Body Composition Evaluation and Clinical Markers of Cardiometabolic Risk in Patients with Phenylketonuria. *Nutrients* **2023**, *15*, 5133. [CrossRef]
11. Guyatt, G.; Oxman, A.D.; Akl, E.A.; Kunz, R.; Vist, G.; Brozek, J.; Norris, S.; Falck-Ytter, Y.; Glasziou, P.; DeBeer, H.; et al. GRADE guidelines: 1. Introduction—GRADE evidence profiles and summary of findings tables. *J. Clin. Epidemiol.* **2011**, *64*, 383–394. [CrossRef] [PubMed]

12. Guyatt, G.H.; Oxman, A.D.; Kunz, R.; Atkins, D.; Brozek, J.; Vist, G.; Alderson, P.; Glasziou, P.; Falck-Ytter, Y.; Schünemann, H.J. GRADE guidelines: 2. Framing the question and deciding on important outcomes. *J. Clin. Epidemiology* **2011**, *64*, 395–400. [CrossRef] [PubMed]
13. Morgan, R.L.; Whaley, P.; Thayer, K.A.; Schünemann, H.J. Identifying the PECO: A framework for formulating good questions to explore the association of environmental and other exposures with health outcomes. *Environ. Int.* **2018**, *121*, 1027–1031. [CrossRef] [PubMed]
14. National Heart, Lung, and Blood Institute (NHLBI) Quality Assessment Tool for Observational Cohort and Cross-Sectional Studies. Available online: https://www.nhlbi.nih.gov/health-topics/study-quality-assessment-tools (accessed on 23 February 2022).
15. Page, M.J.; McKenzie, J.E.; Bossuyt, P.M.; Boutron, I.; Hoffmann, T.C.; Mulrow, C.D.; Shamseer, L.; Tetzlaff, J.M.; Akl, E.A.; Brennan, S.E.; et al. he PRISMA 2020 statement: An updated guideline for reporting systematic reviews Systematic reviews and Meta-Analyses. *BMJ* **2021**, *372*, 71. [CrossRef] [PubMed]
16. Alghamdi, N.; Alfheeaid, H.; Cochrane, B.; Adam, S.; Galloway, P.; Cozens, A.; Preston, T.; Malkova, D.; Gerasimidis, K. Mechanisms of obesity in children and adults with phenylketonuria on contemporary treatment. *Clin. Nutr. ESPEN* **2021**, *46*, 539–543. [CrossRef] [PubMed]
17. Barta, A.G.; Becsei, D.; Kiss, E.; Sumánszki, C.; Simonová, E.; Reismann, P. The Impact of Phenylketonuria on Body Composition in Adults. *Ann. Nutr. Metab.* **2021**, *78*, 98–105. [CrossRef] [PubMed]
18. Jani, R.; Coakley, K.; Douglas, T.; Singh, R. Protein intake and physical activity are associated with body composition in individuals with phenylalanine hydroxylase deficiency. *Mol. Genet. Metab.* **2017**, *121*, 104–110. [CrossRef] [PubMed]
19. Mezzomo, T.R.; Dias, M.R.M.G.; Pereira, R.M. Adults with early diagnosis of phenylketonuria have higher resting energy expenditure than adults with late diagnosis. *Clin. Nutr. ESPEN* **2023**, *56*, 166–172. [CrossRef] [PubMed]
20. Montanari, C.; Ceccarani, C.; Corsello, A.; Zuvadelli, J.; Ottaviano, E.; Cas, M.D.; Banderali, G.; Zuccotti, G.; Borghi, E.; Verduci, E. Glycomacropeptide Safety and Its Effect on Gut Microbiota in Patients with Phenylketonuria: A Pilot Study. *Nutrients* **2022**, *14*, 1883. [CrossRef] [PubMed]
21. Rocha, J.C.; van Spronsen, F.J.; Almeida, M.F.; Soares, G.; Quelhas, D.; Ramos, E.; Guimarães, J.T.; Borges, N. Dietary treatment in phenylketonuria does not lead to increased risk of obesity or metabolic syndrome. *Mol. Genet. Metab.* **2012**, *107*, 659–663. [CrossRef]
22. Rojas-Agurto, E.; Leal-Witt, M.J.; Arias, C.; Cabello, J.F.; Bunout, D.; Cornejo, V. Muscle and Bone Health in Young Chilean Adults with Phenylketonuria and Different Degrees of Compliance with the Phenylalanine Restricted Diet. *Nutrients* **2023**, *15*, 2939. [CrossRef] [PubMed]
23. Stroup, B.M.; Hansen, K.E.; Krueger, D.; Binkley, N.; Ney, D.M. Sex differences in body composition and bone mineral density in phenylketonuria: A cross-sectional study. *Mol. Genet. Metab. Rep.* **2018**, *15*, 30–35. [CrossRef] [PubMed]
24. Weng, H.-L.; Yang, F.-J.; Chen, P.-R.; Hwu, W.-L.; Lee, N.-C.; Chien, Y.-H. Dietary intake and nutritional status of patients with phenylketonuria in Taiwan. *Sci. Rep.* **2020**, *10*, 14537. [CrossRef] [PubMed]
25. Tansek, M.Z.; Bertoncel, A.; Sebez, B.; Zibert, J.; Groselj, U.; Battelino, T.; Stefanija, M.A. Anthropometry and bone mineral density in treated and untreated hyperphenylalaninemia. *Endocr. Connect.* **2020**, *9*, 649–657. [CrossRef] [PubMed]
26. Ney, D.M.; Stroup, B.M.; Clayton, M.K.; Murali, S.G.; Rice, G.M.; Rohr, F.; Levy, H.L. Glycomacropeptide for nutritional management of phenylketonuria: A randomized, controlled, crossover trial. *Am. J. Clin. Nutr.* **2016**, *104*, 334–345. [CrossRef] [PubMed]
27. McCully, K.S.; Wilson, R.B. Homocysteine theory of arteriosclerosis. *Atherosclerosis* **1975**, *22*, 215–227. [CrossRef] [PubMed]
28. Clarke, R.; Daly, L.; Robinson, K.; Naughten, E.; Cahalane, S.; Fowler, B.; Graham, I. Hyperhomocysteinemia: An Independent Risk Factor for Vascular Disease. *N. Engl. J. Med.* **1991**, *324*, 1149–1155. [CrossRef] [PubMed]
29. Verhoef, P.; Stampfer, M.J. Prospective Studies of Homocysteine and Cardiovascular Disease. *Nutr. Rev.* **2009**, *53*, 283–288. [CrossRef] [PubMed]
30. Mayer, E.L.; Jacobsen, D.W.; Robinson, K. Homocysteine and coronary atherosclerosis. *Circ.* **1996**, *27*, 517–527. [CrossRef] [PubMed]
31. Tsai, J.C.; A Perrella, M.; Yoshizumi, M.; Hsieh, C.M.; Haber, E.; Schlegel, R.; E Lee, M. Promotion of vascular smooth muscle cell growth by homocysteine: A link to atherosclerosis. *Proc. Natl. Acad. Sci. USA* **1994**, *91*, 6369–6373. [CrossRef]
32. Hirano, K.; Ogihara, T.; Miki, M.; Yasuda, H.; Tamai, H.; Kawamura, N.; Mino, M. Homocysteine Induces Iron-Catalyzed Lipid Peroxidation of Low-Density Lipoprotein that is Prevented by Alpha-Tocopherol. *Free. Radic. Res.* **1994**, *21*, 267–276. [CrossRef] [PubMed]
33. Di Minno, G.; Davì, G.; Margaglione, M.; Cirillo, F.; Grandone, E.; Ciabattoni, G.; Catalano, I.; Strisciuglio, P.; Andria, G.; Patrono, C. Abnormally high thromboxane biosynthesis in homozygous homocystinuria. Evidence for platelet involvement and probucol-sensitive mechanism. *J. Clin. Investig.* **1993**, *92*, 1400–1406. [CrossRef] [PubMed]
34. Magner, M.; Krupková, L.; Honzík, T.; Zeman, J.; Hyánek, J.; Kožich, V. Vascular presentation of cystathionine beta-synthase deficiency in adulthood. *J. Inherit. Metab. Dis.* **2010**, *34*, 33–37. [CrossRef] [PubMed]
35. Wald, D.S.; Morris, J.K.; Wald, N.J. Reconciling the Evidence on Serum Homocysteine and Ischaemic Heart Disease: A Meta-Analysis. *PLoS ONE* **2011**, *6*, e16473. [CrossRef] [PubMed]
36. Wald, D.S.; Law, M.; Morris, J.K. Homocysteine and cardiovascular disease: Evidence on causality from a meta-analysis. *BMJ* **2002**, *325*, 1202–1206. [CrossRef] [PubMed]

37. Rake, J.; Visser, G.; Labrune, P.; Leonard, J.V.; Ullrich, K.; Smit, P.G. Glycogen storage disease type I: Diagnosis, management, clinical course and outcome. Results of the European Study on Glycogen Storage Disease Type I (ESGSD I). *Eur. J. Pediatr.* **2002**, *161*, S20–S34. [CrossRef] [PubMed]
38. Bandsma, R.H.; Smit, P.G.; Kuipers, F. Disturbed lipid metabolism in glycogen storage disease type 1. *Eur. J. Pediatr.* **2002**, *161*, S65–S69. [CrossRef]
39. Wierzbicki, A.S.; Watts, G.F.; Lynas, J.; Winder, A.F.; Wray, R. Very low-density lipoprotein apolipoprotein B-100 turnover in glycogen storage disease type Ia (von Gierke disease). *J. Inherit. Metab. Dis.* **2001**, *24*, 527–534. [CrossRef]
40. Bernier, A.V.; Correia, C.E.; Haller, M.J.; Theriaque, D.W.; Shuster, J.J.; Weinstein, D.A. Vascular Dysfunction in Glycogen Storage Disease Type I. *J. Pediatr.* **2009**, *154*, 588–591. [CrossRef]
41. Xue, Y.; Petrovic, N.; Cao, R.; Larsson, O.; Lim, S.; Chen, S.; Feldmann, H.M.; Liang, Z.; Zhu, Z.; Nedergaard, J.; et al. Hypoxia-Independent Angiogenesis in Adipose Tissues during Cold Acclimation. *Cell Metab.* **2009**, *9*, 99–109. [CrossRef]
42. Després, J.-P. Body Fat Distribution and Risk of Cardiovascular Disease: An update. *Circulation* **2012**, *126*, 1301–1313. [CrossRef] [PubMed]
43. Recinella, L.; Orlando, G.; Ferrante, C.; Chiavaroli, A.; Brunetti, L.; Leone, S. Adipokines: New Potential Therapeutic Target for Obesity and Metabolic, Rheumatic, and Cardiovascular Diseases. *Front. Physiol.* **2020**, *11*, 578966. [CrossRef] [PubMed]
44. Farkhondeh, T.; Llorens, S.; Pourbagher-Shahri, A.M.; Ashrafizadeh, M.; Talebi, M.; Shakibaei, M.; Samarghandian, S. An Overview of the Role of Adipokines in Cardiometabolic Diseases. *Molecules* **2020**, *25*, 5218. [CrossRef] [PubMed]
45. Smekal, A.; Vaclavik, J. Adipokines and cardiovascular disease: A comprehensive review. *Biomed. Pap.* **2017**, *161*, 31–40. [CrossRef] [PubMed]
46. Shibata, R.; Ouchi, N.; Ohashi, K.; Murohara, T. The role of adipokines in cardiovascular disease. *J. Cardiol.* **2017**, *70*, 329–334. [CrossRef]
47. Javed, A.; Jumean, M.; Murad, M.H.; Okorodudu, D.; Kumar, S.; Somers, V.K.; Sochor, O.; Lopez-Jimenez, F. Diagnostic performance of body mass index to identify obesity as defined by body adiposity in children and adolescents: A systematic review and meta-analysis. *Pediatr. Obes.* **2014**, *10*, 234–244. [CrossRef]
48. Zimmet, P.; Magliano, D.; Matsuzawa, Y.; Alberti, G.; Shaw, J. The Metabolic Syndrome: A Global Public Health Problem and A New Definition. *J. Atheroscler. Thromb.* **2005**, *12*, 295–300. [CrossRef] [PubMed]
49. Wei, M.; Gaskill, S.P.; Haffner, S.M.; Stern, M.P. Waist Circumference as the Best Predictor of Noninsulin Dependent Diabetes Mellitus (NIDDM) Compared to Body Mass Index, Waist/hip Ratio and Other Anthropometric Measurements in Mexican Americans—A 7-Year Prospective Study. *Obes. Res.* **1997**, *5*, 16–23. [CrossRef] [PubMed]
50. Van Der Kooy, K.; Leenen, R.; Seidell, J.C.; Deurenberg, P.; Visser, M. Abdominal diameters as indicators of visceral fat: Comparison between magnetic resonance imaging and anthropometry. *Br. J. Nutr.* **1993**, *70*, 47–58. [CrossRef] [PubMed]
51. De La Torre, M.L.; Guerrero, D.B.; Cortada, J.V.; González, A.S.; Malpartida, K.G.; Hernandez-Mijares, A. Distribución de la circunferencia de la cintura y de la relación circunferencia de la cintura con respecto a la talla según la categoría del índice de masa corporal en los pacientes atendidos en consultas de endocrinología y nutrición. *Endocrinol. Nutr.* **2010**, *57*, 479–485. [CrossRef]
52. Rodea-Montero, E.R.; Evia-Viscarra, M.L.; Apolinar-Jiménez, E. Waist-to-Height Ratio Is a Better Anthropometric Index than Waist Circumference and BMI in Predicting Metabolic Syndrome among Obese Mexican Adolescents. *Int. J. Endocrinol.* **2014**, *2014*, 195407. [CrossRef]
53. Woolcott, O.O.; Bergman, R.N. Relative fat mass (RFM) as a new estimator of whole-body fat percentage—A cross-sectional study in American adult individuals. *Sci. Rep.* **2018**, *8*, 10980. [CrossRef] [PubMed]
54. Corrêa, C.R.; Formolo, N.P.S.; Dezanetti, T.; Speretta, G.F.F.; Nunes, E.A. Relative fat mass is a better tool to diagnose high adiposity when compared to body mass index in young male adults: A cross-section study. *Clin. Nutr. ESPEN* **2020**, *41*, 225–233. [CrossRef] [PubMed]
55. Amato, M.C.; Giordano, C.; Pitrone, M.; Galluzzo, A. Cut-off points of the visceral adiposity index (VAI) identifying a visceral adipose dysfunction associated with cardiometabolic risk in a Caucasian Sicilian population. *Lipids Health Dis.* **2011**, *10*, 183. [CrossRef] [PubMed]
56. Lu, Y.; Ge, L.; Yang, H.; He, Y.; Wang, Y. Chinese Visceral Adipose Index Shows Superior Diagnostic Performance in Predicting the Risk of Metabolic Dysfunction Associated Fatty Liver Disease in Early Postmenopausal Chinese Women. *Diabetes Metab. Syndr. Obes. Targets Ther.* **2023**, *2023*, 607–617. [CrossRef] [PubMed]
57. Fosbøl, M.O.; Zerahn, B. Contemporary methods of body composition measurement. *Clin. Physiol. Funct. Imaging* **2015**, *35*, 81–97. [CrossRef]
58. Ceniccola, G.D.; Castro, M.G.; Piovacari, S.M.F.; Horie, L.M.; Corrêa, F.G.; Barrere, A.P.N.; Toledo, D.O. Current technologies in body composition assessment: Advantages and disadvantages. *Nutrition* **2018**, *62*, 25–31. [CrossRef]
59. Mulasi, U.; Kuchnia, A.J.; Cole, A.J.; Earthman, C.P. Bioimpedance at the Bedside. *Nutr. Clin. Pract.* **2015**, *30*, 180–193. [CrossRef] [PubMed]
60. Price, K.L.; Earthman, C.P. Update on body composition tools in clinical settings: Computed tomography, ultrasound, and bioimpedance applications for assessment and monitoring. *Eur. J. Clin. Nutr.* **2018**, *73*, 187–193. [CrossRef]
61. García-Almeida, J.M.; García-García, C.; Vegas-Aguilar, I.M.; Pomar, M.D.B.; Cornejo-Pareja, I.M.; Medina, B.F.; Román, D.A.d.L.; Guerrero, D.B.; Lesmes, I.B.; Madueño, F.J.T. Nutritional ultrasound®: Conceptualisation, technical considerations and standardisation. *Endocrinol. Diabetes Y Nutr.* **2023**, *70*, 74–84. [CrossRef]

62. Walker, F. Neuromuscular ultrasound. *Neurol. Clin.* **2004**, *22*, 563–590. [CrossRef] [PubMed]
63. Mayans, D.; Cartwright, M.S.; Walker, F.O. Neuromuscular Ultrasonography: Quantifying Muscle and Nerve Measurements. *Phys. Med. Rehabil. Clin. N. Am.* **2012**, *23*, 133–148. [CrossRef]
64. Casey, P.; Alasmar, M.; McLaughlin, J.; Ang, Y.; McPhee, J.; Heire, P.; Sultan, J. The current use of ultrasound to measure skeletal muscle and its ability to predict clinical outcomes: A systematic review. *J. Cachex Sarcopenia Muscle* **2022**, *13*, 2298–2309. [CrossRef]
65. Hernández-Socorro, C.R.; Saavedra, P.; López-Fernández, J.C.; Ruiz-Santana, S. Assessment of Muscle Wasting in Long-Stay ICU Patients Using a New Ultrasound Protocol. *Nutrients* **2018**, *10*, 1849. [CrossRef]
66. Figueiredo, P.; Marques, E.A.; Gudnason, V.; Lang, T.; Sigurdsson, S.; Jonsson, P.V.; Aspelund, T.; Siggeirsdottir, K.; Launer, L.; Eiriksdottir, G.; et al. Computed tomography-based skeletal muscle and adipose tissue attenuation: Variations by age, sex, and muscle. *Exp. Gerontol.* **2021**, *149*, 111306. [CrossRef]
67. Amini, B.; Boyle, S.P.; Boutin, R.D.; Lenchik, L. Approaches to Assessment of Muscle Mass and Myosteatosis on Computed Tomography: A Systematic Review. *J. Gerontol. Ser. A* **2019**, *74*, 1671–1678. [CrossRef]
68. Correa-De-Araujo, R.; Addison, O.; Miljkovic, I.; Goodpaster, B.H.; Bergman, B.C.; Clark, R.V.; Elena, J.W.; Esser, K.A.; Ferrucci, L.; Harris-Love, M.O.; et al. Myosteatosis in the Context of Skeletal Muscle Function Deficit: An Interdisciplinary Workshop at the National Institute on Aging. *Front. Physiol.* **2020**, *11*, 963. [CrossRef] [PubMed]
69. Rosenquist, K.J.; Pedley, A.; Massaro, J.M.; Therkelsen, K.E.; Murabito, J.M.; Hoffmann, U.; Fox, C.S. Visceral and Subcutaneous Fat Quality and Cardiometabolic Risk. *JACC Cardiovasc. Imaging* **2013**, *6*, 762–771. [CrossRef] [PubMed]
70. Brennan, D.D.; Whelan, P.F.; Robinson, K.; Ghita, O.; O'Brien, J.M.; Sadleir, R.; Eustace, S.J. Rapid Automated Measurement of Body Fat Distribution from Whole-Body MRI. *Am. J. Roentgenol.* **2005**, *185*, 418–423. [CrossRef]
71. Borga, M.; West, J.; Bell, J.D.; Harvey, N.C.; Romu, T.; Heymsfield, S.B.; Leinhard, O.D. Advanced body composition assessment: From body mass index to body composition profiling. *J. Investig. Med.* **2018**, *66*, 1–9. [CrossRef]
72. Zaffina, C.; Wyttenbach, R.; Pagnamenta, A.; Grasso, R.F.; Biroli, M.; Del Grande, F.; Rizzo, S. Body composition assessment: Comparison of quantitative values between magnetic resonance imaging and computed tomography. *Quant. Imaging Med. Surg.* **2022**, *12*, 1450–1466. [CrossRef] [PubMed]
73. Lehr, S.; Hartwig, S.; Lamers, D.; Famulla, S.; Müller, S.; Hanisch, F.-G.; Cuvelier, C.; Ruige, J.; Eckardt, K.; Ouwens, D.M.; et al. Identification and Validation of Novel Adipokines Released from Primary Human Adipocytes. *Mol. Cell. Proteom.* **2012**, *11*. [CrossRef]
74. Kahn, C.R.; Wang, G.; Lee, K.Y. Altered adipose tissue and adipocyte function in the pathogenesis of metabolic syndrome. *J. Clin. Investig.* **2019**, *129*, 3990–4000. [CrossRef] [PubMed]
75. van de Woestijne, A.P.; Monajemi, H.; Kalkhoven, E.; Visseren, F.L.J. Adipose tissue dysfunction and hypertriglyceridemia: Mechanisms and management. *Obes. Rev.* **2011**, *12*, 829–840. [CrossRef] [PubMed]
76. Luengo-Pérez, L.M.; Ambrojo, A.; Fernández-Bueso, M.; Guijarro, M.; Ferreira, A.; Luzes, G.; Pereira, M.; Calhau, C.; Rocha, J.C. Muscle Quality and Risk of Metabolic Syndrome in Adult Patients with Inherited Metabolic Diseases. *Endocr. Metab. Immune Disord. Drug Targets* **2023**, *24*, 1–2. [CrossRef] [PubMed]
77. Sena, B.d.S.; de Andrade, M.I.S.; da Silva, A.P.F.; Dourado, K.F.; Silva, A.L.F. Overweight and associated factors in children and adolescents with phenylketonuria: A systematic review. *Rev. Paul. Pediatr.* **2020**, *38*, e2018201. [CrossRef]
78. Aldámiz-Echevarría, L.; Bueno, M.A.; Couce, M.L.; Lage, S.; Dalmau, J.; Vitoria, I.; Andrade, F.; Blasco, J.; Alcalde, C.; Gil, D.; et al. Anthropometric characteristics and nutrition in a cohort of PAH-deficient patients. *Clin. Nutr.* **2013**, *33*, 702–717. [CrossRef] [PubMed]
79. Burrage, L.C.; McConnell, J.; Haesler, R.; O'Riordan, M.A.; Sutton, V.R.; Kerr, D.S.; McCandless, S.E. High prevalence of overweight and obesity in females with phenylketonuria. *Mol. Genet. Metab.* **2012**, *107*, 43–48. [CrossRef] [PubMed]
80. Camatta, G.C.; Kanufre, V.d.C.; Alves, M.R.A.; Soares, R.D.L.; Norton, R.D.C.; de Aguiar, M.J.B.; Starling, A.L.P. Body fat percentage in adolescents with phenylketonuria and associated factors. *Mol. Genet. Metab. Rep.* **2020**, *23*, 100595. [CrossRef]
81. Couce, M.L.; Vitoria, I.; Aldámiz-Echevarría, L.; Fernández-Marmiesse, A.; Roca, I.; Llarena, M.; Sánchez-Pintos, P.; Leis, R.; Hermida, A. Lipid profile status and other related factors in patients with Hyperphenylalaninaemia. *Orphanet J. Rare Dis.* **2016**, *11*, 123. [CrossRef]
82. Daly, A.; Evans, S.; Pinto, A.; Jackson, R.; Ashmore, C.; Rocha, J.C.; MacDonald, A. The Impact of the Use of Glycomacropeptide on Satiety and Dietary Intake in Phenylketonuria. *Nutrients* **2020**, *12*, 2704. [CrossRef] [PubMed]
83. Dios-Fuentes, E.; Marin, M.G.; Remón-Ruiz, P.; Avila, R.B.; Delgado, M.A.B.; Alonso, J.B.; Gamgaram, V.K.D.; Olveira, G.; Soto-Moreno, A.; Venegas-Moreno, E. Cardiometabolic and Nutritional Morbidities of a Large, Adult, PKU Cohort from Andalusia. *Nutrients* **2022**, *14*, 1311. [CrossRef] [PubMed]
84. Enns, G.; Koch, R.; Brumm, V.; Blakely, E.; Suter, R.; Jurecki, E. Suboptimal outcomes in patients with PKU treated early with diet alone: Revisiting the evidence. *Mol. Genet. Metab.* **2010**, *101*, 99–109. [CrossRef] [PubMed]
85. Ozel, H.G.; Ahring, K.; Bélanger-Quintana, A.; Dokoupil, K.; Lammardo, A.; Robert, M.; Rocha, J.; Almeida, M.; van Rijn, M.; MacDonald, A. Overweight and obesity in PKU: The results from 8 centres in Europe and Turkey. *Mol. Genet. Metab. Rep.* **2014**, *1*, 483–486. [CrossRef]
86. Gramer, G.; Haege, G.; Langhans, C.-D.; Schuhmann, V.; Burgard, P.; Hoffmann, G.F. Long-chain polyunsaturated fatty acid status in children, adolescents and adults with phenylketonuria. *Prostaglandins Leukot. Essent. Fat. Acids* **2016**, *109*, 52–57. [CrossRef] [PubMed]

87. Hochuli, M.; Bollhalder, S.; Thierer, C.; Refardt, J.; Gerber, P.; Baumgartner, M.R. Effects of Inadequate Amino Acid Mixture Intake on Nutrient Supply of Adult Patients with Phenylketonuria. *Ann. Nutr. Metab.* **2017**, *71*, 129–135. [CrossRef] [PubMed]
88. Htun, P.; Nee, J.; Ploeckinger, U.; Eder, K.; Geisler, T.; Gawaz, M.; Bocksch, W.; Fateh-Moghadam, S. Fish-Free Diet in Patients with Phenylketonuria Is Not Associated with Early Atherosclerotic Changes and Enhanced Platelet Activation. *PLoS ONE* **2015**, *10*, e0135930. [CrossRef]
89. Leiva, C.; Bravo, P.; Arias, C.; Cabello, J.; Leal-Witt, M.; Salazar, F.; Cornejo, V. 25 Hydroxy Vitamin D Level, Bone Health, Vitamin D and Calcium Intake in Chilean Patients with Phenylketonuria and Hyperphenylalaninemias. *J. Inborn Errors Metab. Screen.* **2021**, *9*. [CrossRef]
90. MacLeod, E.L.; Gleason, S.T.; van Calcar, S.C.; Ney, D.M. Reassessment of phenylalanine tolerance in adults with phenylketonuria is needed as body mass changes. *Mol. Genet. Metab.* **2009**, *98*, 331–337. [CrossRef]
91. Mazzola, P.N.; Teixeira, B.C.; Schirmbeck, G.H.; Reischak-Oliveira, A.; Derks, T.G.; van Spronsen, F.J.; Dutra-Filho, C.S.; Schwartz, I.V.D. Acute exercise in treated phenylketonuria patients: Physical activity and biochemical response. *Mol. Genet. Metab. Rep.* **2015**, *5*, 55–59. [CrossRef]
92. Okano, Y.; Hattori, T.; Fujimoto, H.; Noi, K.; Okamoto, M.; Watanabe, T.; Watanabe, R.; Fujii, R.; Tamaoki, T. Nutritional status of patients with phenylketonuria in Japan. *Mol. Genet. Metab. Rep.* **2016**, *8*, 103–110. [CrossRef] [PubMed]
93. van Calcar, S.C.; MacLeod, E.L.; Gleason, S.T.; Etzel, M.R.; Clayton, M.K.; A Wolff, J.; Ney, D.M. Improved nutritional management of phenylketonuria by using a diet containing glycomacropeptide compared with amino acids. *Am. J. Clin. Nutr.* **2009**, *89*, 1068–1077. [CrossRef] [PubMed]
94. Vazquez-Agra, N.; Fernandez-Crespo, S.; Marques-Afonso, A.-T.; Cruces-Sande, A.; Barbosa-Gouveia, S.; Martinez-Olmos, M.-A.; Hermida-Ameijeiras, A. The correlation of lipid profile and waist circumference with phenylalanine levels in adult patients with classical phenylketonuria. *Med. Clin.* **2023**, *160*, 385–391. [CrossRef] [PubMed]
95. Viau, K.; Wessel, A.; Martell, L.; Sacharow, S.; Rohr, F. Nutrition status of adults with phenylketonuria treated with pegvaliase. *Mol. Genet. Metab.* **2021**, *133*, 345–351. [CrossRef] [PubMed]
96. Wernlund, P.G.; Hvas, C.L.; Dahlerup, J.F.; Bahl, M.I.; Licht, T.R.; Knudsen, K.E.B.; Agnholt, J.S. Casein glycomacropeptide is well tolerated in healthy adults and changes neither high-sensitive C-reactive protein, gut microbiota nor faecal butyrate: A restricted randomised trial. *Br. J. Nutr.* **2021**, *125*, 1374–1385. [CrossRef] [PubMed]
97. de Castro, M.-J.; Sánchez-Pintos, P.; Abdelaziz-Salem, N.; Leis, R.; Couce, M.L. Evaluation of Body Composition, Physical Activity, and Food Intake in Patients with Inborn Errors of Intermediary Metabolism. *Nutrients* **2021**, *13*, 2111. [CrossRef] [PubMed]
98. Doulgeraki, A.; Skarpalezou, A.; Theodosiadou, A.; Monopolis, I.; Schulpis, K. Body Composition Profile of Young Patients With Phenylketonuria and Mild Hyperphenylalaninemia. *Int. J. Endocrinol. Metab.* **2014**, *12*, e16061. [CrossRef]
99. Evans, M.; Truby, H.; Boneh, A. The relationship between dietary intake, growth and body composition in Phenylketonuria. *Mol. Genet. Metab.* **2017**, *122*, 36–42. [CrossRef]
100. Evans, M.; Nguo, K.; Boneh, A.; Truby, H. The Validity of Bioelectrical Impedance Analysis to Measure Body Composition in Phenylketonuria. *JIMD Rep.* **2018**, *42*, 37–45. [CrossRef]
101. Mazzola, P.N.; Nalin, T.; Castro, K.; van Rijn, M.; Derks, T.G.; Perry, I.D.; Mainieri, A.S.; Schwartz, I.V.D. Analysis of body composition and nutritional status in Brazilian phenylketonuria patients. *Mol. Genet. Metab. Rep.* **2016**, *6*, 16–20. [CrossRef]
102. Alfheeaid, H.; Gerasimidis, K.; Năstase, A.-M.; Elhauge, M.; Cochrane, B.; Malkova, D. Impact of phenylketonuria type meal on appetite, thermic effect of feeding and postprandial fat oxidation. *Clin. Nutr.* **2018**, *37*, 851–857. [CrossRef] [PubMed]
103. Rocha, J.C.; van Spronsen, F.J.; Almeida, M.F.; Ramos, E.; Guimarães, J.T.; Borges, N. Early dietary treated patients with phenylketonuria can achieve normal growth and body composition. *Mol. Genet. Metab.* **2013**, *110*, S40–S43. [CrossRef] [PubMed]

nutrients

MDPI

Article

Malnutrition-Related Liver Steatosis, CONUT Score and Poor Clinical Outcomes in an Internal Medicine Department

Nicoletta Miano, Giorgia Todaro, Maurizio Di Marco, Sabrina Scilletta, Giosiana Bosco, Francesco Di Giacomo Barbagallo, Roberto Scicali, Salvatore Piro, Francesco Purrello and Antonino Di Pino *

Department of Clinical and Experimental Medicine, University of Catania, 95122 Catania, Italy; nicoletta.miano@gmail.com (N.M.); giorgia.todaro92@gmail.com (G.T.); maurizio.dimarco@studium.unict.it (M.D.M.); sabrinascilletta@gmail.com (S.S.); giosiana.bosco@gmail.com (G.B.); fdigiacomobarbagallo@gmail.com (F.D.G.B.); roberto.scicali@unict.it (R.S.); salvatore.piro@unict.it (S.P.); francesco.purrello@unict.it (F.P.)

* Correspondence: antonino.dipino@unict.it; Tel.: +39-0957598401

Abstract: Fatty liver disease has been identified as a marker of malnutrition in different clinical settings. Recently, the COntrolling NUTritional status score (CONUT score) emerged as a promising tool for malnutrition assessment. Our aim was to evaluate short-term outcomes among patients with malnutrition-related liver steatosis in an Internal Medicine department. Furthermore, we evaluated the association of the CONUT score with malnutrition-related liver steatosis. Data from 247 patients hospitalized in an Internal Medicine department were retrospectively collected. The study population was stratified into three groups based on hepatic radiodensity assessed with computed tomography: mild steatosis (≥56.1 HU), moderate steatosis (between 49.7 and 56 HU), and severe steatosis (≤49.6 HU). We then calculated the CONUT score. Severe steatosis patients had higher in-hospital mortality (18.2 vs. 15.5%) and longer in-hospital stays compared with the mild steatosis group (length of in-hospital stay longer than 12 days: 45% vs. 40%). Logistic regression analysis showed that severe steatosis was not significantly associated with in-hospital all-cause death, while a high CONUT score was an independent risk factor for sepsis. We found an independent relationship between malnutrition-associated liver steatosis and the CONUT score. These results identified the CONUT score as a tool for nutritional assessment of hospitalized patients.

Keywords: malnutrition; hepatic steatosis; CONUT score; in-hospital outcomes; internal medicine

1. Introduction

Malnutrition (MN) is a condition developing from inadequate nutrient intake or absorption that results in altered body composition, reduced physical and mental function, and poor clinical outcomes [1,2].

One-third to one-half of patients hospitalized in medical or surgical departments suffer from protein–energy undernutrition, and the prognosis of the patients during hospitalization, in the short, medium, and long term, is significantly affected by nutrient deficiency, leading to worse outcomes [3,4].

The current evidence indicates that undernutrition can trigger the development of a type of liver steatosis different from conventional nonalcoholic fatty liver disease (NAFLD), which is basically related to overnutrition and obesity. This form of liver steatosis associated with malnutrition often arises in the context of an inadequate intake of essential nutrients, such as proteins, calories, and certain vitamins. The primary pathogenetic processes include deficiency in nutrients with hepatoprotective properties that support hepatic lipid metabolism, deficiency in chemicals required for the output of very low-density lipoprotein (VLDL), and modifications in the makeup and role of the intestinal microbiota [5–7]. It seems that malnutrition is linked to chronic liver disease, particularly in hospitalized patients, because of insufficient intake of macro- and micronutrients, which increases mortality and complications [8,9]. In fact, it has been found that a patient's nutritional state might predict their prognosis if they have liver disease [10,11]. However, nutritional assessment is often neglected, and nutritional challenges in patients with liver steatosis and other chronic diseases are underestimated. Abdominal ultrasonography is the instrument of choice for hepatic examinations. Nevertheless, over the past 20 years, computed tomography (CT) has become more frequently used for the non-invasive evaluation of fatty liver disease, offering an accurate measurement of the liver's fat content [12,13].

As concerns the diagnosis of malnutrition, there is not a validated gold standard approach yet, and the ones that are available are generally inadequate for routine clinical practice [14]. Accordingly, we evaluated the association of the CONUT score, a simple and easy-to-calculate clinical score, with malnutrition-related hepatic steatosis. The COntrolling NUTritional status score (CONUT score), which was recently introduced, seems to have a promising predictive impact in various clinical scenarios [15]. It was developed as an assessment tool for the early identification of low nutritional status and depends on the total peripheral lymphocyte count, serum albumin concentration, and levels of total cholesterol (TC). Protein reserves are shown by albumin; caloric depletion is shown by TC; and immunological defense is shown by lymphocyte count. An increased score paired with a lower level of nutrients is linked to a decline in each factor. The CONUT score was initially developed and evaluated in Surgical and Oncology departments to predict acute worsening during hospitalization. However, recently, it has also been analyzed in patients hospitalized in Internal Medicine departments, demonstrating that it has a significant prognostic impact for various clinical conditions such as chronic disease, cancer, and cardiac disorders [16–18]. The aim of this study was to evaluate short-term complications among patients with malnutrition-related liver steatosis admitted to an internal medicine department. Furthermore, given the clinical relevance of prompt recognition of patients with malnutrition, we evaluated the association of the CONUT score, a simple and easy way to calculate clinical scores with malnutrition-related hepatic steatosis.

2. Materials and Methods

2.1. Patients

We retrospectively acquired clinical and radiological data through the medical records of patients that underwent abdominal CT while admitted to the Internal Medicine and Geriatric departments of the Azienda Ospedaliera di Alta Specializzazione Garibaldi Nesima, Catania, Italy, from the months of September to December 2021. The data included the following: (1) age, gender, comorbidities (the presence of hypertension, diabetes mellitus, chronic heart failure, chronic kidney failure, neoplasm, previous stroke, chronic obstructive pulmonary disease (COPD), and chronic liver disease); (2) clinical occurrences during in-hospital stay (mortality, length of stay, diagnosis of sepsis, blood transfusions needed); (3) patients' clinical and biochemical features at the time of admission, such as systolic and diastolic blood pressure, glycemia, creatinine, estimated glomerular filtration rate (eGFR), TC, high-density lipoprotein cholesterol (HDL-c), low-density lipoprotein cholesterol (LDL-c), triglycerides, total proteins, albumin, glutamic oxaloacetic transaminase, glutamic pyruvic transaminase, N-terminal fragment brain natriuretic peptide (NT-pro-BNP), procalcitonin, high-sensitivity C-reactive protein (hs-CRP), erythrocyte sedimentation rate (ESR), complete blood count, hemoglobin, hematocrit, and international normalized ratio (INR); (4) values of liver radiodensity on abdomen CT without contrast medium. We excluded all patients with a previous diagnosis of MAFLD in their clinical records, including those with alcoholic liver disease, autoimmune hepatitis, chronic liver disease of viral etiology, toxic damage associated with drugs, genetic accumulation of metals, or other genetically based liver diseases.

2.2. Evaluation of Liver Steatosis

Liver radiodensity was calculated on the basis of the X-ray attenuation, expressed in Hounsfield Units (HUs) and in agreement with the recent literature, by placing three circular regions of interest (ROIs) of 300 $mm^2 \pm 10$ mm^2 in peripheral areas of the liver parenchyma, avoiding vessels, bile ducts, focal lesions, areas of parenchymal inhomogeneity or artifacts caused by the ribs or by the air present in the gastrointestinal tract: in particular, one ROI circle was positioned on the right anterior lobe, one on the right posterior lobe and one on the left lobe, on CT section where the right portal branch enters the liver; the mean of the three attenuation values, quantitative index of the liver fat content, was then calculated [12].

2.3. Calculations

The CONUT score was determined, in accordance with the first study results [15], from the serum albumin concentration, total peripheral lymphocyte count, and total cholesterol concentration. Albumin concentrations $\geq$ 3.5 g/dL, 3.0–3.49 g/dL, 2.5–2.99 g/dL, and $\leq$2.5 g/dL were scored as 0, 2, 4, and 6, respectively. Total lymphocyte counts $\geq$ 1600/mm^3, 1200–1599/mm^3, 800–1199/mm^3, and $\leq$800/mm^3 were scored as 0, 1, 2, and 3, respectively. Total cholesterol concentrations $\geq$ 180 mg/dL, 140–179 mg/dL, 100–139 mg/dL, and $\leq$100 mg/dL were scored as 0, 1, 2, and 3, respectively. The three scores were added together, resulting in the CONUT score. Patients were divided into two categories according to the degree of undernutrition as follows: low (0–4) and high (5–12) CONUT scores. The Chronic Kidney Disease Epidemiology Collaboration (CKD-EPI) formula was used to calculate the eGFR [19]. According to the original study, the Padua Prediction Score for the risk of venous thromboembolism was estimated [20]. We evaluated the high/low cut-offs of NT-proBNP, procalcitonin, AST, ALT, and high-sensitivity C-reactive protein according to upper laboratory limits as follows: NT-proBNP, 260 pg/mL; procalcitonin, 0.5 µg/L; AST, 34 UI/L; ALT, 55 UI/L; and hs-CRP, 0.5 mg/dL.

Our population was stratified into three equal-sized groups based on the values of hepatic radiodensity expressed in Hounsfield Units as an index of the hepatic fat content.

We identified two points within the data set: the first tertile (or lower tertile) and the second tertile (or upper tertile). These points corresponded to the following values: 56.1 and 49.7, so that one-third of the data lies below the first tertile and two-thirds below the second tertile. Thus, we defined three groups as follows: mild steatosis ($\geq$56.1 HU), moderate steatosis (between 49.7 and 56 HU), and severe steatosis ($\leq$49.6 HU). The three groups were composed as follows: 82 patients with mild steatosis, 82 patients with moderate steatosis, and 83 patients with severe steatosis.

2.4. Statistical Analysis

Statistical analyses of clinical and biological variables were conducted with Stat View 6.0 for Windows. The data are presented as median (IQR), means, or SD. The distributional properties of each variable, including normality, were evaluated using the Kolmogorov–Smirnov test. Group comparisons were conducted using ANOVA for continuous variables and the Chi-square test for non-continuous variables. We used a multinomial logistic regression model, setting the CONUT score as the independent variable and the group of steatosis as the dependent variable, to verify a possible association between the CONUT score and each category of steatosis. We applied logistic regression to investigate the independent association between fatty liver disease and clinical outcomes. We adjusted for the following variables: age, sex, cardiovascular disease, history of stroke, COPD, diabetes mellitus, chronic kidney disease, and tumors. A statistically significant finding was defined as a p value of less than 0.05. When required, logarithmic transformation was applied to numerical variables to lessen skewness; values are reported as the median and interquartile range.

2.5. Ethics

The Ethical Board Catania 2 approved this retrospective study (N° Protocol 370/CE; approval date of 21 May 2021). Every method performed in research projects involving human subjects complied with the Declaration of Helsinki and the ethical guidelines established by national and/or institutional research committees. Data collection was conducted retrospectively; thus, informed consent was not necessary.

3. Results

3.1. Baseline Characteristics, Medical History, and Comorbidities of the Patients

In total, data from 247 patients, 112 men and 135 women, were retrospectively collected based on clinical. Our population was separated into three groups according to the values of hepatic radiodensity expressed in HU as an index of the hepatic fat content: 82 patients with mild steatosis ($\geq$56.1 HU), 82 patients with moderate steatosis (between 49.7 and 56 HU), and 83 patients with severe steatosis ($\leq$49.6 HU).

The clinical and biochemical characteristics of the study population according to liver steatosis are shown in Table 1. The three groups were homogeneous for age, while a higher percentage of men was found in the mild steatosis group in comparison with those with severe steatosis (51.2% mild steatosis vs. 32.5% severe steatosis, $p = 0.01$).

Table 1. Clinical characteristics and blood test parameters at admission to an Internal Medicine department according to mean liver density tertiles.

	Mild Steatosis (n = 82)	Moderate Steatosis (n = 82)	Severe Steatosis (n = 83)
Age, years	71.9 ± 16.2	72.2 ± 14.4	71.9 ± 14.4
Sex, female %	51.2	45.1	27 *
Drugs in home therapy, n	6.2 ± 5.1	5.3 ± 3.9	6.2 ± 4.1
VTE risk (Padua Score)	3.6 ± 1.8	3.3 ± 1.9	4.2 ± 1.7 †
SBP, mmHg	123.5 ± 18.3	126.2 ± 23.0	127.6 ± 18.8
DBP, mmHg	69.1± 11.8	70.7 ± 10.7	71.7± 10.0
CONUT score	5.0 ± 3.0	5.9 ± 2.7	6.2 ± 2.9 *,†
Mean liver density, HUs	61.5 ± 5.4	52.9 ± 1.8	43.6 ± 4.9
Fasting Glucose, mg/dL	111.1 ± 46.9	110.1± 46.6	105.4 ± 51.0
Urea mg/dL	62.0 ± 43.0	67.9 ± 59.1	62.5 ± 50.7
eGFR, mL/min/1.73 m^2	68.8 ± 33.9	67.4 ± 31.3	70.1 ± 31.6
Albumin, g/dL	3.2 ± 0.6	3.0 ± 0.6 *	2.9 ± 0.6 *
Total bilirubin, mg/dL	0.9 ± 0.7	1.3± 2.3	1.6 ± 2.4
AST, UI/L	23.5 (19–37)	20 (15–31)	27 (19–47) †
ALT, UI/L	15 (10–37)	14 (6–28)	18 (8–29)
GGT UI/L	29 (18–44)	37 (18–77)	34 (20–111)
ALP UI/L	70 (58.2–86)	74.5 (60–115)	74 (61–122)
NT-proBNP > 260 pg/mL, %	35.3	18.2	13.5
hs-CRP > 0.5 mg/dL, %	80.5	88.5	79 *,†
Procalcitonin > 0.5 μg/L, %	23.5	26.0	32.4
WBC, 10^3/μL	9.4 ± 4.9	8.9 ± 4.1	11.4 ± 10.2
Neutrophils, 10^3/μL	7.1 ± 4.7	6.4 ± 3.8	8.7 ± 8.6
Lymphocites, 10^3/μL	1.5 ± 1.6	1.4 ± 0.8	1.5 ± 1.3
Platelets, 10^3/μL	249.5 ± 122.5	225.8 ± 113.0	227.9 ± 119.5
HB, g/dL	11.4 ± 2.7	10.7 ± 1.8	10.9 ± 2.2
INR	1.3 ± 0.2	1.3 ± 0.2	1.4 ± 06
Total cholesterol, mg/dL	150.9 ± 42.1	147.5 ± 52.3	140.3 ± 59.3
LDL cholesterol, mg/dL	89.5 ± 36.6	91.2 ± 43.2	87.3 ± 55.8
HDL cholesterol, mg/dL	36.9 ± 15.5	32.8 ± 13.6 *	25.7 ± 13.6 *,†
Triglycerides, mg/dL	113 (81–142)	118 (92–154)	111 (78–159)

Data are presented as percentage, mean ± SD, or median (IQR). VTE: venous thromboembolism; SBP: systolic blood pressure; DBP: diastolic blood pressure; CONUT: controlling nutritional status; HUs: Hounsfield Units; eGFR: estimated glomerular filtration rate; AST: aspartate aminotransferase; ALT: alanine aminotransferase; GGT: Gamma Glutamyl Transpeptidase; ALP: Alkaline Phosphatase; NT-proBNP: N-terminal pro-brain natriuretic peptide; hs-CRP: high-sensitivity C-reactive protein; WBC: white blood cells; HB: hemoglobin; INR: international normalized ratio; LDL: low-density lipoprotein; HDL: high-density lipoprotein. * $p < 0.05$ vs. mild steatosis; † $p < 0.05$ vs. moderate steatosis.

Patients in the severe steatosis group showed a significantly higher thromboembolic risk (4.2 ± 1.7 severe steatosis vs. 3.6 ± 1.8 mild steatosis; $p = 0.16$; 4.2 ± 1.7 severe steatosis vs. 3.3 ± 1.9 mild steatosis, $p = 0.03$). Moreover, patients with severe steatosis were more likely to have lower HDL cholesterol (25.7 ± 13.6 severe steatosis vs. 36.9 ± 15.5 mild steatosis; $p < 0.0001$) and albumin values (2.9 ± 06 severe steatosis vs. 3.2 ± 0.6 mild steatosis; $p = 0.009$), whereas they showed higher ESR values (68.4 ± 29.3 severe steatosis vs. 48.6 ± 30.5 mild steatosis; $p = 0.007$) and C-reactive protein (CRP) (97.5% severe steatosis vs. 80.5% mild steatosis; $p = 0.0006$). Furthermore, those with severe steatosis had higher values of white blood cells (WBC) (11.4 ± 10.2 severe steatosis vs. 9.4 ± 4.9 mild steatosis, $p < 0.07$; 11.4 ± 10.2 severe steatosis vs. 8.9 ± 4.1 mild steatosis, $p < 0.02$). Patients in the severe steatosis group showed higher INR values (1.4 ± 0.6 severe steatosis vs. 1.3 ± 0.2 mild steatosis; $p < 0.09$). Patients in the severe steatosis group had a higher CONUT score compared to those in the mild and moderate steatosis groups (6.2 ± 2.9 vs. 5.0 ± 3.0 $p = 0.009$, and 6.2 ± 2.9 vs. 5.9 ± 2.7 $p < 0.0001$, respectively).

Furthermore, we noted that the total bilirubin levels, as well as the levels of AST, ALT, and procalcitonin > 0.5 microg/L, increased from the mild steatosis group to the severe steatosis group, however, without statistical significance.

The medical history and comorbidities of the patients are shown in Table 2. Patients in the severe steatosis group were more frequently affected by oncological disease (40.5% severe steatosis vs. 24.7% mild steatosis, $p = 0.03$). Furthermore, patients in the severe steatosis group had a higher probability of having a stroke history, healthcare-related infections from multidrug-resistant germs, type 2 diabetes, neoplasms, and the need for blood transfusion during in-hospital stays, without statistical significance compared with those in the mild steatosis and moderate steatosis groups.

Table 2. Comorbidities according to mean liver density tertiles.

	Mild Steatosis (n = 82)	Moderate Steatosis (n = 82)	Severe Steatosis (n = 83)
Cardiovascular disease, %	67.9	75	64.5
History of stroke, %	2.7	4.6	11.3
COPD, %	27.5	29.1	28.8
Diabetes mellitus, %	29.6	26.6	32.5
CKD, %	21.0	25.6	22.7
Neoplasms, %	24.7	36.6	40.5 *
MDR germs isolation, %	15.8	15.6	20.4
Patient needing blood transfusions, %	15.8	15.6	27.3

Data are presented as percentage. COPD: chronic obstructive pulmonary disease; CKD: chronic kidney disease; MDR: multidrug resistant; * $p < 0.05$ vs. mild steatosis.

3.2. Multinomial Logistic Regression Analysis to Assess the Association of CONUT Score to Each Steatosis Group

We performed a multinomial logistic regression using the CONUT score as the independent variable and the categories of steatosis (i.e., mild steatosis, moderate steatosis, and severe steatosis) as the dependent variable. We found that with an increasing CONUT score, the odds of being in the group with severe steatosis were significantly higher (OR 1.15, 95%CI 1.04–1.29, $p = 0.01$). However, the odds of being in the group with moderate steatosis were higher, but without reaching statistical significance (OR 1.11, 95%CI 0.99–1.24, $p = 0.06$).

3.3. Clinical Outcomes According to Steatosis Groups

In-hospital all-cause death occurred in 14 patients (18.2%) in the severe steatosis group vs. 11 patients (15.5%) in the mild steatosis group (Table 3). We showed that people with moderate steatosis were more likely to have sepsis compared to those in the mild steatosis group (42.1% moderate steatosis vs. 38.7% mild steatosis, $p = 0.27$).

Table 3. In-hospital outcomes according to mean liver density tertiles.

	Mild Steatosis (n = 82)	Moderate Steatosis (n = 82)	Severe Steatosis (n = 83)
In-hospital mortality, %	15.5	17.7	18.2
Length of in-hospital stay >12 days, %	45.5	43	44.6
Diagnosis of sepsis, %	38.7	42.1	31.6

Data are presented as percentage.

The in-hospital stay was longer in the severe steatosis group compared with the mild steatosis group (length of in-hospital stay longer than 12 days: 45% severe steatosis vs. 40% mild steatosis).

3.4. Subgroup Analysis for the Primary Outcome Measure

We then performed logistic regression analysis and, after adjusting for confounders, found that severe steatosis was not significantly associated with in-hospital all-cause death [OR 0.94, 95%CI (0.87–1.01), $p = 0.11$]. Moreover, we demonstrated that a high CONUT score was an independent risk factor for sepsis [OR 1.34, CI 1.08–1.64), $p = 0.005$], while it was not significantly associated with in-hospital all-cause death [OR 1.26, 95%CI (0.96–1.63), $p = 0.08$].

To estimate the relationship between malnutrition-associated liver steatosis and the CONUT score, we performed multivariate logistic analysis, considering the mean liver density as a dependent variable and a number of clinical parameters as independent variables: age, sex, cardiovascular disease, history of stroke, chronic obstructive pulmonary disease, diabetes mellitus, chronic kidney disease, neoplasms, and CONUT score (Table 4). We found that mean liver density was inversely and independently related to the CONUT score ($\beta = -0.26$, $p = 0.01$).

Table 4. Multiple regression analysis evaluating major determinants of mean liver density.

Independent Variables	Coefficient β	p
Age	−0.07	n.s.
Male sex	−0.08	n.s.
Cardiovascular disease	0.09	n.s.
History of stroke	−0.19	0.03
COPD	0.12	n.s.
Diabetes mellitus	−0.13	n.s.
CKD	0.04	n.s.
Neoplasms	−0.07	n.s.
CONUT score	−0.26	0.01

COPD: Chronic obstructive pulmonary disease; CKD: chronic kidney disease; CONUT: controlling nutritional status; n.s.: not significant.

4. Discussion

The aim of this study was to evaluate short-term in-hospital outcomes among patients with malnutrition related to liver steatosis admitted to an Internal Medicine Department.

We found that severe steatosis was not significantly associated with in-hospital all-cause death after adjustment for multiple confounders. Most of the studies in the literature have focused on the role of a high-calorie diet in the pathogenesis of hepatic steatosis. Although this assumption is undoubtedly valid, in recent decades, numerous pathogenic mechanisms responsible for excessive lipid accumulation in the liver of undernourished subjects have been recognized. Indeed, it appears that fatty liver disease depends on many nutritional factors, and micronutrient deficiency (MND) seems to play a crucial role [5–7]. The association between liver disease and severe hypoalimentation was previously demonstrated in other clinical contexts. Hanachi M et al. demonstrated that a BMI < 12 was the sole independent risk factor for hepatic cytolysis in a study conducted in patients with anorexia nervosa [21]; furthermore, other studies have shown that increased caloric consumption and weight gain can lead to a rapid improvement in liver function tests [22]. Liver abnormalities have been reported as complications of other clinical conditions associated with impairment of nutrient absorption, such as bariatric surgery and intestinal failure [23,24]. These results support evidence from previous observations: chronic liver disease, ranging from steatosis (fatty liver) to steatohepatitis, acute alcohol-associated hepatitis, and liver cirrhosis, is associated with malnutrition, especially among hospitalized patients due to an inadequate intake of both macro- and micro-nutrients, leading to higher mortality and complications [8,9]. Currently, an unmet clinical need is the identification of a screening tool that could quickly identify patients who are more likely to have poorer clinical outcomes, primarily in the hospitalized population. Considering that patients admitted to Internal Medicine departments frequently suffer from malnutrition, it is crucial to find a simple score with a high predictive value to properly treat patients' nutritional needs. Currently, several clinical tools have been proposed for nutritional evaluation; however, numerous difficulties have arisen in their clinical application. In this context, a straightforward, impartial measure of inflammation and nutritional status, which is gaining more reliability, is the CONUT score. The CONUT score is a comprehensive index that uses standard blood biochemical tests that are typically performed at admission for hospitalized patients in Internal Medicine units [15]. In a previous study, we demonstrated that patients hospitalized in an internal medicine department should be evaluated using the CONUT score to assess their nutritional status and, consequently, the risk of adverse outcomes due to malnutrition [16]. Furthermore, the utility of the CONUT score in identifying hospitalized malnourished patients with inadequate clinical results has been shown in other clinical settings. Our findings indicated that the CONUT score could be useful in assessing the nutritional state of patients admitted to an Internal Medicine ward. These results show that patients who are more prone to have negative in-hospital outcomes can be identified using the CONUT score as a nutritional screening tool. Moreover, this study highlighted an independent association between the CONUT score and malnutrition-related liver steatosis. To our knowledge, this is the first study in the literature to analyze this association. Indeed, previous studies explored the possible association between liver steatosis and malnutrition through different food frequency questionnaires. Petermann-Rocha et al. [25] showed that patients with higher scores at the 14-Item Mediterranean Diet Adherence Screener (MEDAS-14) and other scores, such as the Mediterranean Diet Score [26] and the Healthy Diet Indicator, strictly linked with better diet quality, had a significantly lower risk of severe liver steatosis compared with patients with worse nutrition habits. Furthermore, Matsui M. et al. [27] found that the prognostic nutritional index (PNI) was a predictor of nutritional status in patients with chronic liver disease, liver steatosis included. In particular, a PNI score of <40 was beneficial in predicting clinical outcomes for those suffering from long-term liver disease.

People suffering from liver disease frequently experience malnourishment and are unable to have a proper oral food intake. Poor body composition and biological function can result from insufficient consumption and poor gastrointestinal absorption [25,27,28]. Nutritional status has been identified as a prognostic predictor for patients with liver disease [10,11]. Nevertheless, while treating patients with liver steatosis and other chronic diseases, nutritional evaluation is frequently overlooked, and nutritional problems in these patients are underestimated. Nutritional therapy interventions are therefore frequently underused for this group of patients [29]. This study has several strengths. Our study is the first, to our knowledge, to investigate the short-term prognostic value of the CONUT score in a cohort of patients with different grades of hepatic steatosis in an internal medicine department. Indeed, patients who are at risk for unfavorable outcomes and could benefit from nutritional supplementation could be easily identified thanks to the predictive value of a high CONUT score at admission. There are a few limitations that should be noted. Firstly, the study's statistical power is limited due to the retrospective nature of this work and a small sample size. In addition, even though we adjusted for the measured confounders, other variables such as drugs and nosocomial infections were not taken into consideration. Third, we were unable to make any deductions regarding the patients' long-term prognosis (i.e., re-hospitalization rate, death within the first month, loss of autonomy in daily living activities, etc.) since no information is currently given concerning the nutritional status or clinical outcomes of the patients after discharge. Finally, even if patients with a previous diagnosis of MAFLD in their clinical records were not included, we do not exclude that there may be an overlap between MAFLD and malnutrition-related liver steatosis, given the inclusive nature of the new definition of MAFLD.

5. Conclusions

The CONUT score is strictly associated with liver steatosis. Thus, the CONUT score can be used as a tool for nutritional assessment to recognize patients who require careful monitoring while hospitalized.

Author Contributions: Conceptualization, N.M. and G.T.; methodology, N.M., M.D.M. and S.S.; software, S.S.; validation, N.M., G.T., S.S. and M.D.M.; formal analysis, G.B. and F.D.G.B.; investigation, N.M.; resources, R.S., A.D.P., S.P. and F.P.; data curation, N.M.; writing—original draft preparation, N.M.; writing—review and editing, N.M.; visualization, S.S. and M.D.M.; supervision, A.D.P.; project administration, A.D.P. All authors have read and agreed to the published version of the manuscript.

Funding: This research received no external funding.

Institutional Review Board Statement: The study was conducted in accordance with the Declaration of Helsinki and approved by the Ethics Committee Catania 2 (No. Prot 370/CE, 21 May 2021).

Informed Consent Statement: Informed consent was obtained from all subjects involved in the study.

Data Availability Statement: Data from this study are available upon request from corresponding author. Data are not publicly available due to privacy.

Acknowledgments: This study was in keeping with the objectives of the project "DEGENER-action", Department of Clinical and Experimental Medicine, University of Catania.

Conflicts of Interest: The authors declare no conflicts of interest.

References

1. Lim, S.L.; Ong, K.C.B.; Chan, Y.H.; Loke, W.C.; Ferguson, M.; Daniels, L. Malnutrition and its impact on cost of hospitalization, length of stay, readmission and 3-year mortality. *Clin. Nutr.* **2012**, *31*, 345–350. [CrossRef]
2. Cederholm, T.; Barazzoni, R.; Austin, P.; Ballmer, P.; Biolo, G.; Bischoff, S.C.; Compher, C.; Correia, I.; Higashiguchi, T.; Holst, M.; et al. ESPEN guidelines on definitions and terminology of clinical nutrition. *Clin. Nutr.* **2017**, *36*, 49–64. [CrossRef] [PubMed]
3. Barker, L.A.; Gout, B.S.; Crowe, T.C. Hospital Malnutrition: Prevalence, Identification and Impact on Patients and the Healthcare System. *Int. J. Environ. Res. Public Health* **2011**, *8*, 514–527. [CrossRef] [PubMed]
4. Dent, E.; Hoogendijk, E.O.; Visvanathan, R.; Wright, O.R.L. Malnutrition Screening and Assessment in Hospitalised Older People: A Review. *J. Nutr. Health Aging* **2019**, *23*, 431–441. [CrossRef]
5. Veraldi, S.; Pietrobattista, A.; Liccardo, D.; Basso, M.S.; Mosca, A.; Alterio, T.; Cardile, S.; Benedetti, S.; Della Corte, C.; Candusso, M. Fat soluble vitamins deficiency in pediatric chronic liver disease: The impact of liver transplantation. *Dig. Liver Dis.* **2020**, *52*, 308–313. [CrossRef]
6. Ullah, R.; Rauf, N.; Nabi, G.; Ullah, H.; Shen, Y.; Zhou, Y.-D.; Fu, J. Role of Nutrition in the Pathogenesis and Prevention of Non-alcoholic Fatty Liver Disease: Recent Updates. *Int. J. Biol. Sci.* **2019**, *15*, 265–276. [CrossRef]
7. Allen, L. *Guidelines on Food Fortification with Micronutrients*; World Health Organization: Geneva, Switzerland; Food and Agriculture Organization of the United Nations: Rome, Italy, 2006.
8. Starekova, J.; Hernando, D.; Pickhardt, P.J.; Reeder, S.B. Quantification of Liver Fat Content with CT and MRI: State of the Art. *Radiology* **2021**, *301*, 250–262. [CrossRef]
9. Chalasani, N.; Younossi, Z.; LaVine, J.E.; Charlton, M.; Cusi, K.; Rinella, M.; Harrison, S.A.; Brunt, E.M.; Sanyal, A.J. The diagnosis and management of nonalcoholic fatty liver disease: Practice guidance from the American Association for the Study of Liver Diseases. *Hepatology* **2018**, *67*, 328–357. [CrossRef] [PubMed]
10. Cederholm, T.; Bosaeus, I.; Barazzoni, R.; Bauer, J.; Van Gossum, A.; Klek, S.; Muscaritoli, M.; Nyulasi, I.; Ockenga, J.; Schneider, S.; et al. Diagnostic criteria for malnutrition—An ESPEN Consensus Statement. *Clin. Nutr.* **2015**, *34*, 335–340. [CrossRef]

11. De Ulíbarri, J.I.; González-Madroño, A.; de Villar, N.G.; González, P.; González, B.; Mancha, A.; Rodríguez, F.; Fernández, G. CONUT: A tool for controlling nutritional status. First validation in a hospital population. *Nutr. Hosp.* **2005**, *20*, 38–45.
12. Miano, N.; Di Marco, M.; Alaimo, S.; Coppolino, G.; L'episcopo, G.; Leggio, S.; Scicali, R.; Piro, S.; Purrello, F.; Di Pino, A. Controlling Nutritional Status (CONUT) Score as a Potential Prognostic Indicator of In-Hospital Mortality, Sepsis and Length of Stay in an Internal Medicine Department. *Nutrients* **2023**, *15*, 1554. [CrossRef] [PubMed]
13. Wada, H.; Dohi, T.; Miyauchi, K.; Doi, S.; Konishi, H.; Naito, R.; Tsuboi, S.; Ogita, M.; Kasai, T.; Okazaki, S.; et al. Prognostic impact of nutritional status assessed by the Controlling Nutritional Status score in patients with stable coronary artery disease undergoing percutaneous coronary intervention. *Clin. Res. Cardiol.* **2017**, *106*, 875–883. [CrossRef] [PubMed]
14. Li, W.; Li, M.; Wang, T.; Ma, G.; Deng, Y.; Pu, D.; Liu, Z.; Wu, Q.; Liu, X.; Zhou, Q. Controlling Nutritional Status (CONUT) score is a prognostic factor in patients with resected breast cancer. *Sci. Rep.* **2020**, *10*, 6633. [CrossRef] [PubMed]
15. Inker, L.A.; Eneanya, N.D.; Coresh, J.; Tighiouart, H.; Wang, D.; Sang, Y.; Crews, D.C.; Doria, A.; Estrella, M.M.; Froissart, M.; et al. New Creatinine- and Cystatin C–Based Equations to Estimate GFR without Race. *N. Engl. J. Med.* **2021**, *385*, 1737–1749. [CrossRef] [PubMed]
16. Barbar, S.; Noventa, F.; Rossetto, V.; Ferrari, A.; Brandolin, B.; Perlati, M.; DE Bon, E.; Tormene, D.; Pagnan, A.; Prandoni, P. A risk assessment model for the identification of hospitalized medical patients at risk for venous thromboembolism: The Padua Prediction Score. *J. Thromb. Haemost.* **2010**, *8*, 2450–2457. [CrossRef] [PubMed]
17. Hanachi, M.; Melchior, J.C.; Crenn, P. Hypertransaminasemia in severely malnourished adult anorexia nervosa patients: Risk factors and evolution under enteral nutrition. *Clin. Nutr.* **2013**, *32*, 391–395. [CrossRef]
18. Jones, S.C.; Pieri, L.F.; Losowsky, M.S. Abnormalities of liver function in severe anorexia nervosa. *Eur. Eat. Disorders Rev.* **1999**, *7*, 28–36. [CrossRef]
19. Cavicchi, M.; Beau, P.; Crenn, P.; Degott, C.; Messing, B. Prevalence of Liver Disease and Contributing Factors in Patients Receiving Home Parenteral Nutrition for Permanent Intestinal Failure. *Ann. Intern. Med.* **2000**, *132*, 525–532. [CrossRef] [PubMed]
20. Anandacoomarasamy, A.; Caterson, I.; Sambrook, P.; Fransen, M.; March, L. The impact of obesity on the musculoskeletal system. *Int. J. Obes.* **2008**, *32*, 211–222. [CrossRef]
21. McNeice, A.; Scott, R.; Rafferty, G.P.; Cash, W.J.; Turner, G.B. The hepatobiliary complications of malnutrition and nutritional support in adults. *Ir. J. Med. Sci.* **2018**, *188*, 109–117. [CrossRef]
22. Shah, N.D.; Barritt, A.S. Nutrition as Therapy in Liver Disease. *Clin. Ther.* **2022**, *44*, 682–696. [CrossRef] [PubMed]
23. Petermann-Rocha, F.; Carrasco-Marin, F.; Boonpor, J.; Parra-Soto, S.; Shannon, O.; Malcomson, F.; Phillips, N.; Jain, M.; Deo, S.; Livingstone, K.M.; et al. Association of five diet scores with severe NAFLD incidence: A prospective study from UK Biobank. *Diabetes Obes. Metab.* **2024**, *26*, 860–870. [CrossRef] [PubMed]
24. Piccirillo, F.; Miano, N.; Goffredo, C.; Nusca, A.; Mangiacapra, F.; Khazrai, Y.M.; De Gara, L.; Ussia, G.P.; Grigioni, F. Impact of Mediterranean diet on metabolic and inflammatory status of patients with polyvascular atherosclerotic disease. *Nutr. Metab. Cardiovasc. Dis.* **2022**, *32*, 117–124. [CrossRef] [PubMed]
25. Matsui, M.; Asai, A.; Ushiro, K.; Onishi, S.; Nishikawa, T.; Ohama, H.; Tsuchimoto, Y.; Kim, S.K.; Nishikawa, H. Prognostic Nutritional Index Correlates with Liver Function and Prognosis in Chronic Liver Disease Patients. *Diagnostics* **2023**, *14*, 49. [CrossRef] [PubMed]
26. Lieber, C.S. Relationships between nutrition, alcohol use, and liver disease. *Alcohol. Res. Health* **2003**, *27*, 220–231. [PubMed]
27. Traub, J.; Reiss, L.; Aliwa, B.; Stadlbauer, V. Malnutrition in Patients with Liver Cirrhosis. *Nutrients* **2021**, *13*, 540. [CrossRef] [PubMed]
28. Koretz, R.L.; Avenell, A.; Lipman, T.O. Nutritional support for liver disease. *Cochrane Database Syst. Rev.* **2012**, *5*, CD008344. [CrossRef]
29. Kawaguchi, T.; Charlton, M.; Kawaguchi, A.; Yamamura, S.; Nakano, D.; Tsutsumi, T.; Zafer, M.; Torimura, T. Effects of Mediterranean Diet in Patients with Nonalcoholic Fatty Liver Disease: A Systematic Review, Meta-Analysis, and Meta-Regression Analysis of Randomized Controlled Trials. *Semin. Liver Dis.* **2021**, *41*, 225–234. [CrossRef]

nutrients

MDPI

Article

Malnutrition in Amyotrophic Lateral Sclerosis: Insights from Morphofunctional Assessment and Global Leadership Initiative on Malnutrition Criteria

María Teresa Zarco-Martín [1,2,*], Carmen Freire [3,4,5], María Carmen Andreo-López [1,4,*], Socorro Leyva-Martínez [1] and María Luisa Fernández-Soto [1,4,6]

1 Endocrinology and Nutrition Unit, San Cecilio University Hospital, 18016 Granada, Spain
2 Fundación para la Investigación Biosanitaria en Andalucía Oriental-Alejandro Otero (FIBAO), 18012 Granada, Spain
3 Department of Legal Medicine, Toxicology and Physical Anthropology, University of Granada, 18006 Granada, Spain
4 Instituto de Investigación Biosanitaria de Granada (Ibs. Granada), 18012 Granda, Spain
5 CIBER de Epidemiología y Salud Pública, 28029 Madrid, Spain
6 Department of Medicine, University of Granada, 18016 Granada, Spain
* Correspondence: terezarco@correo.ugr.es (M.T.Z.-M.); mcandreo21@gmail.com (M.C.A.-L.)

Abstract: Amyotrophic Lateral Sclerosis (ALS) is a progressive neurodegenerative disease frequently accompanied by malnutrition due to weight loss, increased energy expenditure, and muscle mass loss. This study aimed to evaluate morphofunctional assessment tools as predictors of malnutrition and to investigate their relationship with muscle status and disease severity in ALS patients. A cross-sectional study was conducted with 45 ALS patients at the San Cecilio University Hospital in Granada. Malnutrition was assessed using the Global Leadership Initiative on Malnutrition (GLIM) criteria. Morphofunctional assessment was performed using Bioimpedance Vectorial Analysis (BIVA), handgrip strength (HGS), and Short Physical Performance Battery (SPPB). Malnutrition prevalence was 38% according to GLIM criteria. Significant differences were observed between malnourished and non-malnourished groups in age (70 ± 9 vs. 62 ± 10 years, $p = 0.01$), sex (female prevalence: 58.8% vs. 25.0%, $p = 0.02$), dysphagia prevalence (83% vs. 29%, $p < 0.001$), PEG/PRG use (35.3% vs. 3.6%, $p = 0.01$), and ALSFRS-R scores (30 ± 12 vs. 34 ± 12, $p = 0.02$). Malnourished patients had lower values in anthropometric measurements, muscle mass obtained by BIVA, and phase angle (PA) (4.05 ± 0.8° vs. 5.09 ± 0.8°, $p < 0.001$). No significant differences were found in muscle strength or functional status. PA showed significant correlations with muscle strength (r = 0.52, $p < 0.001$) and muscle mass measures (r = 0.48, $p < 0.001$). Moreover, PA was associated with poorer disease progression and physical performance. In our sample, BIVA metrics such as PA (<4.3°), SPA (<−0.8), body cell mass (<9.2 kg/m), and extracellular water (>49.75%) were identified as malnutrition risk factors. The study underscores the critical importance of comprehensive morphofunctional assessment and the use of advanced diagnostic criteria, for early identification and intervention in malnutrition among people with ALS. Further research is warranted to validate these findings and develop targeted nutritional strategies into routine clinical practice.

Keywords: ALS; malnutrition; phase angle; body composition

1. Introduction

Amyotrophic Lateral Sclerosis (ALS) is a progressive neurodegenerative disease characterized by the selective loss of motor neurons in the brain and spinal cord, leading to muscle weakness. The incidence of ALS is estimated to be about 2–3 cases per 100,000 people, with some variation across different regions [1]. The most common symptoms are muscle weakness, fatigue, atrophy, fasciculation, dysarthria, dysphagia, sialorrhea, and emotional instability [2].

In addition, ALS patients are at high risk of malnutrition due to weight loss, eating difficulties, increased energy needs, and muscle mass loss, affecting their quality of life and survival [3,4]. In fact, nutritional status is considered a significant prognostic factor and, specifically, muscle mass loss also aggravates the loss of spinal motor neurons [5].

Malnutrition prevalence in ALS patients ranges from 15 to 55% [6]. Its diagnosis is particularly challenging due to the heterogeneity in criteria and tools, leading to ambiguous assessment of nutritional state and the implementation of effective nutritional therapy [7].

Traditionally, BMI has been used for the diagnosis of malnutrition and has been considered as a clinical outcome predictor [8]; however, it does not allow us to detect changes in body composition or muscle mass loss. Some tools used in morphofunctional assessment, such as bioelectrical impedance analysis, have been described in ALS patients [9]. However, there is a lack of evidence on the use of functional and muscle assessment tools in this population. Therefore, there is a need of a holistic approach of these patients, including a morphofunctional assessment. This approach involves assessing body composition and muscle and functional state, focusing on both the quantity and quality of the body compartments for nutritional and physical intervention [10].

The hypothesis of this study is that morphofunctional assessment tools, including BIVA, HGS, and SPPB, can provide accurate and early identification of malnutrition in ALS patients when used alongside the GLIM criteria.

This study aims to evaluate morphofunctional assessment tools as predictors of malnutrition and their relationship with muscle status and disease progression in ALS patients.

2. Materials and Methods

2.1. Study Design and Population

A single-center cross-sectional observational study of people with ALS who attended the nutrition consultation in the multidisciplinary team of ALS (UMELA) at San Cecilio University Hospital in Granada was conducted between March 2022 and January 2023.

The sample size was determined using an a priori power analysis with G*Power. A power level of 0.80 (80%) and an alpha level of 0.05 were set as thresholds for detecting significant differences and associations. The analysis indicated that a minimum of 36 patients was required to achieve sufficient power.

A total of 45 patients were included in the study; 29 patients (64%) were attended to for the first time at the time of data collection during UMELA. The inclusion criteria were patients diagnosed with ALS according to El Escorial criteria, who were aged over 18 years old, and who agreed to participate in the study and signed the informed consent. The exclusion criteria were people with neurodegenerative diseases other than ALS. The study was approved by the Biomedical Research Ethics Committee of Granada (approval no. 1770-N-21), approval date: 25 February 2022.

2.2. Clinical Variables

Clinical variables included data on sex (male/female), age (years), evolution of the disease since ALS diagnosis (months), dysphagia diagnosed by the volume and viscosity test (MECV-V) [11], use of percutaneous endoscopic or radiologic gastrostomy (PEG or PRG), type of symptomatology onset (bulbar/spinal), and use of non-invasive mechanic ventilation (NIMV).

2.2.1. Anthropometric Measurements

Habitual weight (kg) in the last 6–12 months was reported by the patients. Actual weight (kg) was assessed using a scale (SECA, Birmingham, UK). Height (m) was obtained using a stadiometer (SECA, Birmingham, UK). Weight loss (habitual weight-actual weight/habitual weight × 100) and body mass index (actual weight/height × height (kg/m^2) were calculated.

Arm circumference (AC) was obtained at the midpoint between the acromion and olecranon with a measuring tape (SECA 201, Birmingham, UK), in cm. Triceps skinfold (TS) was obtained with a skinfold caliper (Holtain LTD, Crymych, UK), in mm. Arm muscle circumference (AMC) was calculated with the formula AC (cm) − (0.314 × TS (mm)).

Calf circumference (CC) was obtained at the widest section of the calf area with a measuring tap, in cm. We calculated the appendicular skeletal mass index (ASMI) with a predictive equation using calf circumference (in cm), age (in years), height (in m), and sex [12].

2.2.2. Phase Angle and Body Composition Parameters

Phase angle and body composition analyses were obtained using Nutrilab®, a 50 kHz phase-sensitive impedance analyzer (Akern, Florence, Italy [13]). The PA was expressed in degrees as arctan (Xc/R) × (180°/p). An individual standardized PA value (SPA) was determined by adjusting it by sex and age. Data obtained using BIVA for body composition were categorized as fat-free mass (FFM/height, kg/m), fat mass (FM/height, kg/m), total body water (TBW/height, kg/m), extracellular water (% ECW of TBW), body cellular mass (BCM/height, kg/m), skeletal muscle mass index (SMI, kg/m^2), and appendicular skeletal muscle mass (ASMM, kg), obtained from predictive equations [14,15]. Normality values from Nutrilab® were used [16].

BIVA was conducted following established guidelines to ensure accuracy and reproducibility. Participants were positioned in a supine position with their limbs slightly apart to prevent skin contact, which could interfere with the electrical impedance measurement and to ensure stability. A five-minute rest period in the supine position was ensured prior to measurements to minimize the impact of fluid shifts caused by changes in posture. The BIVA device was calibrated daily according to the manufacturer's instructions, and the accuracy of the BIVA measurements was verified using a precision circuit provided by the manufacturer.

2.2.3. Muscle Strength

Muscle strength was assessed using an adult dynamometer (Jamar handgrip dynamometry, Asimow Engineering Co., Los Angeles, CA, USA) and measurements were performed in the dominant limb, repeated on three occasions, and the highest value was used to represent HGS.

To classify normality, we used the cut-off points proposed by the EWGSOP2 (males > 27 kg and females > 16 kg) [17].

2.2.4. Biochemical Analysis

Serum albumin and high-sensitivity C-reactive protein (hs-CRP) levels were measured using standard laboratory techniques.

2.3. *Physical Performance*

Physical performance was analyzed using the SPPB [18], which includes 3 domains: balance, walking speed, and getting up from and sitting down on a chair 5 times.

In the balance test, the participant tries to hold 3 positions: feet together, semi-tandem, and tandem for 10 s each. These subtests follow a hierarchical sequence. In the walking speed test, the participant walks a distance of 4 m at his/her usual pace. This test is performed and the time is recorded in seconds. Finally, in the stand up and sit down on a chair 5 times test, the participant stands up and sits down on a chair 5 times, as fast as possible, and the total time taken is recorded.

Each test is scored from 0 (worst performance) to 4 (best performance). A total score is obtained which is the sum of the 3 tests and ranges from 0 to 12. The cut-off point to assess poor physical performance is $\leq$8 [17].

2.4. *Malnutrition Disease Related Diagnosis*

Malnutrition diagnosis was based on the GLIM criteria [19] whereby patients need to meet the sum of at least two criteria: a phenotypic criterion, i.e., weight loss, BMI, and the decrease in muscle mass; and an etiological criterion decrease in the intake of the requirements and the presence of inflammatory biomarkers. To assess muscle mass, we used ASMI calculated using a predictive equation. To classify normality, the cut-off points used were males > 7 kg/m^2 and females > 6 kg/m^2. The severity of malnutrition was defined: moderate cases included a BMI < 20 kg/m^2 at age < 70 or BMI $\leq$ 22 kg/m^2 at age $\geq$ 70, weight loss between 5 and 10% in the last 6 months. Severe cases included a BMI < 18.5 kg/m^2 at age < 70 or BMI $\leq$ 20 kg/m^2 at age $\geq$ 70, weight loss $\geq$ 10% in the last 6 months.

2.5. Disease Progression

The ALSFRS-R (Revised Amyotrophic Lateral Sclerosis Functional Rating Scale) score was used to assess ALS severity [20]. It is 12-item scale that assesses activities of daily living affected during the course of the disease. The total score ranges from 0 to 48, in which higher scores indicate better physical function [21].

2.6. Statistical Analysis

Data statistical analyses were carried out using IBM SPSS 25.0 (IBM, New York, NY, USA), and graphic representation was performed using R v.3.5.1 software (Integrated Development for R. RStudio, PBC, Boston, MA, USA).

Normality of the distribution of quantitative variables was verified using the Shapiro–Wilk test. Quantitative variables are presented as the mean and standard deviation, and differences between paired observations according to the nutritional status (malnutrition diagnosis or not) were determined using Student's t-test (or the Wilcoxon test in the absence of normality). The qualitative variables are described as proportions, and the differences between groups were analyzed via the Chi-square test, using Fisher's exact test when necessary. Pearson correlation coefficients between quantitative variables were obtained.

Logistic regression analysis was used to calculate the association between malnutrition and morphofunctional measurements, using as independent variables those with significant differences in Student's *t*-test ($p < 0.05$) between malnourished and well-nourished groups, and clinical relevance. The model was adjusted for sex and age due to the possible interference of these parameters with the variables of interest owing to physiological factors.

The predictive capability of morphofunctional variables was assessed using the receiver operating characteristic (ROC) curves and the area under the curve (AUC). Statistical significance was set at $p < 0.05$.

3. Results

3.1. General Characterization of the Population Study

A total of 45 patients were included in the study, 28 (62.2%) males and 17 (37.8%) females. Mean age of the participants was 65 $\pm$ 10 years. Mean disease evolution time was 32 $\pm$ 27 months. Dysphagia prevalence was 49%. A total of 16% of the patients used PRG/PEG and 20% NIMV. A total of 44.4% had bulbar onset, 40% spinal onset, 11.1% had primary lateral sclerosis, and 4.4% had flail arm. The ALSFRS-R median was 32.

According to GLIM criteria, 17 patients (38%) were malnourished, of which 24.4% (11) were classified as moderate malnutrition and 6 (13.3%) as severe malnutrition.

Table 1 shows that malnourished ALS patients had significatively higher age, female prevalence, dysphagia diagnosis, and PEG/PRG use, and a lower ALSFRS-R.

No significant differences were found between non-malnourished and malnourished groups in serum albumin levels (4.2 $\pm$ 0.4 mg/dL vs. 4.0 $\pm$ 0.4 mg/dL, $p = 0.2$) and hs-CRP (4.5 $\pm$ 5.2 mg/L vs. 4.1 $\pm$ 3.9 mg/L, $p = 0.8$).

Table 1. Clinical characteristics of the population according to malnutrition diagnosis.

	Total (n = 45)	Non-Malnutrition (n = 28/62%)	Malnutrition (n = 17/38%)	p-Value
Sex				0.02
Male	62.2	75.0	41.2	
Female	37.8	25.0	58.8	
Age (years)	65 ± 9.9	62 ± 10	70 ± 9	0.01
Disease evolution (months)	32 ± 27	37 ± 31	23 ± 19	0.15
Dysphagia diagnosis (%)	49	29	83	<0.001
PRG/PEG use (%)	15.6	3.6	35.3	0.01
NIMV (%)	20	14.3	29.4	0.40
ALSFRS-R (points)	32	34	30	0.02

Results are expressed as mean ± SD (numeric variables) or % (categorical variables). ALSFRS-R: Revised Amyotrophic Lateral Sclerosis Functional Rating Scale (0–48); NIMV: non-invasive mechanical ventilation; PEG: percutaneous endoscopic gastrostomy; PRG: percutaneous radiologic gastrostomy.

3.2. Morphofunctional Status

Morphofunctional assessment variables and differences between patients with and without a diagnosis of malnutrition are shown in Table 2. The mean percentage of weight loss (WL) was 9.5 ± 8.2%. There were significant differences between groups, with higher values of % WL in the malnourished group (11.8 ± 9.6% vs. 5.8 ± 2.5%, p = 0.03) over the last 6–12 months.

Table 2. Morphofunctional assessment variables and differences by malnutrition diagnosis.

	Total (n = 45)	Non-Malnutrition (n = 28, 62%)	Malnutrition (n = 17, 38%)	p-Value
Anthropometric measures				
Weight (kg)	69.3 ± 13.7	75.1 ± 10.2	59.6 ± 13.5	<0.001
Weight loss (%)	9.5 ± 8.2	5.8 ± 2.5	11.8 ± 9.6	0.03
BMI (kg/m^2)	25.16 ± 4.64	27.4 ± 4.1	24.2 ± 2.8	<0.001
AC (cm)	27.8 ± 4	29.35 ± 3.7	25.4 ± 3.3	0.001
TS (mm)	15 ± 3.6	15.7 ± 7.7	13.8 ± 7	0.43
AMC (cm)	23.1 ± 3.4	24.3 ± 2.7	21 ± 3.4	0.001
CC (cm)	34.7 ± 3.6	33.3 ± 2.6	32.6 ± 2.3	0.39
ASMI (kg/m^2)	6.4 ± 1.4	6.9 ± 1.4	5.6 ± 1.2	0.01
BIVA				
Rz (Ohm)	593.6 ± 106.1	549.8 ± 77.1	651.9 ± 113.6	0.01
Xc (Ohm)	48.6 ± 8.8	50.4 ± 9.2	46.2 ± 7.8	0.17
PA (°)	4.63 ± 0.96	5.09 ± 0.8	4.05 ± 0.8	<0.001
SPA	−0.85 ± 1.19	−0.55 ± 0.94	−1.26 ± 1.38	0.08
TBW (kg/m)	21.5 ± 3.4	23.1 ± 2.7	19.5 ± 3.3	0.001
ECW (%/TBW)	53.1 ± 6	50.3 ± 4.4	56.7 ± 6	0.001
ECW/ICW	1.17 ± 0.32	1.03 ± 0.18	1.36 ± 0.36	0.01
FFM (kg/m)	29 ± 4.4	31.2 ± 3.1	26.2 ± 3.8	<0.001
FM (kg/m)	11.9 ± 5.5	13.7 ± 5.7	9.5 ± 3.4	0.02
BCM (kg/m)	13.3 ± 3.6	15.2 ± 3.0	10.8 ± 2.8	<0.001
ASMM (kg)	17.4 ± 4.3	19.4 ± 3.4	14.8 ± 4.1	0.001
SMI (kg^2/m^2)	7.9 ± 1.7	8.7 ± 1.3	6.9 ± 1.6	<0.001
Functional status				
HGS max (kg)	20 ± 10.3	22 ± 9.8	17 ± 10.9	0.18
SPPB	5	7	4	0.19

Results are expressed as mean ± SD (numeric variables). AC: arm circumference; AMC: arm muscle circumference; ASMI: appendicular skeletal mass index; BMI: body mass index; BCM: body cell mass; BIVA: Bioimpedance Vectorial Analysis; CC: calc circumference; ECW: extracellular water; FFM: fat-free mass; FM: fat mass; HGS: hand grip strength; PA: phase angle; SMI: skeletal muscle index; SPA: standardized phase angle; SPPB: Short Physical Performance Battery; TBW: total body water; TS: tricipital skinfold.

There was a statistically significant difference in anthropometric parameters, showing lower values in the malnourished group for all measurements except TS and CC. Significant differences were found in mean BIVA variables based on malnutrition diagnosis. Specifically, the malnutrition group showed notably lower values of PA, TBW, FFM, FM, BCM, ASMM, and SM, alongside higher values of Rz, ECW, and ECW/ICW.

Regarding HGS values, 82.2% had values lower than the 50th percentile, 55.6% lower than the 10th percentile, and 57.8% lower than the cut-off point for sarcopenia diagnosis.

Based on the classification for the SPPB, 42.2% were classified as disabled, 6.7% as frail, 24.4% as prefrail, and 26.7% as autonomous. Using the EWGSOP2 cut-off point, 69% exhibited impairment of functional status. However, no significant differences were found in strength or functional status according to the diagnosis of malnutrition.

3.3. Correlation between Nutritional Parameters

There was significant correlation between PA and anthropometric measurements (AMC: r = 0.53, p = 0.001; ASMI: r = 0.54, p < 0.001) and muscle strength (HGS: r = 0.54, p = 0.001).

BCM had a significant correlation with anthropometric measurements (AMC: r = 0.77, p < 0.001; CC: r = 0.58, p < 0.001; ASMI: r = 0.60, p < 0.001) and HGS (r = 0.69, p < 0.001).

Disease progression measured by ALSFRS-r showed a significant correlation with morphofunctional parameters such as the functional test SPPB (r = 0.67, p< 0.001), muscle mass values (ASMM: r = 0.40, p = 0.02; SMI: r = 0.46, p = 0.01; BCM: r = 0.49, p = 0.01), PA (r = 0.38, p = 0.01), and HGS (r = 0.46, p = 0.003). All these results are detailed in Figure 1.

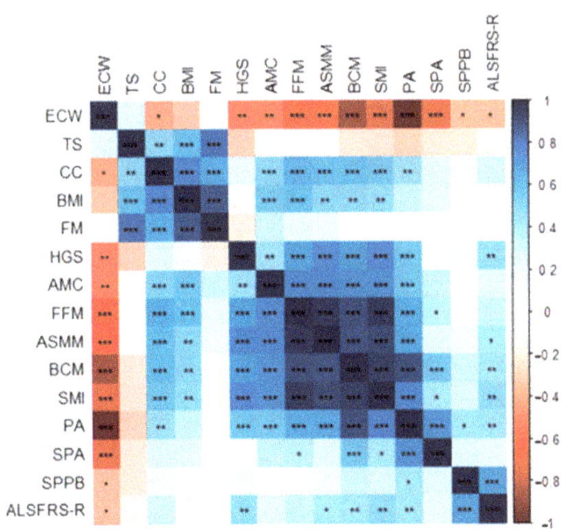

Figure 1. Pearson's correlation plot of morphofunctional and disease evolution scores. Red colors indicate negative correlation, while blue colors positive correlations. Color intensity represents the strength of the correlation, with deeper shades signifying stronger relationships. Asterisks (*) indicate significant correlation between variables according to the Pearson's correlation test (* p < 0.05; ** p < 0.01; *** p < 0.001).

3.4. Malnutrition Risk Factors and Related Morphofunctional Parameter Cut-Off Values

We found that BIVA variables were associated with malnutrition risk. Specifically, an increase in PA was associated with a 75% decreased risk, an increase in SPA was associated with a 77% lower risk, an increase in BCM was associated with a 40% decreased risk, and an increase in %ECW increased the risk of malnutrition by 30% (results are detailed in Table 3).

Table 3. Logistic regression for the association between morphofunctional variables and malnutrition status.

	OR_c (95%CI)	*p*-Value	OR_{adj} (95% CI)	*p*-Value
Rz	1.01 (1.00–1.02)	0.01	1.01 (0.99–1.02)	0.07
Xc	0.94 (0.86–1.03)	0.17	0.94 (0.84–1.06)	0.36
PA	0.21 (0.07–0.60)	0.004	0.25 (0.08–0.80)	0.02
SPA	0.56 (0.30–1.10)	0.10	0.23 (0.06–0.90)	0.03
%ECW	1.30 (1.06–1.55)	0.01	1.23 (0.99–1.50)	0.051
BCM/h	0.60 (0.43–0.93)	0.02	0.60 (0.43–0.90)	0.001
SMI	0.39 (0.20–0.73)	0.004	0.39 (0.14–1.07)	0.07
FM/h	0.80 (0.70–0.94)	0.03	0.80 (0.60–0.98)	0.04
ALSFRS-R	0.92 (0.85–0.99)	0.02	0.93 (0.86–1.02)	0.12
SPPB	0.90 (0.80–1.04)	0.17	0.94 (0.80–1.10)	0.45
HGS	0.58 (0.04–4.50)	0.60	0.19 (0.01–2.01)	0.17

OR_c: crude Odds Ratio, OR_{adj}: Odds Ratio adjusted by sex and age. 95% CI: 95% confidence interval.

The cut-off value obtained for the prediction of malnutrition for PA was 4.3° with an AUC of 0.801, a sensitivity of 82%, and specificity of 59%; the value for SPA was −0.8 with an AUC of 0.663, a sensitivity of 80%, and specificity of 60%; the value for ECW was 49.8% with an AUC of 0.787, a sensitivity of 93%, and specificity of 55%; and the value for BCM was 9.2 kg/m with an AUC of 0.850, a sensitivity of 96%, and specificity of 70% (Figure 2).

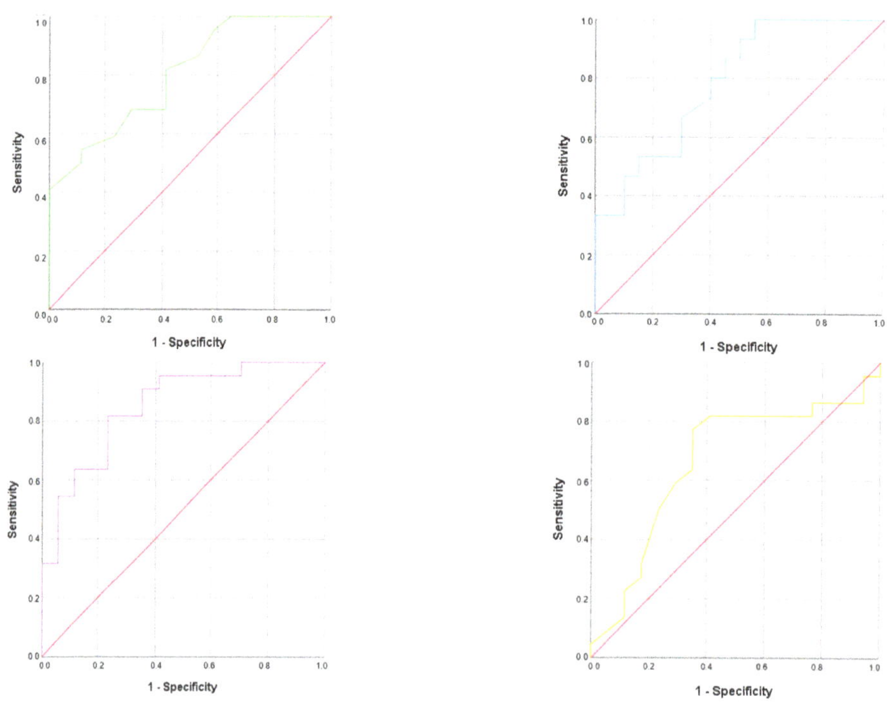

Figure 2. ROC curve of PA (**upside left**), SPA (**upside right**), ECW (**downside right**), and BCM (**downside left**).

4. Discussion

This study showed a high prevalence of malnutrition (38%) in a sample of patients with ALS who were attended to at UMELA. According to GLIM criteria, malnourished

ALS patients had lower PA and muscle and fat mass parameters. However, ECW values were higher in the malnutrition group. No significant differences were found in muscle strength and physical performance between both groups. PA was significantly associated with muscle strength and with muscle mass parameters measured by classic anthropometry. Additionally, PA was associated with worse disease evolution and physical performance. BIVA values such as PA, SPA, BCM, and ECW were independent prognostic factors for malnutrition in our sample.

The reported prevalence of malnutrition among ALS patients is heterogeneous, mainly due to diagnostic criteria used. According to the BMI, the malnutrition prevalence documented was 12% in a French ALS register of 117 patients (mean BMI: 24.6 ± 4.6 kg/m^2) and 14.7% in a study performed in Brazil with 34 ALS patients (mean BMI: unknown) [22,23]. This differs from our results, as we found a higher malnutrition prevalence (38%) with a similar BMI (mean BMI: 25.2 kg/m^2). Using the same criteria, a higher malnutrition prevalence (45%), has been described in a Brazilian study, which may be explained by a lower mean BMI (21.7 kg/m^2) [24].

On the other hand, López-Gómez et al. studied the nutritional status of 93 ALS patients in Spain according to VGS and GLIM criteria, finding a higher prevalence when they considered VGS (71%) compared with GLIM criteria diagnosis (48%). Compared with these results, we detected a slightly lower prevalence (38% vs. 48%) with our sample having a comparable mean BMI (25.6 kg/m^2 vs. 24.4 kg/m^2) and mean age (65 vs. 67 years) [25]. Nakamura et al. found a 36% malnutrition prevalence in 48 Japanese subjects with ALS; defining it as % ideal body weight <0.9 [26]. Although there was a similar malnutrition prevalence, the results are not comparable because their sample had a lower mean BMI, the patients were older, and there was a higher proportion of females. Controversy remains concerning weight and BMI as useful tools to diagnose malnutrition in persons with ALS, due to the disease's intrinsic characteristics. These include muscle atrophy and hypermetabolism, which complicate accurate assessments. Although the GLIM criteria are considered practical and comprehensive for diagnosing malnutrition across various clinical settings, their application in ALS requires further validation and reliable techniques. The criteria's broad applicability and incorporation of multiple indicators provide a robust framework for assessing malnutrition, but they must be adapted to account for the unique challenges presented by ALS [27].

Beyond weight loss and BMI, we found significant differences between malnourished and non-malnourished patients in muscle mass parameters measured by anthropometry, with significantly lower values in malnourished patients in AC, AMC, and ASMI. These have been considered useful tools to detect malnutrition in ALS patients [28]. Salvioni et al. revealed a significant positive correlation between disease progression and AMC [24], supporting our results that muscle mass measurements are related to malnutrition and disease severity.

BIVA can indirectly estimate body composition, representing an useful, non-invasive, and validated assessment tool in people with ALS [9]. In our study, the muscle mass parameters measured by BIVA (FFM, BCM, ASMM, and SMI) showed significantly lower values in malnourished patients compared with those without malnutrition. Therefore, this tool could be useful for measuring active muscle mass and monitoring nutritional treatment in patients with. We also found lower FM in the malnourished group. Li et al. reported results which showed that patients with a significant weight loss (>5%) at diagnosis had a significantly lower BMI, FM, and FFM than those without weight loss [29].

Although in our study we detected a lower FM in the ALS malnourished group, no differences were found in the TS measurement. This could be due to the decreased visceral fat mass with no decrease in the subcutaneous fat mass. This is supported by a study by Choi et al. (2023) which analyzed using the subcutaneous fat volume index (FVI) and visceral FVI from abdominal CT, finding that visceral FVI declined during the disease progression while subcutaneous FVI did not [30].

When analyzing hydration status, in our sample, the malnourished group had a lower TBW and a higher ECW value and ECW/ICW ratio. Malnutrition often results in lower muscle mass, therefore the ICW is reduced as well, leading to an increase in the ECW [31]. The ratio ECW/BCM has been proposed as a potential biomarker for disease onset in pre-symptomatic ALS gene carriers [32]. Our results showed a negative correlation of ECW with muscle mass, functionality, and disease severity, suggesting that an increase in ECW might be a useful marker of malnutrition. It highlights the importance of evaluating changes in hydration status.

We used BIVA not only to assess body composition but also to evaluate body bioelectrical properties, reflected by PA [33]. PA has been associated with poor survival [22]. The PA mean value in our work was slightly lower than the one recently reported by López-Gómez et al. in a similar ALS sample [34]. Our sample showed lower PA values in the malnourished group compared to well-nourished people. Desport J.C. et al. presented similar results, although mean PA in both groups (malnourished and non-malnourished) was remarkably lower than ours [35]. This difference could be due to the higher disease severity of the patients, measured by ALSFRS-R, since our mean value was higher than theirs. Similarly, Barone M. et al. compared PA values between groups categorized by BMI, finding lower PA values in the underweight group compared to the normal weight group [36]. No differences in PA values were observed between spinal or bulbar onset groups [25].

In a recent study, PA and body composition were investigated as biomarkers, finding that pre-symptomatic ALS mutation carriers exhibited lower PA compared to non-carriers [32]. This finding underscores the potential of using body composition as a non-invasive tool for future biomarker research.

Despite BIVA not being universally regarded as the gold standard for morphofunctional assessment, it offers valuable insights into body composition and fluid distribution. However, it is important to recognize that other tools can provide complementary or more detailed assessments of morphofunctional status. One complementary tool widely used in morphofunctional assessment is Nutritional Ultrasound®. It has gained prominence for its ability to assess muscle and fat tissue directly [37]. In fact, a recent study found direct correlations between muscle mass parameters measured by ultrasonography (quadriceps thickness) and muscle mass markers from BIVA (e.g., BCMI, FFMI, ASMI) [34].

Our study showed a significantly positive correlation between PA and HGS. Consistent with this finding, the literature has evidenced the relationship between PA and muscle strength (HGS) in healthy adults, as well as in individuals with cancer, kidney disease, chronic obstructive pulmonary disease, and heart failure disease [38].

However, there is no existing evidence assessing muscle strength using HGS in subjects with ALS to compare with our results, since muscle strength in ALS patients has typically been evaluated using the Medical Research Council Scale [29,39] and knee extension strength [40]. We observed that the mean HGS value (20 ± 10.3 kg) was significantly lower compared to the cut-off points proposed by the EWGSOP2 [17]. Nevertheless, in studies from different populations, HGS has demonstrated an association with nutritional status [41]. We did not find these results in our sample. However, we found significant correlations with other nutritional values, such as muscle mass measurements.

We also found a correlation of HGS with ALSFRS-R. Supporting our results, ALSFRS-R has been correlated with muscle mass in other studies [29,30]. We assessed functionality with the SPPB, which has demonstrated its value as a predictor of all-cause mortality [42]. However, there is no evidence of the assessment in physical function using SPPB in ALS populations. In our sample, we found a high prevalence of impairment of physical function, with only 27% of patients with ALS showing a normal result in the test (SPPB > 10). In a study conducted by Montes J. et al. using a Timed Up and Go (TUG) test, an association was found between the TUG test and the risk of falls [43]. Furthermore, SPPB had a positive and significant correlation with ALSFRS-R and PA.

In the assessment of the capacity of morphofunctional tools as prognostic factors for malnutrition, we highlight the results of the ECW, whose increase raised the risk of malnutrition. In the case of BCM, FM, PA, and SPA, their decrease raised the risk of malnutrition. Additionally, we identified cut-off points for ECW (>49.75%), PA (<4.3°), SPA (<−0.8), and BCM (9.2 kg/m) that could distinguish malnourished ALS patients. These specific cut-off points within the GLIM criteria tailored for the diagnosis of malnutrition in patients with ALS. Traditional reliance on standard metrics like weight and BMI often fails to accurately reflect the nutritional status of ALS patients due to the disease's characteristic muscle atrophy and altered metabolism.

To our knowledge, this is the first study that analyses body composition and its association with malnutrition diagnosed by GLIM criteria in ALS patients. Another strength of this study is that assesses not only nutritional status and body composition but also their interaction with functionality. Despite the absence of a standardized protocol for assessing the nutritional status of patients with ALS, guidelines recommend evaluating weight loss, and, if possible, body composition by DEXA or BIA, in addition to BMI. We used BIVA to assess body composition that has been validated in this population compared to gold standard body composition tools. However, this study has several limitations, such as the modest sample size and the differences in timing between nutritional assessment and diagnosis, which may lead to a heterogeneous sample. Moreover, it was conducted in a single center, and the results could be biased by our routine clinical practices. We also used general cut-off points for assessing nutritional status, as there is a lack of cut-off points specific for ALS. Therefore, it is important to register all clinical characteristics evaluated to compare our results within each clinical population.

5. Conclusions

Patients with ALS showed a significant impairment of nutrition status according to GLIM criteria. Malnourished ALS patients exhibited declines in body compartments, evidenced by lower muscle mass, lower fat mass, and higher extracellular water. Malnutrition was also associated with worse ALSFRS-R scores. Despite the deterioration of functional status, there were no differences in functional measurements according to malnutrition diagnosis. BIVA values such as PA, SPA, and ECW are useful for detecting malnutrition risk in ALS patients. Future lines of research are needed to test which cut-off points of morphofunctional tools best identify clinical outcomes and survival in ALS.

Author Contributions: Conceptualization, M.T.Z.-M. and M.L.F.-S.; methodology, M.T.Z.-M. and M.L.F.-S.; software, M.T.Z.-M. and C.F.; validation, M.T.Z.-M., M.L.F.-S. and C.F.; formal analysis, M.T.Z.-M. and C.F.; investigation, M.T.Z.-M., M.C.A.-L. and S.L.-M.; resources, M.L.F.-S.; data curation, M.T.Z.-M. and C.F.; writing—original draft preparation, M.T.Z.-M.; writing—review and editing, M.T.Z.-M., M.L.F.-S., C.F. and M.C.A.-L.; visualization, M.T.Z.-M.; supervision, M.L.F.-S.; project administration, M.L.F.-S.; funding acquisition, M.T.Z.-M. All authors have read and agreed to the published version of the manuscript.

Funding: María Teresa Zarco-Martín was funded by a pre-doctoral fellowship from Instituto de Investigación Biosanitaria de Granada (Ibs. Granada) (74-2022).

Institutional Review Board Statement: The study was conducted in accordance with the Declaration of Helsinki, and approved by the Ethics Committee of San Cecilio University Hospital (1770-N-21), approval date: 25 February 2022.

Informed Consent Statement: Informed consent was obtained from all subjects involved in the study.

Data Availability Statement: The data presented in this study will be made available upon request to the corresponding author.

Conflicts of Interest: The authors declare no conflicts of interest.

References

1. Couratier, P.; Corcia, P.; Lautrette, G.; Nicol, M.; Preux, P.M.; Marin, B. Epidemiology of amyotrophic lateral sclerosis: A review of literature. *Rev. Neurol.* **2016**, *172*, 37–45. [CrossRef] [PubMed]
2. Almeida, C.S.; Stanich, P.; Salvioni, C.C.S.; Diccini, S. Assessment and nutrition education in patients with amyotrophic lateral sclerosis. *Arq. Neuropsiquiatr.* **2016**, *74*, 902–908. [CrossRef] [PubMed]
3. Mitchell, J.D.; Borasio, G.D. Amyotrophic lateral sclerosis. *Lancet* **2007**, *369*, 2031–2041. [CrossRef] [PubMed]
4. Chiò, A.; Logroscino, G.; Hardiman, O.; Swingler, R.; Mitchell, D.; Beghi, E.; Traynor, B.G.; Eurals Consortium. Prognostic factors in ALS: A critical review. *Amyotroph. Lateral Scler.* **2009**, *10*, 310–323. [CrossRef] [PubMed]
5. Ferri, A.; Coccurello, R. What is 'Hyper' in the ALS Hypermetabolism? *Mediat. Inflamm.* **2017**, *2017*, 7821672. [CrossRef] [PubMed]
6. Del Olmo García, M.D.; Virgili Casas, N.; Cantón Blanco, A.; Lozano Fuster, F.M.; Wanden-Berghe, C.; Avilés, V.; Ashbaugh Enguídanos, R.; Ferrero López, I.; Molina Soria, J.B.; Montejo González, J.C.; et al. [Nutritional management of amyotrophic lateral sclerosis: Summary of recommendations]. *Nutr. Hosp.* **2018**, *35*, 1243–1251. [CrossRef] [PubMed]
7. Essat, M.; Coates, E.; Clowes, M.; Beever, D.; Hackney, G.; White, S.; Stavroulakis, T.; Halliday, V.; McDermott, C. Understanding the current nutritional management for people with amyotrophic lateral sclerosis—A mapping review. *Clin. Nutr. ESPEN* **2022**, *49*, 328–340. [CrossRef] [PubMed]
8. Burgos, R.; Bretón, I.; Cereda, E.; Desport, J.C.; Dziewas, R.; Genton, L.; Gomes, F.; Jésus, P.; Leischker, A.; Muscaritoli, M.; et al. ESPEN guideline clinical nutrition in neurology. *Clin. Nutr.* **2018**, *37*, 354–396. [CrossRef] [PubMed]
9. Desport, J.C.; Preux, P.M.; Bouteloup-Demange, C.; Clavelou, P.; Beaufrère, B.; Bonnet, C.; Couratier, P.P. Validation of bioelectrical impedance analysis in patients with amyotrophic lateral sclerosis. *Am. J. Clin. Nutr.* **2003**, *77*, 1179–1185. [CrossRef]
10. García Almeida, J.M.; García García, C.; Vegas Aguilar, I.M.; Bellido Castañeda, V.; Bellido Guerrero, D. Morphofunctional assessment of patient's nutritional status: A global approach. *Nutr. Hosp.* **2021**, *38*, 592–600.
11. Rofes, L.; Arreola, V.; Clavé, P. The volume-viscosity swallow test for clinical screening of dysphagia and aspiration. *Nestle Nutr. Inst. Workshop Ser.* **2012**, *72*, 33–42. [PubMed]
12. Santos, L.P.; Gonzalez, M.C.; Orlandi, S.P.; Bielemann, R.M.; Barbosa-Silva, T.G.; Heymsfield, S.B.; COCONUT Study Group. New Prediction Equations to Estimate Appendicular Skeletal Muscle Mass Using Calf Circumference: Results from NHANES 1999–2006. *J. Parenter. Enter. Nutr.* **2019**, *43*, 998–1007. [CrossRef] [PubMed]
13. Piccoli, A.; Rossi, B.; Pillon, L.; Bucciante, G. A new method for monitoring body fluid variation by bioimpedance analysis: The RXc graph. *Kidney Int.* **1994**, *46*, 534–539. [CrossRef] [PubMed]
14. Janssen, I.; Heymsfield, S.B.; Baumgartner, R.N.; Ross, R. Estimation of skeletal muscle mass by bioelectrical impedance analysis. *J. Appl. Physiol.* **2000**, *89*, 465–471. [CrossRef] [PubMed]
15. Kyle, U.G.; Genton, L.; Karsegard, L.; Slosman, D.O.; Pichard, C. Single prediction equation for bioelectrical impedance analysis in adults aged 20–94 years. *Nutrition* **2001**, *17*, 248–253. [CrossRef] [PubMed]
16. Piccoli, A.; Nigrelli, S.; Caberlotto, A.; Bottazzo, S.; Rossi, B.; Pillon, L.; Maggiore, Q. Bivariate normal values of the bioelectrical impedance vector in adult and elderly populations. *Am. J. Clin. Nutr.* **1995**, *61*, 269–270. [CrossRef] [PubMed]
17. Cruz-Jentoft, A.J.; Bahat, G.; Bauer, J.; Boirie, Y.; Bruyère, O.; Cederholm, T.; Cooper, C.; Landi, F.; Rolland, Y.; Sayer, A.A.; et al. Sarcopenia: Revised European consensus on definition and diagnosis. *Age Ageing* **2019**, *48*, 16–31. [CrossRef] [PubMed]
18. Guralnik, J.M.; Simonsick, E.M.; Ferrucci, L.; Glynn, R.J.; Berkman, L.F.; Blazer, D.G.; Scherr, P.A.; Wallace, R.B. A short physical performance battery assessing lower extremity function: Association with self-reported disability and prediction of mortality and nursing home admission. *J. Gerontol.* **1994**, *49*, M85–M94. [CrossRef]
19. Baptista, G.; Barazzoni, R.; Blaauw, R.; Coats, A.; Crivelli, A.; Evans, D.; Gramlich, L.; Fuchs-Tarlovsky, V.; Keller, H.; Llido, L.; et al. GLIM criteria for the diagnosis of malnutrition—A consensus report from the global clinical nutrition community. *Clin. Nutr.* **2019**, *38*, 1–9.
20. Campos, T.S.; Rodríguez-Santos, F.; Esteban, J.; Vázquez, P.C.; Mora Pardina, J.S.; Carmona, A.C. Spanish adaptation of the revised Amyotrophic Lateral Sclerosis Functional Rating Scale (ALSFRS-R). *Amyotroph. Lateral Scler.* **2010**, *11*, 475–477. [CrossRef]
21. Cedarbaum, J.M.; Stambler, N.; Malta, E.; Fuller, C.; Hilt, D.; Thurmond, B.; Nakanishi, A. The ALSFRS-R: A revised ALS functional rating scale that incorporates assessments of respiratory function. BDNF ALS Study Group (Phase III). *J. Neurol. Sci.* **1999**, *169*, 13–21. [CrossRef] [PubMed]
22. Roubeau, V.; Blasco, H.; Maillot, F.; Corcia, P.; Praline, J. Nutritional assessment of amyotrophic lateral sclerosis in routine practice: Value of weighing and bioelectrical impedance analysis. *Muscle Nerve* **2015**, *51*, 479–484. [CrossRef] [PubMed]
23. Salvioni, C.; Oda, A.L.; Orsini, M.; Pauli, M.; Frabasile, L.M.; Alves, P.C.L.; Borges, R.M.; Sierra, H.N.M.; Menegatti, G.; Pinho, M.O.; et al. Association between Body Composition and Dysphagia in Patients with Amyotrophic Lateral Sclerosis. *Neurol. Int.* **2021**, *13*, 315–327. [CrossRef]
24. Salvioni, C.C.D.S.; Stanich, P.; Oliveira, A.S.B.; Orsini, M. Anthropometry of Arm: Nutritional Risk Indicator in Amyotrophic Lateral Sclerosis. *Neurol. Int.* **2015**, *7*, 5952. [CrossRef]
25. López-Gómez, J.J.; Ballesteros-Pomar, M.D.; Torres-Torres, B.; De la Maza, B.P.; Penacho-Lázaro, M.Á.; Palacio-Mures, J.M.; Abreu-Padín, C.; López-Guzmán, A.; De Luis-Román, D.A. Malnutrition at diagnosis in amyotrophic lateral sclerosis (als) and its influence on survival: Using glim criteria. *Clin. Nutr.* **2021**, *40*, 237–244. [CrossRef]

26. Nakamura, R.; Kurihara, M.; Ogawa, N.; Kitamura, A.; Yamakawa, I.; Bamba, S.; Sanada, M.; Sasaki, M.; Urushitani, M. Prognostic prediction by hypermetabolism varies depending on the nutritional status in early amyotrophic lateral sclerosis. *Sci. Rep.* **2021**, *11*, 17943. [CrossRef]
27. Barone, M.; Leo, A.D.; de van der Schueren, M.A.E. Malnutrition assessment by Global Leadership Initiative on Malnutrition criteria in patients with amyotrophic lateral sclerosis. *Nutrition* **2023**, *109*, 111997. [CrossRef] [PubMed]
28. Kasarskis, E.J.; Berryman, S.; English, T.; Nyland, J.; Vanderleest, J.G.; Schneider, A.; Berger, R.; McClain, C. The use of upper extremity anthropometrics in the clinical assessment of patients with amyotrophic lateral sclerosis. *Muscle Nerve* **1997**, *20*, 330–335. [CrossRef]
29. Li, J.Y.; Sun, X.H.; Cai, Z.Y.; Shen, D.C.; Yang, X.Z.; Liu, M.S.; Cui, L.Y. Correlation of weight and body composition with disease progression rate in patients with amyotrophic lateral sclerosis. *Sci. Rep.* **2022**, *12*, 13292. [CrossRef]
30. Choi, S.J.; Yoon, S.H.; Sung, J.J.; Lee, J.H. Association Between Fat Depletion and Prognosis of Amyotrophic Lateral Sclerosis: CT-Based Body Composition Analysis. *Ann. Neurol.* **2023**, *94*, 1116–1125. [CrossRef]
31. Lukaski, H.C.; Kyle, U.G.; Kondrup, J. Assessment of adult malnutrition and prognosis with bioelectrical impedance analysis: Phase angle and impedance ratio. *Curr. Opin. Clin. Nutr. Metab. Care* **2017**, *20*, 330–339. [CrossRef]
32. Dorst, J.; Weydt, P.; Brenner, D.; Witzel, S.; Kandler, K.; Huss, A.; Herrmann, C.; Wiesenfarth, M.; Knehr, A.; Günther, K.; et al. Metabolic alterations precede neurofilament changes in presymptomatic ALS gene carriers. *eBioMedicine* **2023**, *90*, 104521. [CrossRef] [PubMed]
33. Lukaski, H.C.; Talluri, A. Phase angle as an index of physiological status: Validating bioelectrical assessments of hydration and cell mass in health and disease. *Rev. Endocr. Metab. Disord.* **2023**, *24*, 371–379. [CrossRef]
34. López-Gómez, J.J.; Izaola-Jauregui, O.; Almansa-Ruiz, L.; Jiménez-Sahagún, R.; Primo-Martín, D.; Pedraza-Hueso, M.I.; Ramos-Bachiller, B.; González-Gutiérrez, J.; De Luis-Román, D. Use of Muscle Ultrasonography in Morphofunctional Assessment of Amyotrophic Lateral Sclerosis (ALS). *Nutrients* **2024**, *16*, 1021. [CrossRef]
35. Desport, J.C.; Marin, B.; Funalot, B.; Preux, P.M.; Couratier, P. Phase angle is a prognostic factor for survival in amyotrophic lateral sclerosis. *Amyotroph. Lateral Scler.* **2008**, *9*, 273–278. [CrossRef]
36. Barone, M.; Viggiani, M.T.; Introna, A.; D'errico, E.; Scarafino, A.; Iannone, A.; Di Leo, A.; Simone, I.L. Nutritional prognostic factors for survival in amyotrophic lateral sclerosis patients undergone percutaneous endoscopic gastrostomy placement. *Amyotroph. Lateral Scler. Front. Degener.* **2019**, *20*, 490–496. [CrossRef] [PubMed]
37. García-Almeida, J.M.; García-García, C.; Vegas-Aguilar, I.M.; Ballesteros Pomar, M.D.; Cornejo-Pareja, I.M.; Fernández Medina, B.; de Luis Román, D.A.; Bellido Guerrero, D.; Bretón Lesmes, I.; Tinahones Madueño, F.J. Nutritional ultrasound®: Conceptualisation, technical considerations and standardisation. *Endocrinol. Diabetes Nutr.* **2023**, *70* (Suppl. 1), 74–84. [CrossRef]
38. Kawakami, W.; Umehara, T.; Iwamoto, Y.; Takahashi, M.; Katayama, N. Phase Angle Is Associated with Handgrip Strength in Older Patients with Heart Failure. *Ann. Rehabil. Med.* **2023**, *47*, 129–137. [CrossRef]
39. Miller, R.G.; Mitchell, J.D.; Moore, D.H. Riluzole for amyotrophic lateral sclerosis (ALS)/motor neuron disease (MND). *Cochrane Database Syst. Rev.* **2012**, *2012*, CD001447. [CrossRef]
40. Kato, N.; Hashida, G.; Kobayashi, M.; Konaka, K. Physical therapy improves lower limb muscle strength but not function in individuals with amyotrophic lateral sclerosis: A case series study. *Ann. Phys. Rehabil. Med.* **2018**, *61*, 108–110. [CrossRef]
41. Victoria-Montesinos, D.; García-Muñoz, A.M.; Navarro-Marroco, J.; Lucas-Abellán, C.; Mercader-Ros, M.T.; Serrano-Martínez, A.; Abellán-Aynés, O.; Barcina-Pérez, P.; Hernández-Sánchez, P. Phase Angle, Handgrip Strength, and Other Indicators of Nutritional Status in Cancer Patients Undergoing Different Nutritional Strategies: A Systematic Review and Meta-Analysis. *Nutrients* **2023**, *15*, 1790. [CrossRef]
42. Pavasini, R.; Guralnik, J.; Brown, J.C.; Di Bari, M.; Cesari, M.; Landi, F.; Vaes, B.; Legrand, D.; Verghese, J.; Wang, C.; et al. Short Physical Performance Battery and all-cause mortality: Systematic review and meta-analysis. *BMC Med.* **2016**, *14*, 215. [CrossRef]
43. Montes, J.; Cheng, B.; Diamond, B.; Doorish, C.; Mitsumoto, H.; Gordon, P.H. The Timed Up and Go test: Predicting falls in ALS. *Amyotroph. Lateral Scler.* **2007**, *8*, 292–295. [CrossRef] [PubMed]

nutrients MDPI

Systematic Review

Practical Guidelines by the Andalusian Group for Nutrition Reflection and Investigation (GARIN) on Nutritional Management of Patients with Chronic Obstructive Pulmonary Disease: A Review

Alicia Justel Enríquez [1], Juana M. Rabat-Restrepo [2,3,*], Francisco J. Vilchez-López [4], Carmen Tenorio-Jiménez [5], José M. García-Almeida [6,7], José-Antonio Irles Rocamora [3,8], José L. Pereira-Cunill [3,9,10], María J. Martínez Ramírez [11,12], María J. Molina-Puerta [13,14], Juan B. Molina Soria [15], María I. Rebollo-Pérez [16], Gabriel Olveira [7,17,18,19,*] and Pedro P. García-Luna [3,9,10]

1 Servicio de Endocrinología y Nutrición, Hospital Universitario de la Princesa, 28006 Madrid, Spain
2 Servicio de Endocrinología y Nutrición, Hospital Universitario Virgen Macarena, 41009 Sevilla, Spain
3 Departamento de Medicina, Facultad de Medicina, Universidad de Sevilla, 41009 Sevilla, Spain; irles@us.es (J.-A.I.R.); garcialunapp@yahoo.es (P.P.G.-L.)
4 Servicio de Endocrinología y Nutrición, Hospital Puerta del Mar, 11009 Cádiz, Spain
5 Endocrinology and Nutrition Clinical Management Unit, University Hospital Virgen de las Nieves, 18014 Granada, Spain
6 Unidad de Gestión Clínica de Endocrinología y Nutrición, Hospital Universitario Virgen de la Victoria, 29010 Málaga, Spain
7 Instituto de Investigación Biomédica de Málaga/Plataforma Bionand, 29010 Málaga, Spain
8 UGC Endocrinología y Nutrición, Hospital Universitario Valme, 41014 Sevilla, Spain
9 Unidad de Gestión Clínica de Endocrinología y Nutrición, Hospital Universitario Virgen del Rocío, 41013 Sevilla, Spain
10 Endocrine Diseases Research Group, Institute of Biomedicine of Seville (IBIS), 41007 Sevilla, Spain
11 Servicio de Endocrinología y Nutrición, Complejo Hospitalario de Jaén, 23007 Jaén, Spain
12 Facultad de Medicina, Universidad de Jaén, 23071 Jaén, Spain
13 UGC Endocrinología y Nutrición, Hospital Universitario Reina Sofía, 14004 Córdoba, Spain
14 Instituto Maimónides de Investigación Biomédica de Córdoba (IMIBIC), 14004 Córdoba, Spain
15 Unidad de Nutrición y Dietética, Hospital General, 23700 Linares, Spain
16 Servicio de Endocrinología y Nutrición, Hospital Juan Ramón Jiménez, 21005 Huelva, Spain
17 Unidad de Gestión Clínica de Endocrinología y Nutrición, Hospital Regional Universitario de Málaga, 29010 Málaga, Spain
18 Centro de Investigación Biomédica en Red de Diabetes y Enfermedades Metabólicas Asociadas (CIBERDEM), Instituto de Salud Carlos III, 28029 Madrid, Spain
19 Departamento de Medicina y Dermatología, Facultad de Medicina, Universidad de Málaga, 29010 Málaga, Spain
* Correspondence: juanamariarabat@gmail.com (J.M.R.-R.); gabrielm.olveira.sspa@juntadeandalucia.es (G.O.); Tel.: +34-954-45-4493 (J.M.R.-R.); +34-951-29-0343 (G.O.)

Abstract: Malnutrition is common in chronic obstructive pulmonary disease (COPD) patients and is associated with worse lung function and greater severity. This review by the Andalusian Group for Nutrition Reflection and Investigation (GARIN) addresses the nutritional management of adult COPD patients, focusing on Morphofunctional Nutritional Assessment and intervention in clinical practice. A systematic literature search was performed using the Preferred Reporting Items for Systematic Reviews and Meta-Analyses (PRISMA) methodology, followed by critical appraisal based on Scottish Intercollegiate Guidelines Network (SIGN) guidelines. Recommendations were graded according to the European Society for Clinical Nutrition and Metabolism (ESPEN) system. The results were discussed among GARIN members, with consensus determined using a Likert scale. A total of 24 recommendations were made: 2(A), 6(B), 2(O), and 14(GPP). Consensus exceeded 90% for 17 recommendations and was 75–90% for 7. The care of COPD patients is approached from a nutritional perspective, emphasizing nutritional screening, morphofunctional assessment, and food intake in early disease stages. Nutritional interventions include dietary advice, recommendations on food group intake, and the impact of specialized nutritional treatment, particularly oral nutritional supplements. Other critical aspects, such as physical activity and quality of life, are also analyzed. These recommendations provide practical guidance for managing COPD patients nutritionally in clinical practice.

Keywords: chronic obstructive pulmonary disease; nutrition; diet; enteral nutrition

1. Introduction

Chronic obstructive pulmonary disease (COPD) is the third leading cause of death worldwide, amounting to 3 million in 2016 [1]. It is also associated with morbidity and disability [2,3] and usually presents with other associated comorbidities, including malnutrition [4–7].

The prevalence of malnutrition in these patients is estimated to be between 20 and 45%, depending on the series and the different methods used [5–7], and is often underdiagnosed. The cost of malnutrition in patients with COPD includes an increase in the use of resources, such as a greater number of hospitalizations, longer hospital stays, an increase in emergency department visits, as well as higher medical, pharmacy, and home oxygen therapy expenses. This ultimately translates into a higher expenditure per patient and year, as demonstrated by numerous studies [8–10].

Nutritional care in this pathology is of vital importance in the overall results of the treatment, but even more so in the aspects related to the patient's quality of life throughout their entire disease process [11–18]. However, in most of the clinical practice guidelines (CPG) or reviews of more consolidated organizations [19–25], although they are updated year after year, the nutritional and dietary contents are scarce and do not provide a response tailored to the nutritional needs of these patients.

The objective of this review, therefore, is to respond to relevant questions that arise regarding the nutritional management of adult patients with COPD in terms of Morphofunctional Nutritional Assessment and intervention in routine clinical practice. These recommendations are specifically aimed at doctors, nurses, and dieticians involved in the care of these patients.

2. Methodology

The Andalusian Group for Nutrition Reflection and Investigation (GARIN) recommendations have been developed by a group of physicians specializing in endocrinology and nutrition with recognized expertise in clinical nutrition. Initially, the members of GARIN proposed a series of relevant issues in the clinical practice and nutritional management of patients with COPD. From these, the questions based on patient characteristics, Nutritional Screening and Morphofuntional Assessment, type of intervention, control, and outcome (PICO) were formulated to address the most individualized nutritional therapy according to the clinical characteristics of the patients and their level of risk or complexity. Finally, 24 recommendations were made in response to the PICO questions: 2(A), 6(B), 2(0), and 14(GPP). Of these,17 recommendations reached a consensus above 90% (indicating a strong consensus), and 7 obtained a consensus between ≥75–90%.

To answer the PICO questions, a literature search was conducted in PUBMED and SCOPUS, filtered by systematic reviews, review articles, meta-analyses, and randomized clinical trials (RCTs) from the last 10 years, limited to adult subjects and published in English or Spanish. The keywords were 'COPD' or 'chronic obstructive pulmonary disease' and 'nutrition'. A total of 361 results were obtained, and after eliminating duplicates, articles that did not meet the search criteria, and non-relevant articles, 114 articles were included. Figure 1 specifies the process according to the PRISMA (Preferred Reporting Items for Systematic Reviews and Meta-Analyses) methodology [26]. The critical appraisal of each article was carried out following the SIGN (Scottish Intercollegiate Guidelines Network) methodology [27], and articles were classified according to the checklist for each type of article (Table 1). The articles were reviewed by two independent reviewers (AJE and JMRR). In the case of doubt or discrepancy between reviewers, a third reviewer (MIRP) was consulted.

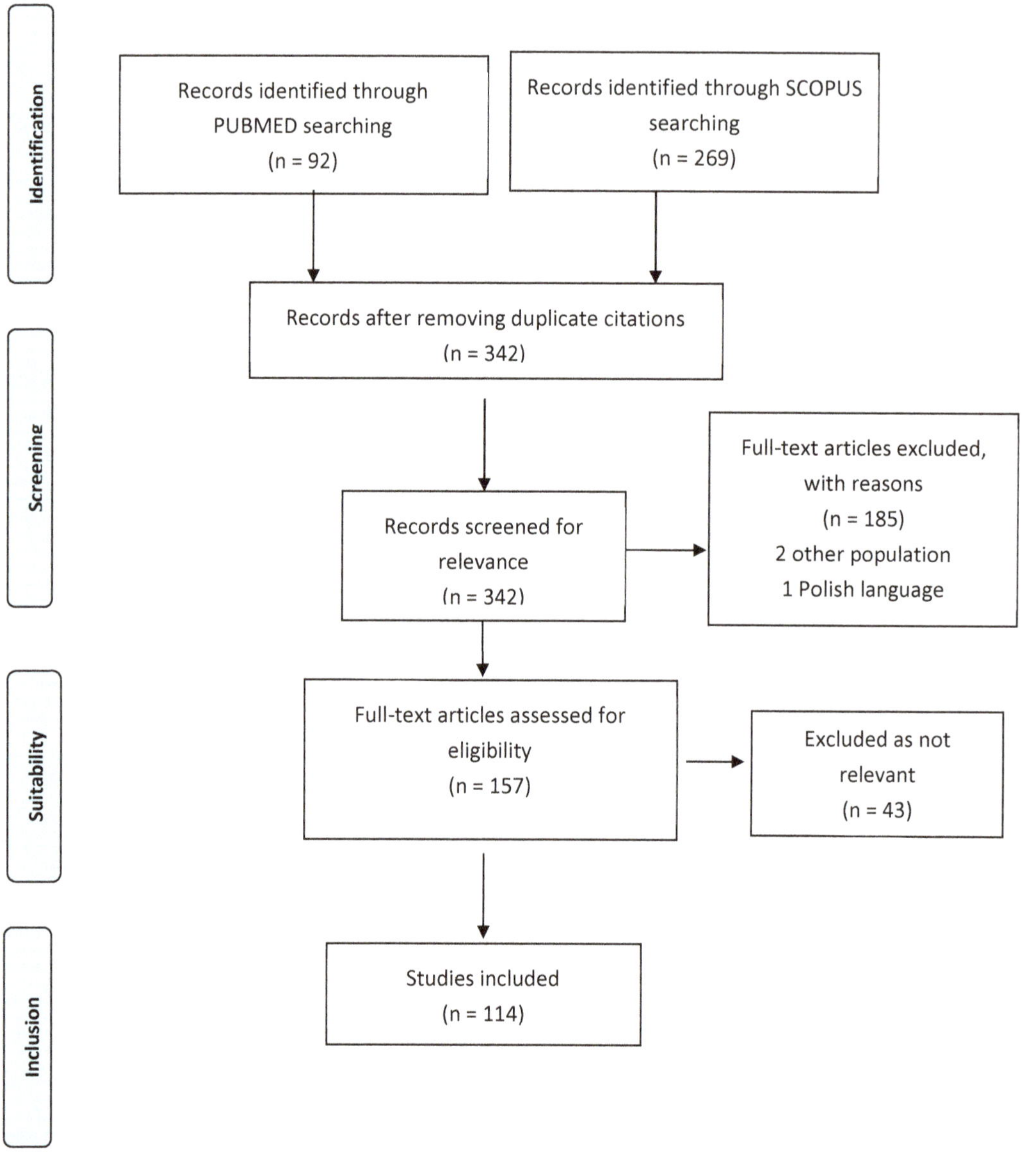

Figure 1. Flowchart following the PRISMA methodology.

Table 1. Levels of evidence (LE) [27].

1++	High-quality meta-analyses, systematic reviews of RCTs, or RCTs with a very low risk of bias
1+	Meta-analyses, systematic reviews of well-conducted RCTs, or RCTs with low risk of bias
1−	Meta-analyses, systematic reviews of well-conducted RCTs, or RCTs at high risk of bias
2++	High-quality systematic reviews of case-control studies; cohort or case-control studies with a low risk of confounding, bias, or chance and a high probability that the relationship is causal
2+	Well-conducted case-control or cohort studies with a low risk of confounding, bias, or chance and a moderate probability that the relationship is causal
2−	Case-control or cohort studies with a high risk of confounding, bias, or chance and a significant risk that the relationship is causal
3	Non-analytical studies, such as case reports and case series
4	Expert opinion

Finally, the draft article was circulated among all members until the final version was completed.

The wording of the recommendations reflects the degrees of evidence (Table 2) [28]; level A is indicated by the word 'Recommend', level B by the word 'Suggest', level 0 by the word 'Advise', and low quality of evidence by 'It is currently not possible to make recommendations'. The 'GPP' recommendations are based on expert opinion because of a lack of studies; in these cases, the drafting was performed by group consensus. The first draft of the document was handed over to the GARIN members in July 2022, and once the document was revised, taking into account the comments and suggestions made by the group, it was sent for online voting in September 2022, applying a Likert scale of 1–5 (Table 3) [29]. The level of consensus for each recommendation was calculated by adding the total value resulting from the responses obtained, dividing it by the maximum value, and then multiplying by 100. Finally, the draft article was circulated among all members until the final version was completed.

Table 2. Grades of recommendation [28].

A	At least one meta-analysis, systematic review, or RCT rated 1++ and directly applicable to the target population; or A body of evidence consisting primarily of studies rated 1+, directly applicable to the target population, and demonstrating the overall consistency of the results
B	A body of evidence that includes studies rated as 2++, directly applicable to the target population; or a body of evidence that includes studies rated as 2+, directly applicable to the target population and demonstrating overall consistency of results; or extrapolated evidence from studies rated 1++ or 1+
O	Level of evidence 3 or 4; or extrapolated evidence from studies rated 2++ or 2+
GPP	Good Practice Point/Expert Consensus: Recommended best practice based on the clinical experience of the expert panel

Table 3. Likert scale [29].

1	Strongly disagree
2	Disagree
3	Neither agree nor disagree
4	Agree
5	Strongly agree

3. Results and Discussion

Four questions were discarded because, in this review, sufficient evidence has not been found to make recommendations in this regard: two on energy requirements, one on the ideal proportion of macronutrients in the diet, and another on the specific use of nutritional supplements. Finally, 24 recommendations were made in response to the PICO questions: 2(A), 6(B), 2(0), and 14(GPP). Of these, 17 recommendations reached a consensus above 90% (indicating a strong consensus), and 7 obtained a consensus between ≥75–90%.

3.1. General

3.1.1. Should Food Intake Be Assessed?

Recommendation 1. *In patients with advanced COPD (GOLD 3 and 4: E), GARIN suggests routinely evaluating daily food intake at all levels of care, integrating dietary advice early that includes increasing the number of meals per day, with a focus on energy-rich foods and proteins, to help improve nutritional status and quality of life.*

Grade of recommendation GPP, (96%) Strong consensus.

Comment:

Decreased food intake is considered one of the main causes of malnutrition in COPD patients [16,30,31]. Malnourished patients have lower intakes and eat fewer meals per day compared with well-nourished patients [12,15,16]. Insufficient intake has been observed during periods of hospitalization [12], especially during exacerbations [32]. Food intake decreases in more advanced stages of COPD [30].

An energy and protein intake below 75% of requirements was considered a predictor of adverse events, and conversely, those patients with higher intakes had a trend of lower mortality risk [12].

Intake has been related to fat-free mass index (FFMI); in the Norden study [33], patients with low FFMI levels, regardless of severity, had a higher symptom burden affecting intake.

3.1.2. When Should COPD Patients' Weight Loss Be Assessed?

Recommendation 2. *GARIN suggests assessing weight loss in all COPD patients from diagnosis and at each visit.*

Grade of recommendation B, (100%) Strong consensus.

Comment:

In COPD patients, progressive weight loss occurs even with adequate caloric intake, possibly conditioned by several circumstances, such as increased work of breathing, a state of systemic inflammation and sustained oxidative stress, acute exacerbations, and infectious complications [11,14,15,30,33].

In COPD, weight loss appears as a dynamic state that accelerates as the disease progresses [17] and is associated with increased morbidity and mortality [8,9,30,34–36]. Increased mortality has been reported in patients with weight loss of >5% in the previous 6 months [15], and weight gain of 2 kg has been found to be associated with improvements in muscle and respiratory strength [32].

In the JO study [8], COPD-related healthcare utilization and medical costs were higher among underweight patients than in the other groups.

3.1.3. Is It Possible to Establish a BMI Range for COPD Patients?

Recommendation 3. *GARIN suggests maintaining a body mass index (BMI) above 21 kg/m^2 and below 30 kg/m^2.*

Grade of recommendation B, (90%) Consensus.

Comment:

In many studies, BMI correlates positively with lung function [8,13,14,35,37,38] and negatively with exacerbations [38]. Patients with a BMI above 22 kg/m^2 have been found to have a better prognosis and fewer exacerbations. Possible reasons include better nutrient intake, better nutritional and muscle status, and less inflammation. In some studies, overweight or obese patients even had better lung function, fewer exacerbations, and less inflammation than those with a BMI of less than 21 kg/m^2 [8,38,39].

Low BMI has been associated with an increased risk of hospital admissions and long-term hospital stays [7] and is considered an independent risk factor for mortality in patients with COPD [7,8,30,34,35]. In the study by WU [38], overweight and obesity were associated with lower mortality rates compared with normal weight among smokers with COPD, but this association was not present among non-smokers with COPD. This could be explained by physiological differences between smoking-associated COPD and COPD in non-smokers [38]. Smoking is a risk factor for COPD and is associated with weight loss and other pathologies that increase the risk of mortality. It is a known central anorectic agent and also conditions the appearance of other cofactors that may influence weight loss [40]. Early implementation of smoking cessation measures can help slow the progression of the disease and reduce the risk of cardiovascular disease and mortality [41,42].

BMI is one of the determining factors of bone mineral density, and the effect of body weight seems to be influenced by both fat mass and lean mass. In addition to a low BMI, patients with COPD often present sarcopenia or low FFMI, and this association is mediated not only by mechanisms such as decreased skeletal load but also by hormonal and other specific factors such as systemic inflammation, vitamin D deficiency, and the use of oral or inhaled corticosteroids [43,44]. A relationship has been found between decreased bone mineral density and low BMI, with significantly high values as BMI and FFMI increase [45].

Despite this, the relationship between obesity and COPD is unclear, and it is difficult to establish whether obesity actually has a detrimental impact on COPD patients. The prevalence of obesity in COPD patients is estimated to range from 10% to 50% [46,47]. Some studies have reported worse respiratory symptoms, increased severe exacerbations, increased comorbidities, worse prognosis, greater restriction of daily activities, worse health-related quality of life, and more use of medical care in obese COPD patients [48,49].

It is clear that the exclusive assessment of BMI does not provide sufficient data to clarify the association of BMI with COPD. Assessing changes in body composition and muscle quality is mandatory. It is also essential for future research to explore the relevance of different phenotypes [15,50,51], taking into account different types of obesity, different symptoms (emphysematous, chronic bronchitis, or both), groups of smokers and non-smokers, and other relevant factors [51].

3.1.4. Should Body Composition Be Assessed in the COPD Patient and When Should It Be Done?

Recommendation 4. *GARIN suggests measuring muscle mass and function, both at diagnosis and at follow-up.*

Grade of recommendation B, (92%) Strong consensus.

Comment:

COPD is characterized by altered body composition, especially increased fat mass and decreased muscle mass [52]. Its influence on disease severity and prognosis has been described in numerous studies [12,14,35,53]. Because it is directly associated with lung function, its loss intensifies as disease severity increases. Morbidity, hospitalization rate, increased readmissions and hospital stay, and the need for ventilatory support are also increased in patients with significant muscle wasting [7,14,22,35,54,55].

Muscle mass is directly related to mortality; for some authors, FFMI is an independent predictor of mortality [7,33,56] and is suggested as a systemic marker of disease severity in COPD staging [35,56].

3.2. *Nutritional Screening and Morphofuntional Assessment*

3.2.1. In Which Patients under Follow-Up for COPD Should Nutritional Screening Be Performed?

Recommendation 5. *GARIN suggests performing nutritional screening in all patients diagnosed with COPD, regardless of the degree of severity and stage of the disease.*

Grade of recommendation GPP, (98%) Strong consensus.

Comment:

Extrapulmonary manifestations in COPD patients due to their chronic inflammatory state, including nutritional status, body composition, and changes in muscle mass, fat mass, and bone mineral density, have been shown to be determinants in the prognosis and severity of the disease, so nutritional screening is recommended for all patients diagnosed with COPD [11,15,35,57–60].

3.2.2. What Nutritional Screening Tool Should Be Used?

Recommendation 6. *GARIN advises the use of any validated screening tool, as there is no specific tool for detecting malnutrition in patients diagnosed with COPD.*

Grade of recommendation O, (98%) Strong consensus.

Comment:

It is essential to determine weight change as a percentage since increased mortality has been reported in patients with weight loss of >5% in the previous 6 months [15].

Validated nutritional screening tools most commonly used in studies of COPD patients include the Mini-Nutritional Assessment (MNA) [15,57,61,62] and MNA-SF [63], Geriatric Nutritional Risk Index (GNRI) in patients >65 years [64], Nutritional Risk Screening (NRS 2002) [35,60,65,66], Malnutrition Universal Screening Tool (MUST) [15], and Icelandic Screening Tool (ISS) [35].

The MNA questionnaire has been widely used in elderly patients for detecting those patients at risk of malnutrition even before weight changes occur, and has been found to be a predictive marker of mortality and hospital costs [62].

An association has been demonstrated with the number of exacerbations and the MNA-SF questionnaire, as well as with other pulmonary assessment parameters, including %FEV1 (forced expiratory volume in 1 s), %VC (vital capacity), %RV (residual volume), %DLCO (diffusing capacity for carbon monoxide) [63].

An association has been found between a low GNRI and a decreased 6 min walk distance (6MWD) value in COPD patients.

A decrease in weight and BMI has been described in those patients with a higher nutritional risk as measured by the NRS 2002 scale, together with worse lung function and lower exercise capacity [60], higher one-year mortality, and higher hospital readmissions (cut-off point < 3 points) [65].

Albumin level (within automated nutritional risk screening) is a good inflammatory marker associated with increased in-hospital mortality (cut-off point < 30.5 g/L) and increased risk of readmission (cut-off point < 30.1 g/L) [65].

3.2.3. How to Establish the Degree of Malnutrition after Screening?

Recommendation 7. *The patient's degree of malnutrition should be previously established according to the latest ESPEN recommendations using the GLIM or SGA criteria (see Appendix A).*

Grade of recommendation A, (98%) Strong consensus.

Comment:

There are many studies in this field that use the Subjective Global Assessment (SGA) for the diagnosis of malnutrition [58,67–72].

GARIN members recommend nutritional diagnosis according to the latest ESPEN consensus guidelines [72], currently the GLIM or SGA criteria [11,35].

Based on the GLIM criteria, the diagnosis of malnutrition is reached when at least one phenotypic criterion (weight loss, age-related BMI, or Fat-Free Mass Index (FFMI)) coexists with another etiological criterion (reduction in intake/nutrient absorption or presence of inflammation/disease). The assessment of muscle mass becomes one of the phenotypic criteria in the diagnosis of malnutrition and the classification of its severity.

The SGA scale is made up of several items that provide a score to predict the patient's nutritional status.

3.2.4. Is It Necessary to Screen for Sarcopenia in These Patients?

Recommendation 8. *GARIN suggests screening for sarcopenia in all patients diagnosed with COPD.*

Grade of recommendation GPP, (98%) Strong consensus.

Comment:

It has been shown that patients with low lung function, even healthy patients without COPD, are associated with decreased muscle mass [73].

The coexistence of COPD/asthma and sarcopenia in the elderly is common, and studies show a prevalence of around 15–25% [11,74]. These associations have been shown to further increase quality of life impairment and reduce the physical capacity for exercise [74].

Further, patients with pulmonary pathology and a higher degree of sarcopenia are associated with a higher percentage of osteoporosis, especially asthma–COPD overlap syndrome [75].

Patients with a low exercise capacity (6MWD < 350 m) and those with a decrease in physical activity (<7128 steps/day) are associated with an increase in exacerbations, a poorer quality of life, higher scores on depression scales, and decreased anthropometric and laboratory parameters related to disease prognosis and mortality [57].

Finally, a statistically significant relationship between the presence of sarcopenia and non-alcoholic fatty liver disease (NAFLD) (highly prevalent in COPD patients) has been determined after multivariate analysis, excluding other risk factors [76], as well as between sarcopenia and the presence of metabolic syndrome, mainly in men with a restrictive pulmonary pattern [77].

The members of GARIN, therefore, propose that, although no literature references have been found in the search, the use of new tools, such as the SARC-F, could be very useful in screening these patients for sarcopenia.

3.2.5. Which Tool Should We Use for the Diagnosis of Sarcopenia?

Recommendation 9. *GARIN suggests making the diagnosis of sarcopenia according to the criteria included in the consensus algorithm established by the European Working Group on Sarcopenia in Older People (EWGSOP2)* [78] *(see Appendix B).*

Grade of recommendation GPP, (92%) Strong consensus.

Comment:

Among the different studies published, the most widely used and validated diagnostic method for determining sarcopenia in this group of patients is the EWGSOP2 algorithm criteria [11,74,79].

According to the EWGSOP2 guideline, the diagnosis of sarcopenia requires a decrease in muscle strength and mass associated with a lack of exercise resistance. Therefore, to establish it, it is necessary to assess muscle strength, mass, and functionality.

3.2.6. How Should Muscle Function Be Assessed?

Recommendation 10. *GARIN suggests the use of tests for the assessment of physical activity and exercise capacity, as they are useful for determining muscle function in COPD patients and offer reliable and comparable measurements over time and between individuals.*

Grade of recommendation GPP, (90%) Consensus.

Comment:

Within the COPD patient population, validated tests for the assessment of physical activity include 4 m gait speed (4MGS), 6MWD, and objective measurements of daily physical activity using pedometers or other devices [11,57,59,64]. Several studies have determined a low limit of less than 0.8 m/s for 4MGS [11].

Two-minute walking distance (2MWD) has also been assessed to detect frailer patients who show an increased risk of 18-month mortality, increased risk of dependency, higher rates of malnutrition, increased dyspnoea, and poorer quality of life test scores [80]. A clear correlation has been described between this and BMI, FEV1, the Medical Research Council dyspnoea score (mMRC), and 6MWD, with a cut-off point of $\leq$80 m.

Grip strength through dynamometry [11,37,74,79,81] has shown a positive correlation with muscle mass, lung function measured by spirometry, and the 6MWD test. A negative correlation between mMRC and morbidity and mortality has also been found [81].

Due to its wide use and ease of use, we especially recommend 6MWD and hand dynamometry.

3.2.7. How to Assess Muscle Mass?

Recommendation 11. *GARIN suggests assessing muscle mass using any of the following techniques depending on the availability and feasibility of each medical equipment.*

Grade of recommendation GPP, (82%) Consensus.

Depending on the techniques available, we can carry out a basic, intermediate, or advanced study of the patient's muscle mass at both diagnosis and follow-up (Table 4).

Table 4. Muscle mass assessment techniques according to the degree of complexity and availability.

	Level of Study
Dual-energy X-ray absorptiometry (DEXA)	***
Magnetic resonance imaging (MRI)	**
Computed tomography (CT)	**
Muscle ultrasound	**
Bioelectric impedance analysis	**
Anthropometry	*

*** Advanced; ** Intermediate; * Basic.

Comment:

The gold standard for the assessment of bone mineral density and body composition is DEXA [15,57,59]. However, there are many studies in which bioelectric impedance analysis has been used, with a good correlation between fat-free mass and physical capacity, as well as a more severe staging of the disease, hospitalization for >7 days, and increased mortality at 6–9 months [11,15,35,79]. A decrease in fat-free mass of <15 kg/m^2 in women and 16/17 kg/m^2 in men or <10th percentile has been associated with increased mortality and morbidity [15,35,58].

Different studies have defined low muscle mass with cut-off points of skeletal muscle mass index (SMI) of $\leq$8.50 kg/m^2 in men and $\leq$5.75 kg/m^2 in women [11]. A significant reduction in phase angle has also been described, especially in patients with sarcopenia [11]. In addition to these two techniques, the assessment of muscle mass has been evaluated in various studies using CT, MRI, and muscle ultrasound [79]. A relationship between decreased fat-free mass/lean mass index and increased disease severity and increased mortality has been reported. Thus, it has been reported in cross-sectional and retrospective studies that the pectoralis major muscle, assessed through CT (in terms of area and density), is associated with various body composition, respiratory, and prognostic variables in COPD. However, further research is required to standardize its use in clinical practice [82–84].

Measurements of the anterior rectus femoris muscle (anteroposterior axis, area, etc.) at different levels (e.g., between the lateral epicondyle and the greater trochanter of the femur) have been performed by ultrasound, showing a significant correlation with the grip strength measured by dynamometry and the fat-free muscle mass by bioelectric impedance analysis [79].

In terms of anthropometry, the most commonly used indices are brachial circumference and calf circumference measured in cm (pathological < 31 cm) [74].

These techniques should always be performed by qualified professionals. In centers without experience in more complex techniques or in those where they are not available, anthropometric measurements such as circumferences and bioimpedance, if accessible, are recommended, in addition to collecting raw bioelectric data.

3.3. Nutritional Requirements

3.3.1. How to Measure Energy Requirements in Adult COPD Patients?

Recommendation 12. *In well-nourished and stable patients, GARIN advises the use of the following:*
WHO or Harris–Benedict Equation × Activity Factor (AF);
Adjusted weight if BMI > 30.
In advanced-stage malnourished patients (GOLD 3 or GOLD 4: E):
Harris–Benedict Equation × FA × Disease Factor (DF) (1.3).
Grade of recommendation GPP, (94%) Strong consensus.

Comment:

Several studies estimate an increase in basal energy expenditure (BEE) of 15–26% above the requirements of healthy individuals [59,85–88]. This increased metabolism has been associated with reduced food intake, weight loss, and muscle wasting and is considered an independent predictor of morbidity and mortality [85].

Although indirect calorimetry (IC) is the recommended method, when it is not available, predictive equations are a good option.

Research that has compared different predictive equations with IC or the doubly labeled water (DWL) method has found that they overestimate or underestimate the REE. Thus, most of those studies recommend the Harris–Benedict and WHO equations as the ones that have best matched the values of the reference method used [59,86]. Rao [86] compared the resting energy expenditure (REE) measured by IC and the Harris–Benedict equation in mechanically ventilated patients. The IC-measured REE was approximately 45.0% higher (49.1% in males; 36.8% in females). In this study, the REE, according to the

Harris–Benedict equation multiplied by 1.5 in men and by 1.4 in women, was close to the values obtained by IC.

GARIN members reaffirm their interest in deepening the morphofunctional assessment of COPD patients and the possibility that, in the future, predictive equations may incorporate body composition data to allow a better adjustment of energy intake in these patients' diets [88–90].

3.3.2. What Are the Protein Requirements of the COPD Patient?

Recommendation 13. *GARIN suggests an intake of 1 g protein/kg body weight/day in stable patients and 1.2–1.5 g/kg for malnourished patients in advanced stages and during exacerbations.*

Grade of recommendation B, (96%) Strong consensus.

Comment:

There is very limited evidence on specific protein requirements in COPD patients. The study by Kao [85] described, using the isotope tracer technique, an increase in protein metabolism that correlated with REE in COPD patients. Protein catabolism was not significantly different between COPD subjects and controls. On the other hand, Jonker et al. [90] found that threshold and anabolic capacity are preserved in clinically and weight-stable COPD patients and, therefore, suggest that there is no disease-related anabolic resistance and/or increased protein requirements [90]. Results obtained from studies on protein metabolism in vivo are inconclusive, and other studies report an increase in both synthesis and catabolism, suggesting an overall increase in protein metabolism compared with healthy subjects, in which the lower leucine concentrations were associated with low FFM in the COPD group [91].

On the other hand, there is some evidence in the reviewed literature on the benefits achieved in terms of increased muscle mass and strength in those patients who consume more protein [14,92–94].

Although the current study has not found any specific recommendations for COPD patients, the members of GARIN, based on the literature reviewed, consider it important to advocate a higher protein intake in the diet of these patients.

3.3.3. What Is the Ideal Macronutrient Ratio in This Patient Group?

There is insufficient evidence to make recommendations.

Comment:

There is limited evidence on the impact of macronutrient distribution on the clinical course of the disease, and there are insufficient metabolic studies to provide an estimate of the ideal percentage distribution of carbohydrates, lipids, and proteins in the COPD patient. A respiratory quotient (RQ) of <1.0 is desirable in these patients, as the patient will exhale less carbon dioxide. However, this review has not found studies that evaluate carbohydrate and fat oxidation separately in COPD patients, and this is critical to understanding the energy metabolism of these individuals. Information on the oxidation of nutritional substrates in this specific population is lacking. In the search conducted, few studies have addressed this issue [14,85,87,90,95].

3.4. Nutritional Management

3.4.1. What Type of Diet Would Be Indicated?

Recommendation 14. *The diet recommendations given by the members of GARIN are shown in Table 5.*

Table 5. The diet recommended by GARIN.

- In stable patients, a varied, healthy and balanced diet, such as the Mediterranean dietary pattern, as in the general population.
- Do not decrease caloric intake to achieve less work of breathing because of the risk of malnutrition associated with a BMI below 21 kg/m^2.
- Eat fish 2–3 times a week.
- Split the intake into several meals (5–6 meals/day) in case of advanced COPD GOLD 3 or 4 and during exacerbations.
- Educate patients on healthy fat choices with a decrease in industrial saturated and trans fats.
- Eat a diet high in fruit and vegetables because of their high antioxidant and fiber content (five servings per day).
- Decrease intake of processed meats and carbonated beverages.

Grade of recommendation GPP, (88%) Consensus

Comment

In general terms, different published reviews recommend the intake of a varied, healthy, and balanced diet for COPD patients without reducing the caloric intake because of the risk of associated malnutrition, trying to divide the intake into several meals to increase the caloric intake [58,96].

A decrease in the risk of developing various pathologies, including COPD, has also been observed in patients with an adequate intake of fish and a low proportion of saturated fats [15,97].

On the other hand, multiple epidemiological studies point to the protective potential of fruit and vegetables due to their high content of antioxidant substances (vitamins A and E) as well as fiber, anti-inflammatory properties, slowing of glucose and starch absorption, decreased lipid oxidation, and increase in anti-inflammatory cytokines by the gut microbiota. Thus, an adequate intake of these to prevent the development of the disease is recommended [58,98,99].

A study of 21,148 patients from the Korean National Health and Nutrition Examination Survey (2007–2014) showed that patients with higher intakes of vitamin A, carotenoids, and vitamin C had significantly higher FEV1 than those with lower intakes, as well as a lower risk of COPD, regardless of smoking status [100].

Another study [101] conducted on this population in 2012, with 3283 adults $\geq$40 years of age, 512 of whom were diagnosed with COPD, described how those with low intakes of nutrients, including potassium, vitamin A, carotenes, retinol, and vitamin C were at significant risk of developing COPD. In the multivariate analysis, gender, older age, smoking, and low vitamin C intake were independent risk factors for developing COPD.

In contrast, a systematic review has shown how a 50 g/week increase in processed red meat intake leads to an increase in COPD risk of 8% [102]. Increased inspiratory limitation has also been reported in patients with higher consumption of carbonated beverages and coffee and increased smoking rates [103].

3.4.2. What Is the Role of Dietary Advice?

Recommendation 15. *GARIN recommends basic dietary advice as it is essential for COPD patients and the basis for proper lifestyle habits, especially in relation to diet.*

Grade of recommendation GPP, (100%) Consensus.

Comment:

Several clinical trials have studied the effect of dietary advice in COPD patients, showing an increase in caloric and protein intake, with an increase in weight and an improvement in SGA scores [70]. An increase in inspiratory strength and quality of life questionnaire scores has also been reported [73]. Several of these studies have also shown an improvement in clinical variables such as 6MWD or grip strength [104] and a significant reduction in the percentage of smokers, as well as better adherence to a Mediterranean diet and an increase in caloric intake with structured meal programs [105,106].

3.4.3. In Patients with COPD and Malnutrition, Is Nutritional Supplementation Associated with an Improvement in Morphofunctional Nutritional Parameters and Disease Progression?

Recommendation 16. *GARIN suggests the use of oral nutritional supplements (ONSs) in malnourished COPD patients to improve nutritional status and disease course (Table 6).*

Table 6. The degree of recommendation according to GARIN's position on each of the aspects under consideration.

Objectives to Be Taken into Account	Grade of Recommendation
Weight increase	***
Lean mass increase	***
Potency of effect in physical exercise	***
Improvement in muscle functionality	**
Improvement in lung function	**
Improvement in quality of life	**
Improvement of laboratory parameters	*
Reduction of post-hospitalisation mortality	*

*** Recommend; ** Suggest; * Advise.

Grade of recommendation B, (96%) Strong consensus.

Comment—Weight and lean mass increase:

The scientific evidence in this area has evolved over time. While more recent authors have reported increases in weight and lean mass, as well as improvements in exercise tolerance, earlier studies did not support these findings.

Ferreira's 2012 Cochrane Review [107] includes a meta-analysis of 17 RCTs with little evidence in favor of those patients receiving nutritional supplements in terms of improvement in weight, lean mass, respiratory muscle strength, and 6MWD, particularly striking in malnourished patients [37].

However, more recent studies show that the use of ONSs is associated with increased intake, improved anthropometric measures, and increased muscle strength [58,67–69,92, 108–112].

A significant improvement in anthropometric measures (fat-free mass, brachial circumference, tricipital fold), 6MWD, ISWT, respiratory muscle strength (maximum inspiratory and expiratory pressure), and grip strength measured by dynamometry is described in the aforementioned studies [15,67,69,92,105,107,109,110,112–115].

Comment—Potency of effect in physical exercise:

Most studies, especially those focused on the assessment of fat-free mass, associate nutritional supplementation with regular physical exercise, so it is known that the association of the two enhances their effect [15,92,108,111,112,116].

Comment—Improved muscle and lung function:

Meta-analyses using different methods have been published, showing a significant association with daily calorie intake, grip strength, and quadriceps muscle strength [11,15,107].

Comment—Improved quality of life:

Improvements have been observed in the Chronic Respiratory Disease Questionnaire (CRQ) (which measures the presence of dyspnoea, fatigue, emotion, and mastery) and quality of life as measured by the St George's Respiratory Questionnaire in undernourished patients with COPD, as well as anxiety and depression scores by HADS and the EQ-5D, in patients with nutritional supplementation [67,69,92,107–110,112–115].

Comment—Improvement in laboratory parameters:

A decrease in blood pressure and triglycerides and an increase in c-HDL have been reported with formulas enriched in omega-3 fatty acids, vitamin D, and high-biological-value proteins [92].

An improvement in laboratory parameters such as vitamin D, eicosapentaenoic acid (EPA) and docosahexaenoic acid (DHA), and inflammatory markers such as highly sensitive C-reactive protein, interleukin-6, interleukin-8, and tumor necrosis factor-alpha, has also been reported [67,112].

Comment—Decreased mortality:

Clinical trials with high protein supplements, some of them enriched in hydroxy methyl butyrate (HMB), have also shown decreased 90-day mortality rates, with a number needed to treat (NNT) of 20.3 [68,93]. A sub-analysis of the EFFORT study showed that these results were consistent in patients with lower respiratory tract infections [66].

3.4.4. Is There a Specific ONS for This Group of Patients?

There is insufficient evidence to make any recommendations about specific supplements in this group of patients.

Comment:

Several supplements have been analyzed that have shown a significant benefit in the variables studied, most of them high-calorie and high-protein supplements enriched with certain micronutrients (omega-3, vitamin D, leucine, HMB) (Table 7).

Enteral nutrition formulas developed with a higher fat content (50–55%) have not shown a clear benefit in hospitalized COPD patients or those on mechanical ventilation [58].

3.4.5. What Is the Role of Enteral and Parenteral Nutrition in Exacerbation Episodes in COPD Patients?

Recommendation 17. *GARIN advises covering the necessary calorie intake in patients admitted for decompensated COPD, using the most physiological route possible at an early stage, as long as this provides adequate coverage of their requirements.*

Grade of recommendation GPP, (98%) Strong consensus.

Comment:

Intake in mechanically ventilated patients is decreased, mainly in those with oral nutrition, longer mechanical ventilation (MV), and higher BMI at admission [117].

In this review, we found only one non-systematic review study analyzing the role of nutritional support during exacerbations. Bordeje Laguna [58] recommends that in patients admitted to intensive care with the need for prolonged MV (>8 days) and high nutritional risk, receiving enteral nutrition and, failing that, total parenteral nutrition is associated with greater survival at 6 months and better recovery 3 months after discharge from the ICU. Likewise, patients with good nutritional coverage are more likely to be discharged home rather than to intermediate rehabilitation centers [58].

On the other hand, it has been determined that ventral decubitus does not contraindicate the use of enteral nutrition and is not associated with an increased risk of gastrointestinal complications or aspiration pneumonia [58].

Table 7. Studies analyzing oral supplementation in patients with COPD.

ONS (kcal/prot)	(*N*) and Time	Grade COPD	Comparator	Effects	References
Normo/Normo Omega-3/6 DHA FOS (Prebiotic fiber)	(99) 3 months	Stable outpatient Mild/moderate/severe	PCB	↑ weight ↑ FEV1 ↑ Grip strength ↑ 6MWT	Benito Martinez et al. [109]
High/High Leucine Omega-3 [111] PUFAs [108] Vitamin D	(81) 4 months [108,111] (45) 3 months [92]	Stable outpatient Moderate/severe +High-intensity exercise	PCB [108,111] Isocaloric formula [92]	↑ Vit D, EPA, DHA, Omega-3 ↑ Weight, ↑ FM ↑ FEV1 ↓ Depression Score without difference with isocaloric formula * [92]	Van de Bool et al. [111] Van Beers et al. [108] Calder et al. [92]
High/High HMB	(652) 3 months [68,69] (214) 3 months [93]	Hospital COPD > 65 years + other pathologies. Up to 90 days post-H	PCB P (comp form 48 kcal standard + Vit C) [68]	↓ 30–60–90 day mortality (NNT 20) ↑ SGA scale ↑ Weight ↑ Vit D ↑ Grip strength ↑ nutritional markers	Deutz et al. [68] Deutz et al. [93] (sub-analysis of [68]) Matheson et al. [69]
Normo/High Whey protein Omega-3 Vitamins A,C,E	(36) 3 months (12) 2 weeks	Stable outpatient Moderate/severe +Low-intensity exercise	PCB [112] Hydrolysed casein [113]	↓ Inflammatory markers ↑ 6MWT ↑ Weight, ↑ FM ↑ Quadriceps strength ↑ Inspiratory pressure max ↑ Emotional Function and Quality of Life score No difference between the two types of protein [113]	Sugawara et al. [112] Jonker et al. [116]
Low (0.45)/High Whey protein Magnesium + Vitamin C	(44) 2 months	Stable outpatient Moderate/severe	PCB	↑ FFM ↑ Vit C ↑ St. George's Respiratory Questionnaire ↓ Inflammatory markers	Ahmadi et al. [67]

Abbreviations: ONS = oral nutritional supplement; N = number of patients included; PCB = placebo (understood as dietary advice); DHA = docosahexaenoic acid; 6MWT = 6 min walking test; EPA = eicosapentaenoic acid; FM = fat mass; FFM = fat-free mass. * milk-based comparator that contained no 25-hydroxy-vitamin D3, milk protein instead of pure whey protein, and sunflower oil in place of omega-3 polyunsaturated fatty acid (PUFA) containing fish oil. ↑ = Increase; ↓ = decrease.

A published clinical trial in 50 hospitalized patients showed that EPA administration at a dose of 1 g/day was not associated with significant benefits in terms of muscle mass preservation or hospital stay [118].

There is insufficient evidence to make specific recommendations on the use of glutamine, branched-chain amino acids, vitamins, or antioxidants in this group of acutely decompensated patients.

3.4.6. Is There Sufficient Evidence to Recommend Any Form of Micronutrient or Trace Element Supplementation?

Recommendation 18. *Grade of recommendation according to GARIN's position on supplementation with micronutrients and trace elements (Table 8).*

Table 8. Grade of recommendation according to GARIN's position on supplementation with micronutrients and trace elements.

	Grade of Recommendation
Monitor levels of ions, especially magnesium, calcium, phosphorus	***
Vit D if deficient (<20 ng/mL)	**
HMB and essential amino acids	*
Omega-3, Vit D and leucine	N
Antioxidant vitamins A, C and E, and selenium	N

*** Recommend; ** Suggest; * Advise; N: Not positioning.

Grade of recommendation GPP, (90%) Consensus.

Comment—HMB and essential amino acids:

Supplements rich in leucine, essential amino acids, HMB, and creatine need further study in critically ill patients.

Supplementation with HMB seems to provide the strongest evidence in this respect, with an improvement in nitrogen balance in patients with high catabolism. Administration of essential amino acids has been shown to improve body composition and nutritional status in other pathologies associated with increased muscle catabolism [119].

Studies conducted in patients with moderate/severe COPD [120] have shown that supplementation with a high proportion of leucine-enriched essential amino acids is associated with increased protein anabolism [32]. Increased physical capacity, fat-free mass, muscle strength, SaO_2, serum albumin, and quality of life scales, as well as a decrease in cognitive impairment progression, have also been observed in patients with severe COPD who do not meet the criteria for participation in pulmonary rehabilitation programs [121].

Comment—Omega-3, Vit D and leucine:

There are numerous published interventions with a very heterogeneous methodology, including supplements enriched in carbohydrates and fatty acids, essential amino acids, whey protein rich in BCAAs, creatine, and polyunsaturated fatty acids (PUFAs) (natural ligands of peroxisome proliferator-activated receptors). Initial studies with fat-enriched supplements do not appear to show a significant benefit; however, more recent studies using carbohydrate and PUFA-enriched formulations appear to show improved physical training in selected patients [15].

In a study of 86 patients with moderate inspiratory limitation, low lung diffusion capacity, adequate protein intake, and decreased levels of vitamin D and DHA, the administration of a supplement enriched in omega-3, vitamin D, and leucine for 4 months in association with physical exercise (in both groups) showed statistically significant differences in the increase in muscle mass, levels of Vit D, EPA, and DHA, and the number of steps achieved [111].

Some studies also show a reduction in exacerbations after vitamin D supplementation in patients with previous deficiency [58,99].

Vitamin D supplementation is, therefore, recommended in patients with deficiency (<20 ng/mL), with a clear benefit in the prevention of falls, especially in association with calcium. A dose of 800 IU with 1 g of calcium is recommended. Supplementation with higher doses requires further study [15,122,123].

The addition of leucine and carbohydrates to protein supplements, either alone or in combination, has not been shown to increase protein anabolism compared with high-protein supplementation alone [94,116].

Comment—Antioxidant vitamins:

Several studies show antioxidant vitamin deficiency rates of up to 81% [58,99,124].

The use of magnesium and vitamin C-enriched whey formulations [67] has shown a decrease in inflammatory markers as well as an increase in fat-free mass, grip strength, and quality of life tests in patients with moderate/severe COPD.

In different systematic reviews, vitamin C supplementation has not demonstrated relevant clinical benefits in patients with pulmonary pathology [99]. However, more recent publications show contradictory results.

According to a published study, the administration of a supplement enriched in α-tocopherol (vitamin E) (30 mg/day), vitamin C (180 mg/day), zinc gluconate (15 mg/day), and selenomethionine (50 μg/day), associated with a physical exercise program, did not show an increase in exercise endurance, although it was associated with an increase in muscle strength and an increase in serum total protein levels [124]. Vitamin E administration in smoking patients showed a reduction in markers related to prostaglandin production, such as urine 8-iso-PGF2α by 21%, not significant compared with in combination with selenium or selenium administration alone [125].

3.5. *Physical Activity*

3.5.1. What Is the Best Strategy in the Rehabilitation of the COPD Patient, Associated with Nutritional Therapy?

Recommendation 19. *GARIN recommends pulmonary rehabilitation, combining aerobic and strength training exercises.*

Grade of recommendation A, (100%) Strong consensus.

Recommendation 20. *GARIN suggests including at least 6–12 weeks of continuous physical training.*

Grade of recommendation GPP, (94%) Strong consensus.

Recommendation 21. *GARIN suggests the interval modality for patients with severe COPD.*

Grade of recommendation B, (93%) Strong consensus.

Comment:

Pulmonary rehabilitation has established itself as one of the key strategies in the management of COPD patients. Pulmonary rehabilitation programs include physical exercise as an essential component of rehabilitation, in addition to other interventions such as education, dietary advice, and psychological support. Studies have shown that a comprehensive and intensive pulmonary rehabilitation program achieves significant improvements in clinical (dyspnoea, fatigue), body composition, physical capacity (exercise tolerance, muscle strength), and quality of life parameters [37,56,104,115,126].

One of the hallmarks of COPD is the progressive decline in physical exercise capacity due to skeletal muscle loss and dysfunction, which is a predictor of morbidity and mortality independent of lung function impairment [15,32,56,60,104,113,126–128]. The COVID-19 pandemic further exacerbated these effects, significantly reducing physical activity levels and potentially worsening muscle loss and dysfunction [129].

Muscle training has been widely shown to be effective in improving exercise tolerance, muscle strength, dyspnoea, fatigue, and quality of life [37,126,130].

Studies are currently focusing on identifying the essential components that achieve the best results in the short and long term, including the type and exercise intensity, frequency and duration of sessions, location (center or home), face-to-face supervision or other innovative strategies (tele rehabilitation), individualized or in groups.

Aerobic or endurance training is the most widely used form of exercise, for which there is the strongest recommendation evidence. A modification of standard aerobic training is interval training, where periods of maximal exertion are regularly alternated with equal periods of rest or lower-intensity exercise. In this way, patients achieve high levels of exertion but with less dyspnoea and fatigue, providing benefits equivalent to those of classical aerobic training [37,126]. Studies consistently show that interval training is one of the best treatments for the most severe COPD patients [124,131].

Muscle strength training has great potential compared with aerobic exercise to increase muscle mass and strength and the advantage of less cardio–respiratory compromise [80, 126,127,132].

Most training programs achieve the best physiological results through a combination of the two types of exercise [115,126].

There is no consistent evidence to define the duration of training programs. Although studies of very variable duration (between 4 and 16 weeks) have been proposed [113, 124,126], most of them consider that substantial benefits can be achieved with a duration between 6 and 12 weeks and with a frequency of 3–4 sessions per week [37,115,126–128,133].

3.5.2. Is It Possible to Make a Specific Recommendation on Physical Exercise?

Recommendation 22. *GARIN recommends regular physical activity according to the WHO guidelines for adults with chronic diseases.*

Grade of recommendation GPP, (96%) Strong consensus.

Recommendation 23. *GARIN advises incorporating behavioral change strategies to increase physical activity engagement in COPD patients.*

Grade of recommendation O, (86%) Consensus.

Comment:

People with COPD are less active than people without COPD. Most reduce their activity levels in the early stages of the disease, walk at a slower pace, and generally do not meet the physical activity criteria recommended by the WHO. Patients avoid activities that involve physical exertion and increased symptoms, thus perpetuating a vicious cycle in which lack of exercise further compromises the physical ability to participate in any activity [30,37,56,104,134–136]. Physical inactivity leads to higher rates of morbidity, increased risk of premature mortality and hospitalization, and decreased quality of life [137]. Therefore, physical activity is identified as a potentially modifiable target that could be related to the patient's disease progression and quality of life [30,113,135,138,139].

Although strategies to increase physical activity have been proposed, some studies have found that these only lead to a 2% increase in the time spent in daily activity, and therefore, recommendations to decrease the time spent in sedentary activities are advocated [137].

The members of GARIN have found no evidence of specific recommendations for physical activity in daily life for COPD patients and, therefore, consider that it is advisable to promote activities following the WHO recommendations for the general population [140].

3.6. *Quality of Life*

What Are the Most Commonly Used Quality of Life Questionnaires?

Recommendation 24. *GARIN suggests the use of the following quality of life, anxiety, and depression questionnaires in the follow-up of COPD patients.*

For the assessment of anxiety and depression [57,108]:

HADS anxiety score;

HADS depression score.

For the evaluation of the quality of life of patients with COPD, GARIN suggests the COPD Assessment Test (CAT) [141] *in clinical practice. The St George's Respiratory Questionnaire in undernourished patients with COPD (SGRQ)* [15,47,70,107,121,142] *and the Health-related quality of life using a validated version of the EuroQol five-dimensional (EQ-5D) questionnaire* [57,75,108,143,144], *such as EQ-5D-5L index value or EQ-5D-5L VAS although they have been validated, are longer and more complex.*

Grade of recommendation GPP, (90%) Consensus.

4. Limitations and Strengths

Limitations: The principal limitation of the study is that only eight recommendations have been made with a high quality of evidence because there are important gaps in methods for assessing nutritional status, the impact of muscles in the process, nutritional requirements, and the most appropriate interventions in terms of nutrition, specific nutrients, and physical activity. The opinion of people with COPD and their caregivers has not been taken into account, nor are there pulmonology specialists in the group. Lastly, the final document was not sent to an external group for validation.

Strengths: A systematic review has been carried out with a methodology following the PRISMA criteria and applying grading of the evidence according to the SIGN (Scottish Intercollegiate Guidelines Network) methodology. In addition, an approximation has been made to the degree of consensus among experts in the area. Questions have been addressed with an eminently practical orientation.

5. Conclusions

Malnutrition is common in COPD patients and is associated with major complications that contribute to the frailty, morbidity, and mortality of COPD patients.

Members of GARIN recommend a multidisciplinary approach to COPD patients, integrating early Morphofunctional Nutritional Assessment and treatment to reduce the occurrence of complications linked to malnutrition and, thus, contribute to the patient's well-being and improved quality of life. In pre-COPD and PRISM clinical presentations, it is important to implement preventive measures that could prevent disease progression or lead to early diagnosis and nutritional treatment [15,51,145,146].

Due to the limitations of the classic parameters for assessing nutritional status, a new global vision of clinical nutrition is necessary, integrating different aspects of the morphofunctional evaluation of patients with COPD, taking into account the different metabolic phenotypes [15,50] and their association with other phenotypes (emphysematous, chronic bronchitis, or both), which allows establishing a more precise diagnosis of the nutritional situation and an individualized therapeutic plan [51], as concluded by recently published studies [147].

These recommendations and suggestions on the nutritional management of the COPD patient have applicability in daily clinical practice; however, there are many questions about energy and nutrient requirements, and there are many uncertainties about the ideal percentage distribution of carbohydrates, lipids, and proteins in COPD patients' diets. There is no consistent evidence to define the duration of training programs and the best strategy to increase physical activity in daily life. Further studies are needed to increase the quality of the evidence and provide specific answers to many of these questions.

Randomized and preferably double-blind clinical trials evaluating the impact of nutritional therapy in different clinical situations in both inpatient and outpatient settings would be desirable. Studies comparing different enteral nutrition formulas in COPD patients should evaluate the efficacy and efficiency (cost-effectiveness) of these formulas on metabolic effects and morbidity/mortality in order to make evidence-based recommendations.

Author Contributions: J.B.M.S.: Writing—original draft. C.T.-J.: Writing—original draft. M.J.M.-P.: Writing—original draft. A.J.E.: Writing—original draft. F.J.V.-L.: Writing—original draft. G.O.: Writing—original draft. P.P.G.-L.: Writing—original draft. J.-A.I.R.: Writing—original draft. J.M.G.-A.: Writing—original draft. J.L.P.-C.: Writing—original draft. M.I.R.-P.: Writing—original draft. M.J.M.R.: Writing—original draft. J.M.R.-R.: Writing—original draft. All authors have read and agreed to the published version of the manuscript.

Funding: This research received no external funding.

Conflicts of Interest: The authors declare no conflicts of interest.

Appendix A. Glim Criteria and SGA

Table A1. GLIM tresholds for severity grading of malnutrition into Stage 1 (Moderate) and Stage 2 (Severe) malnutrition. Adapted from ref. [148].

	Phenotypic Criteria [a]		
	Weight Loss (%)	**Low Body Mass Index (kg/m^2) [b]**	**Reduced Muscle Mass [c]**
Stage 1 (Moderate Malnutrition) (Requires 1 phenotypic criterion that meets this grade)	5–10% within the past 6 mo, or 10–20% beyond 6 mo	<20 if < 70 yr, <22 if ≥70 yr	Mild to moderate deficit (per validated assessment methods—see below)
Stage 2 (Severe Malnutrition) (Requires 1 phenotypic criterion that meets this grade)	>10% within the past 6 mo, or >20% beyond 6 mo	<18.5 if < 70 yr, <20 if ≥70 yr	Severe deficit (per validated assessment methods—see below)

(a) Severity grading is based upon the noted phenotypic criteria while the etiologic criteria described in the text and Figure 1 are used to provide the context to guide intervention and anticipated outcomes.
(b) Further research is needed to secure consensus reference BMI data for Asian populations in clinical settings.
(c) For example appendicular lean mass index (ALMI, kg/m^2) by dual-energy absorptiometry or corresponding standards using other body composition methods like bioelectrical impedance analysis (BIA), CT or MRI. When not available or by regional preference, physical examination or standard anthropometric measures like mid-arm muscle or calf circumferences may be used. Functional assessments like hand-grip strength may be used as a supportive measure.

Table A2. SARC-F SCALE. Adapted from ref. [149].

Component	Question	Scoring
Strength	How much difficulty do you have in lifting and carrying 10 pounds?	None = 0, Some = 1, A lot or unable = 2
Assistance in walking	How much difficulty do you have walking across a room?	None = 0, Some = 1, A lot, use aids, or unable = 2
Rise from a chair	How much difficulty do you have transferring from a chair or bed?	None = 0, Some = 1, A lot or unable without help = 2
Climb stairs	How much difficulty do you have climbing a flight of 10 stairs?	None = 0, Some = 1, A lot or unable = 2
Falls	How many times have you fallen in the past year?	None = 0, 1–3 falls = 1, ≥4 falls = 2

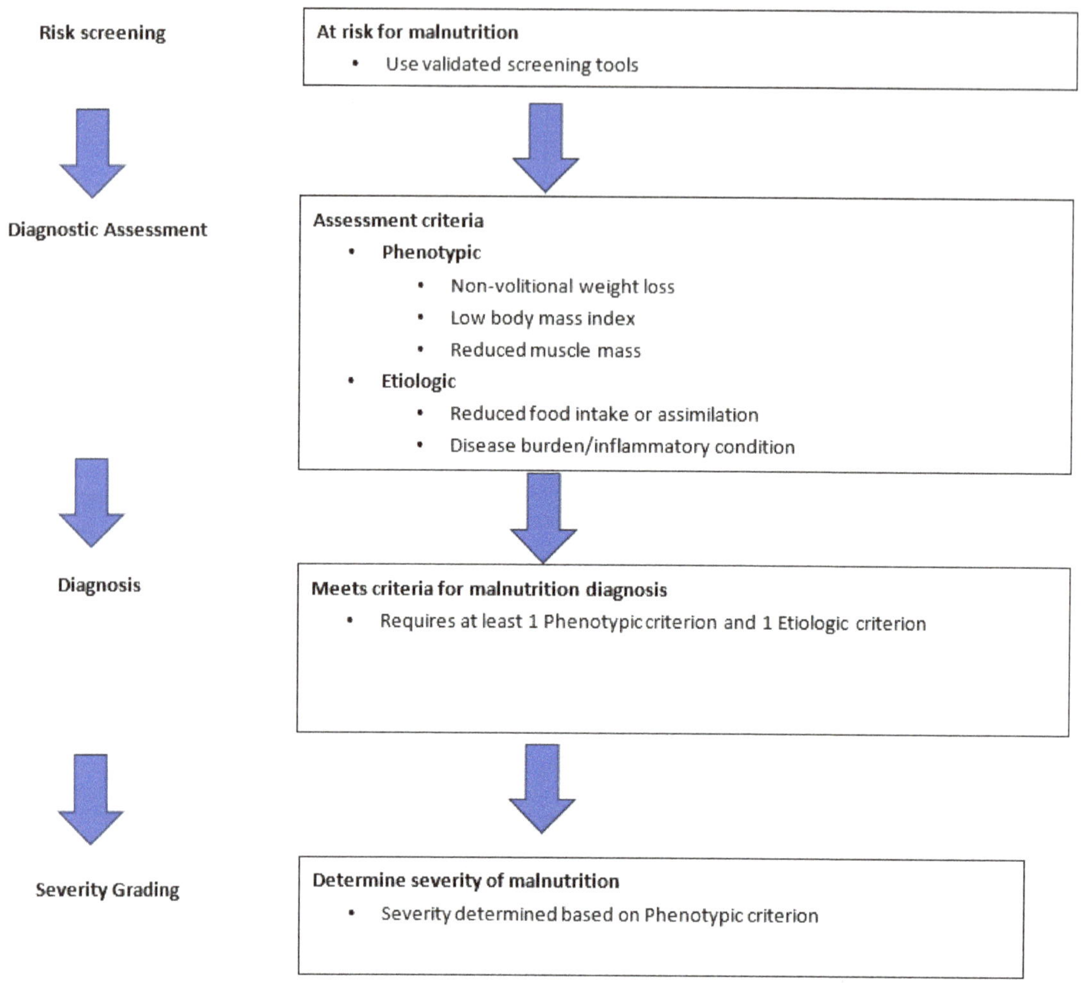

Figure A1. GLIM diagnostic scheme for screening, assessment, diagnosis and grading of malnutrition. Adapted from ref. [148].

A. History

1. Weight change
    - Overall loss in past 6 months: amount = #________kg; % loss = #________
    - Change in past 2 weeks:
        - ________increase,
        - ________no change,
        - ________decrease.
2. Dietary intake change (relative to normal)
    - ________No change,
    - ________Change ________duration = #________weeks
        - Type: ________suboptimal liquid diet,
        - ________full liquid diet
        - ________hypocaloric liquids,
        - ________starvation.
3. Gastrointestinal symptoms (that persisted for >2 weeks)
    - ________ none, ________ nausea, ________ vomiting, ________ diarrhea, ________anorexia.
4. Functional capacity
    - ________No dysfunction (e.g., full capacity),
    - ________Dysfunction ________duration = #________weeks.
        - Type: ________working suboptimally,
        - ________ambulatory,
        - ________bedridden.
5. Disease and its relation to nutritional requirements
    - Primary diagnosis (specify) ____________________________
    - Metabolic demand (stress):
        - ________no stress,
        - ________low stress,
        - ________moderate stress,
        - ________high stress.

B. Physical (for each trait specify: 0 = normal, 1+ = mild, 2+ = moderate, 3+ = severe).

- #________loss of subcutaneous fat (triceps, chest)
- #________muscle wasting (quadriceps, deltoids)
- #________ankle edema
- #________sacral edema
- #________ascites

C. SGA rating (select one)

- ________A = Well nourished
- ________B = Moderately (or suspected of being) malnourished
- ________C = Severely malnourished

Figure A2. Items contained in the Subjective Global Assessment (SGA). Adapted from ref. [148].

Appendix B. EWGSOP2 and SARC-F

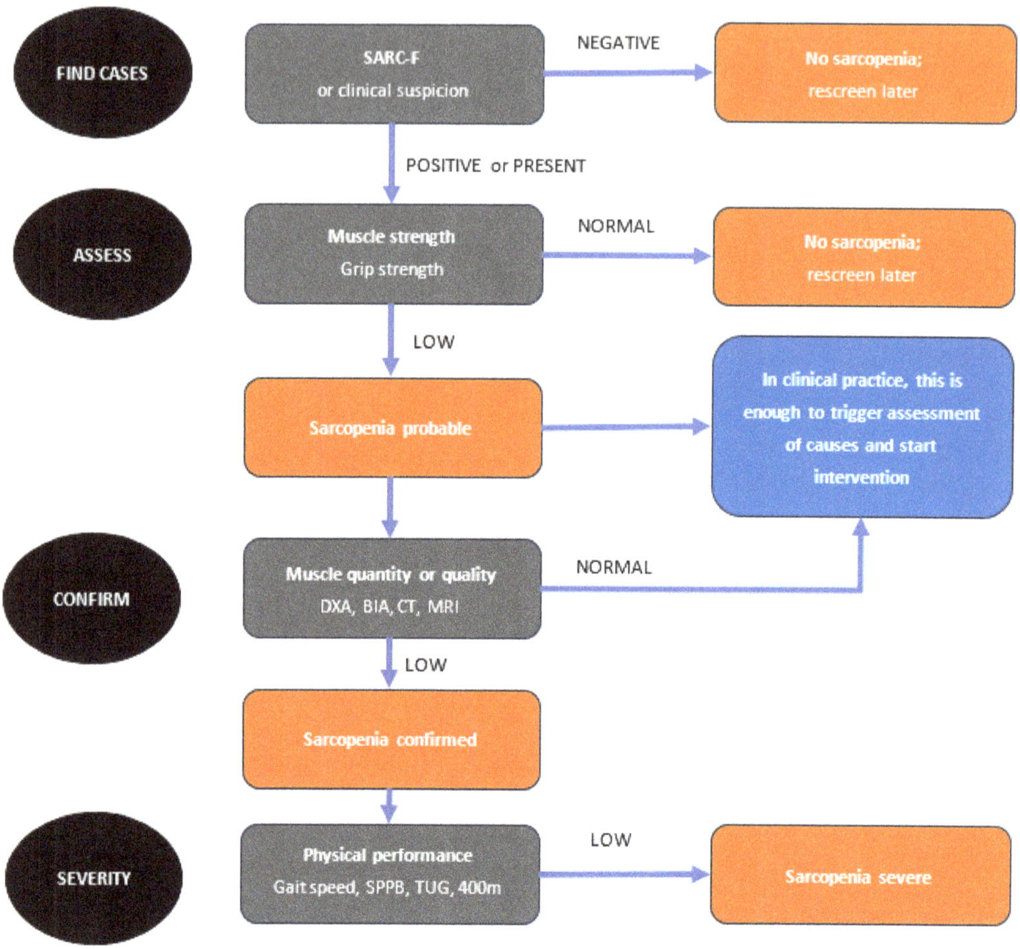

Figure A3. Algorythm for case-finding making a diagnosis and quantifying severity in practice. The steps of the pathway are represented as Find-Assess-Confirm-Severity or F-A-C-S "Consider other reason for low muscle strength (e.g., depression, stroke, balance disorders, peripheral vascular disorders)". Abbrevations: DXA = Dual-energy X-ray absorptiometry; BIA = Bioelectrical impedance analysis; CT = computed tomography; MRI = magnetic resonance imaging; SPPB = short physical performance battery; TUG = timed-up-and-go test. Adapted from ref. [78].

References

1. WHO. The Top 10 Causes of Death. Available online: https://www.who.int/news-room/fact-sheets/detail/the-top-10-causes-of-death (accessed on 23 March 2023).
2. GBD. GBD DALYs Hale Collaborators. Global, regional, and national disability-adjusted life-years (DALYs) for 359 diseases and injuries and healthy life expectancy (HALE) for 195 countries and territories, 1990–2017: A systematic analysis for the Global Burden. *Lancet* **2018**, *392*, 1852–1922.
3. Yang, K.; Wu, Y.; Chen, D.; Liu, S.; Chen, R. The Impact of Lung Function on Extra-Pulmonary Diseases and All-Cause Mortality in US Adult Population with and without COPD. *Clin. Epidemiol.* **2020**, *12*, 997–1005. [CrossRef] [PubMed]
4. Wouters, E.F.M. An update on pulmonary rehabilitation techniques for patients with chronic obstructive pulmonary disease. *Expert Rev. Respir. Med.* **2020**, *14*, 149–161. [CrossRef] [PubMed]

5. Thorsdottir, I.; Gunnarsdottir, I.; Eriksen, B. Screening method evaluated by nutritional status measurements can be used to detect malnourishment in chronic obstructive pulmonary disease. *J. Am. Diet. Assoc.* **2001**, *101*, 648–654. [CrossRef] [PubMed]
6. Vermeeren, M.; Creutzberg, E.; Schols, A.; Postma, D.; Pieters, W.; Roldaan, A.; Wouters, E. Prevalence of nutritional depletion in a large out-patient population of patients with COPD. *Respir. Med.* **2006**, *100*, 1349–1355. [CrossRef]
7. Marco, E.; Sánchez-Rodríguez, D.; Dávalos-Yerovi, V.N.; Duran, X.; Pascual, E.M.; Muniesa, J.M.; Rodríguez, D.A.; Aguilera-Zubizarreta, A.; Escalada, F.; Duarte, E. Malnutrition according to ESPEN consensus predicts hospitalizations and long-term mortality in rehabilitation patients with stable chronic obstructive pulmonary disease. *Clin. Nutr.* **2019**, *38*, 2180–2186. [CrossRef]
8. Jo, Y.S.; Kim, Y.H.; Lee, J.Y.; Kim, K.; Jung, K.S.; Yoo, K.H.; Rhee, C.K. Impact of BMI on exacerbation and medical care expenses in subjects with mild to moderate airflow obstruction. *Int. J. COPD* **2018**, *13*, 2261–2269. [CrossRef]
9. Hoong, J.M.; Ferguson, M.; Hukins, C.; Collins, P.F. Economic and operational burden associated with malnutrition in chronic obstructive pulmonary disease. *Clin. Nutr.* **2017**, *36*, 1105–1109. [CrossRef]
10. Kim, J.; Kim, Y.S.; Kim, K.; Oh, Y.M.; Yoo, K.H.; Rhee, C.K.; Lee, J.H. Socioeconomic impact of asthma, chronic obstructive pulmonary disease and asthma-COPD overlap syndrome. *J. Thorac. Dis.* **2017**, *9*, 1547–1556. [CrossRef]
11. de Blasio, F.; Di Gregorio, A.; de Blasio, F.; Bianco, A.; Bellofiore, B.; Scalfi, L. Malnutrition and sarcopenia assessment in patients with chronic obstructive pulmonary disease according to international diagnostic criteria, and evaluation of raw BIA variables. *Respir. Med.* **2018**, *134*, 1–5. [CrossRef]
12. Ingadottir, A.R.; Beck, A.M.; Baldwin, C.; Weekes, C.E.; Geirsdottir, O.G.; Ramel, A.; Gislason, T.; Gunnarsdottir, I. Association of energy and protein intakes with length of stay, readmission and mortality in hospitalised patients with chronic obstructive pulmonary disease. *Br. J. Nutr.* **2018**, *119*, 543–551. [CrossRef] [PubMed]
13. Benedik, B.; Farkas, J.; Kosnik, M.; Kadivec, S.; Lainscak, M. Mini nutritional assessment, body composition, and hospitalisations in patients with chronic obstructive pulmonary disease. *Respir. Med.* **2011**, *105*, S38–S43. [CrossRef]
14. Mete, B.; Pehlivan, E.; Gülbaş, G.; Günen, H. Prevalence of malnutrition in COPD and its relationship with the parameters related to disease severity. *Int. J. COPD* **2018**, *13*, 3307–3312. [CrossRef] [PubMed]
15. Schols, A.M.; Ferreira, I.M.; Franssen, F.M.; Gosker, H.R.; Janssens, W.; Muscaritoli, M.; Pison, C.; Rutten-Van Mölken, M.; Slinde, F.; Steiner, M.C.; et al. Nutritional assessment and therapy in COPD: A European respiratory society statement. *Eur. Respir. J.* **2014**, *44*, 1504–1520. [CrossRef] [PubMed]
16. Nguyen, H.T.; Collins, P.F.; Pavey, T.G.; Nguyen, N.V.; Pham, T.D.; Gallegos, D.L. Nutritional status, dietary intake, and health-related quality of life in outpatients with COPD. *Int. J. COPD* **2019**, *14*, 215–226. [CrossRef]
17. Gupta, S.S.; Gothi, D.; Narula, G.; Sircar, J. Correlation of BMI and oxygen saturation in stable COPD in Northern India. *Lung India* **2014**, *31*, 29–34. [CrossRef]
18. Lee, H.M.; Liu, M.; Lee, K.; Luo, Y.; Wong, N.D. Does low vitamin D amplify the association of COPD with total and cardiovascular disease mortality? *Clin. Cardiol.* **2014**, *37*, 473–478. [CrossRef]
19. Agustí, A.; Sisó-Almirall, A.; Roman, M.; Vogelmeier, C.F.; Anzueto, A.; Barnes, P.; Bourbeau, J.; Celli, B.R.; Criner, G.J.; Halpin, D.; et al. Gold 2023: Highlights for primary care. *npj Prim. Care Respir. Med.* **2023**, *33*, 28. [CrossRef]
20. Cheng, S.L.; Lin, C.H.; Chu, K.A.; Chiu, K.L.; Lin, S.H.; Lin, H.C.; Ko, H.K.; Chen, Y.C.; Chen, C.H.; Sheu, C.C.; et al. Update on guidelines for the treatment of COPD in Taiwan using evidence and GRADE system-based recommendations. *J. Formos. Med. Assoc.* **2021**, *120*, 1821–1844. [CrossRef]
21. Spruit, M.A.; Singh, S.J.; Garvey, C.; Zu Wallack, R.; Nici, L.; Rochester, C.; Hill, K.; Holland, A.E.; Lareau, S.C.; Man, W.D.C.; et al. An official American thoracic society/European respiratory society statement: Key concepts and advances in pulmonary rehabilitation. *Am. J. Respir. Crit. Care Med.* **2013**, *188*, 889–1042. [CrossRef]
22. Celli, B.R.; Decramer, M.; Wedzicha, J.A.; Wilson, K.C.; Agustí, A.A.; Criner, G.J.; MacNee, W.; Make, B.J.; Rennard, S.I.; Stockley, R.A.; et al. An official American thoracic society/ European respiratory society statement: Research questions in COPD. *Eur. Respir. Rev.* **2015**, *24*, 159–172. [CrossRef] [PubMed]
23. Neumeier, A.; Keith, R. Clinical guideline highlights for the hospitalist: The GOLD and NICE Guidelines for the Management of COPD. *J. Hosp. Med.* **2020**, *15*, 240–241. [CrossRef] [PubMed]
24. Miravitlles, M.; Soler-Cataluña, J.J.; Calle, M.; Molina, J.; Almagro, P.; Quintano, J.A.; Trigueros, J.A.; Cosío, B.G.; Casanova, C.; Riesco, J.A.; et al. Spanish COPD Guidelines (GesEPOC) 2017. Pharmacological Treatment of Stable Chronic Obstructive Pulmonary Disease. *Arch. Bronconeumol.* **2017**, *53*, 324–335. [CrossRef]
25. Soler-Cataluña, J.J.; Piñera, P.; Trigueros, J.A.; Calle, M.; Casanova, C.; Cosío, B.G.; López-Campos, J.L.; Molina, J.; Almagro, P.; Gómez, J.-T.; et al. Actualización 2021 de la guía española de la EPOC (GesEPOC). Diagnóstico y tratamiento del síndrome de agudización de la EPOC. *Arch. Bronconeumol.* **2022**, *58*, 159–170. [CrossRef] [PubMed]
26. Moher, D.; Liberati, A.; Tetzlaff, J.; Altman, D.G. Preferred reporting items for systematic reviews and meta-analyses: The PRISMA statement. *BMJ* **2009**, *339*, 332–336. [CrossRef]
27. Scottish Intercollegiate Guidelines Network. A Guideline Developer's Handbook. (SIGN Publication no. 50) [Internet]. 2019. Available online: http://www.sign.ac.uk (accessed on 14 February 2023).
28. Bischoff, S.C.; Singer, P.; Koller, M.; Barazzoni, R.; Cederholm, T.; van Gossum, A. Standard operating procedures for ESPEN guidelines and consensus papers. *Clin. Nutr.* **2015**, *34*, 1043–1051. [CrossRef]
29. Hartley, J. Some thoughts on Likert-type scales. *Int. J. Clin. Health Psychol.* **2014**, *14*, 83–86. [CrossRef]

30. Jung, J.W.; Yoon, S.W.; Lee, G.E.; Shin, H.G.; Kim, H.; Shin, J.W.; Park, I.W.; Choi, B.W.; Kim, J.Y. Poor nutritional intake is a dominant factor for weight loss in chronic obstructive pulmonary disease. *Int. J. Tuberc. Lung Dis.* **2019**, *23*, 631–637. [CrossRef]
31. Laudisio, A.; Costanzo, L.; Di Gioia, C.; Delussu, A.S.; Traballesi, M.; Gemma, A.; Antonelli Incalzi, R. Dietary intake of elderly outpatients with chronic obstructive pulmonary disease. *Arch. Gerontol. Geriatr.* **2016**, *64*, 75–81. [CrossRef]
32. Collins, P.F.; Yang, I.A.; Chang, Y.C.; Vaughan, A. Nutritional support in chronic obstructive pulmonary disease (COPD): An evidence update. *J. Thorac. Dis.* **2019**, *11*, S2230–S2237. [CrossRef]
33. Nordén, J.; Grönberg, A.M.; Bosaeus, I.; Forslund, H.B.; Hulthén, L.; Rothenberg, E.; Karlsson, J.; Wallengren, O.; Slinde, F. Nutrition impact symptoms and body composition in patients with COPD. *Eur. J. Clin. Nutr.* **2015**, *69*, 256–261. [CrossRef] [PubMed]
34. Park, H.J.; Leem, A.Y.; Lee, S.H.; Song, J.H.; Park, M.S.; Kim, Y.S.; Kim, S.K.; Chang, J.; Chung, K.S. Comorbidities in obstructive lung disease in Korea: Data from the fourth and fifth Korean national health and nutrition examination survey. *Int. J. COPD* **2015**, *10*, 1571–1582. [CrossRef]
35. Ingadottir, A.R.; Beck, A.M.; Baldwin, C.; Weekes, C.E.; Geirsdottir, O.G.; Ramel, A.; Gislason, T.; Gunnarsdottir, I. Two components of the new ESPEN diagnostic criteria for malnutrition are independent predictors of lung function in hospitalized patients with chronic obstructive pulmonary disease (COPD). *Clin. Nutr.* **2018**, *37*, 1323–1331. [CrossRef] [PubMed]
36. Joo, H.; Park, J.; Do Lee, S.; Oh, Y.M. Comorbidities of chronic obstructive pulmonary disease in Koreans: A population-based study. *J. Korean Med. Sci.* **2012**, *27*, 901–906. [CrossRef] [PubMed]
37. Barreiro, E.; Bustamante, V.; Cejudo, P.; Gáldiz, J.B.; Gea, J.; de Lucas, P.; Martínez-Llorens, J.; Ortega, F.; Puente-Maestu, L.; Roca, J.; et al. Guidelines for the Evaluation and Treatment of Muscle Dysfunction in Patients with Chronic Obstructive Pulmonary Disease. *Arch. Bronconeumol.* **2015**, *51*, 384–395. [CrossRef]
38. Wu, T.D.; Ejike, C.O.; Wise, R.A.; McCormack, M.C.; Brigham, E.P. Investigation of the Obesity Paradox in Chronic Obstructive Pulmonary Disease, According to Smoking Status, in the United States. *Am. J. Epidemiol.* **2019**, *188*, 1977–1983. [CrossRef]
39. Hogan, D.; Lan, L.T.T.; Diep, D.T.N.; Gallegos, D.; Collins, P.F. Nutritional status of Vietnamese outpatients with chronic obstructive pulmonary disease. *J. Hum. Nutr. Diet.* **2017**, *30*, 83–89. [CrossRef]
40. Gea, J.; Casadevall, C.; Pascual, S.; Orozco-Levi, M.; Barreiro, E. Respiratory diseases and muscle dysfunction. *Expert Rev. Respir. Med.* **2012**, *6*, 75–90. [CrossRef]
41. Pezzuto, A.; Ricci, A.; D'ascanio, M.; Moretta, A.; Tonini, G.; Calabrò, N.; Minoia, V.; Pacini, A.; De Paolis, G.; Chichi, E.; et al. Short-Term Benefits of Smoking Cessation Improve Respiratory Function and Metabolism in Smokers. *Int. J. COPD* **2023**, *18*, 2861–2865. [CrossRef]
42. Doo, J.H.; Kim, S.M.; Park, Y.J.; Kim, K.H.; Oh, Y.H.; Kim, J.S.; Park, S.M. Smoking cessation after diagnosis of COPD is associated with lower all-cause and cause-specific mortality: A nationwide population-based cohort study of South Korean men. *BMC Pulm. Med.* **2023**, *23*, 237. [CrossRef]
43. Okazaki, R.; Watanabe, R.; Inoue, D. Osteoporosis Associated with Chronic Obstructive Pulmonary Disease. *J. Bone Metab.* **2016**, *23*, 111–120. [CrossRef] [PubMed]
44. Majid, H.; Kanbar-Agha, F.; Sharafkhaneh, A. COPD: Osteoporosis and sarcopenia. *COPD Res. Pract.* **2016**, *2*, 3. [CrossRef]
45. Lee, I.S.; Leem, A.Y.; Lee, S.H.; Rhee, Y.; Ha, Y.; Kim, Y.S. Relationship between pulmonary function and bone mineral density in the Korean National Health and Nutrition Examination Survey. *Korean J. Intern. Med.* **2016**, *31*, 899–909. [CrossRef] [PubMed]
46. Horadagoda, C.; Dinihan, T.; Roberts, M.; Kairaitis, K. Body composition and micronutrient deficiencies in patients with an acute exacerbation of chronic obstructive pulmonary disease. *Intern. Med. J.* **2017**, *47*, 1057–1063. [CrossRef]
47. McDonald, V.M.; Gibson, P.G.; Scott, H.A.; Baines, P.J.; Hensley, M.J.; Pretto, J.J.; Wood, L.G. Should we treat obesity in COPD? The effects of diet and resistance exercise training. *Respirology* **2016**, *21*, 875–882. [CrossRef]
48. Liu, Y.; Pleasants, R.A.; Croft, J.B.; Lugogo, N.; Ohar, J.; Heidari, K.; Strange, C.; Wheaton, A.G.; Mannino, D.M.; Kraft, M. Body mass index, respiratory conditions, asthma, and chronic obstructive pulmonary disease. *Respir. Med.* **2015**, *109*, 851–859. [CrossRef]
49. Park, J.-H.; Lee, J.-K.; Heo, E.Y.; Kim, D.K.; Chung, H.S. The effect of obesity on patients with mild chronic obstructive pulmonary disease: Results from KNHANES 2010 to 2012. *Int. J. Chron. Obstruct. Pulmon. Dis.* **2017**, *12*, 757–763. [CrossRef]
50. Joppa, P.; Tkacova, R.; Franssen, F.M.E.; Hanson, C.; Rennard, S.I.; Silverman, E.K.; McDonald, M.L.N.; Calverley, P.M.A.; Tal-Singer, R.; Spruit, M.A.; et al. Sarcopenic Obesity, Functional Outcomes, and Systemic Inflammation in Patients with Chronic Obstructive Pulmonary Disease. *J. Am. Med. Dir. Assoc.* **2016**, *17*, 712–718. [CrossRef]
51. Venkatesan, P. GOLD COPD report: 2024 update. *Lancet. Respir. Med.* **2024**, *12*, 15–16. [CrossRef]
52. Lei, Y.; Liang, Y.; Chen, Y.; Liu, X.; Liao, X.; Luo, F. Increased circulating obestatin in patients with chronic obstructive pulmonary disease. *Multidiscip. Respir. Med.* **2014**, *9*, 5. [CrossRef]
53. Yee, N.; Locke, E.R.; Pike, K.C.; Chen, Z.; Lee, J.; Huang, J.C.; Nguyen, H.Q.; Fan, V.S. Frailty in chronic obstructive pulmonary disease and risk of exacerbations and hospitalizations. *Int. J. COPD* **2020**, *15*, 1967–1976. [CrossRef] [PubMed]
54. Chua, J.R.; Albay, A.B.; Tee, M.L. Body composition of Filipino chronic obstructive pulmonary disease (COPD) patients in relation to their lung function, exercise capacity and quality of life. *Int. J. COPD* **2019**, *14*, 2759–2765. [CrossRef] [PubMed]
55. Verhage, T.L.; Heijdra, Y.; Molema, J.; Vercoulen, J.; Dekhuijzen, R. Associations of muscle depletion with health status. Another gender difference in COPD? *Clin. Nutr.* **2011**, *30*, 332–338. [CrossRef] [PubMed]

56. Hallin, R.; Janson, C.; Arnardottir, R.H.; Olsson, R.; Emtner, M.; Branth, S.; Boman, G.; Slinde, F. Relation between physical capacity, nutritional status and systemic inflammation in COPD. *Clin. Respir. J.* **2011**, *5*, 136–142. [CrossRef]
57. Matkovic, Z.; Cvetko, D.; Rahelic, D.; Esquinas, C.; Zarak, M.; Miravitlles, M.; Tudoric, N. Nutritional Status of Patients with Chronic Obstructive Pulmonary Disease in Relation to their Physical Performance. *COPD J. Chronic Obstr. Pulm. Dis.* **2017**, *14*, 626–634. [CrossRef]
58. Bordejé Laguna, M.L. Nuestros grandes olvidados, los enfermos respiratorios crónicos. *Nutr. Hosp.* **2017**, *34*, 38–45. [CrossRef]
59. Farooqi, N.; Sandström, T.; Slinde, F.; Håglin, L.; Carlsson, M. Predicting energy requirement with pedometer-determined physical-activity level in women with chronic obstructive pulmonary disease. *Int. J. Chron. Obstruct. Pulmon. Dis.* **2015**, *10*, 1129–1137. [CrossRef]
60. Shan, X.; Liu, J.; Luo, Y.; Xu, X.; Han, Z.; Li, H. Relationship between nutritional risk and exercise capacity in severe chronic obstructive pulmonary disease in male patients. *Int. J. COPD* **2015**, *10*, 1207–1212. [CrossRef]
61. López-López, L.; Torres-Sánchez, I.; González-Jiménez, E.; Díaz-Pelegrina, A.; Merlos-Navarro, S.; Valenza, M.C. Severe chonic obstructive pulmonary disease and malnutrition: Effect on symptoms and function. *Nutr. Hosp.* **2016**, *33*, 319–323. [CrossRef]
62. Battaglia, S.; Spatafora, M.; Paglino, G.; Pedone, C.; Corsonello, A.; Scichilone, N.; Antonelli-Incalzi, R.; Bellia, V. Ageing and COPD affect different domains of nutritional status: The ECCE study. *Eur. Respir. J.* **2011**, *37*, 1340–1345. [CrossRef]
63. Yoshikawa, M.; Fujita, Y.; Yamamoto, Y.; Yamauchi, M.; Tomoda, K.; Koyama, N.; Kimura, H. Mini Nutritional Assessment Short-Form predicts exacerbation frequency in patients with chronic obstructive pulmonary disease. *Respirology* **2014**, *19*, 1198–1203. [CrossRef] [PubMed]
64. Matsumura, T.; Mitani, Y.; Oki, Y.; Fujimoto, Y.; Ohira, M.; Kaneko, H.; Kawashima, T.; Nishio, M.; Ishikawa, A. Comparison of Geriatric Nutritional Risk Index scores on physical performance among elderly patients with chronic obstructive pulmonary disease. *Heart Lung J. Acute Crit. Care* **2015**, *44*, 534–538. [CrossRef] [PubMed]
65. Chen, R.; Xing, L.; You, C.; Ou, X. Prediction of prognosis in chronic obstructive pulmonary disease patients with respiratory failure: A comparison of three nutritional assessment methods. *Eur. J. Intern. Med.* **2018**, *57*, 70–75. [CrossRef] [PubMed]
66. Baumgartner, A.; Hasenboehler, F.; Cantone, J.; Hersberger, L.; Bargetzi, A.; Bargetzi, L.; Kaegi-Braun, N.; Tribolet, P.; Gomes, F.; Hoess, C.; et al. Effect of nutritional support in patients with lower respiratory tract infection: Secondary analysis of a randomized clinical trial. *Clin. Nutr.* **2021**, *40*, 1843–1850. [CrossRef] [PubMed]
67. Ahmadi, A.; Eftekhari, M.H.; Mazloom, Z.; Masoompour, M.; Fararooei, M.; Eskandari, M.H.; Mehrabi, S.; Bedeltavana, A.; Famouri, M.; Zare, M.; et al. Fortified whey beverage for improving muscle mass in chronic obstructive pulmonary disease: A single-blind, randomized clinical trial. *Respir. Res.* **2020**, *21*, 216. [CrossRef]
68. Deutz, N.E.; Matheson, E.M.; Matarese, L.E.; Luo, M.; Baggs, G.E.; Nelson, J.L.; Hegazi, R.A.; Tappenden, K.A.; Ziegler, T.R. Readmission and mortality in malnourished, older, hospitalized adults treated with a specialized oral nutritional supplement: A randomized clinical trial. *Clin. Nutr.* **2016**, *35*, 18–26. [CrossRef]
69. Matheson, E.M.; Nelson, J.L.; Baggs, G.E.; Luo, M.; Deutz, N.E. Specialized oral nutritional supplement (ONS) improves handgrip strength in hospitalized, malnourished older patients with cardiovascular and pulmonary disease: A randomized clinical trial. *Clin. Nutr.* **2021**, *40*, 844–849. [CrossRef]
70. Nguyen, H.T.; Pavey, T.G.; Collins, P.F.; Nguyen, N.V.; Pham, T.D.; Gallegos, D. Effectiveness of Tailored Dietary Counseling in Treating Malnourished Outpatients with Chronic Obstructive Pulmonary Disease: A Randomized Controlled Trial. *J. Acad. Nutr. Diet.* **2020**, *120*, 778–791.e1. [CrossRef]
71. Nogay, N.H. The relationship og subjetive global assessmente with respiratory function and other nutrition parameters in COPD. *Healthmed* **2012**, *6*, 2013–2017.
72. Al-dorzi, H.M.; Aldawood, A.S.; Tamim, H.; Haddad, S.H.; Jones, G.; Mcintyre, L.; Solaiman, O.; Sakhija, M.; Sadat, M.; Afesh, L.; et al. Clinical Nutrition ESPEN Caloric intake and the fat-to-carbohydrate ratio in hypercapnic acute respiratory failure: Post-hoc analysis of the PermiT trial. *Clin. Nutr. ESPEN* **2018**, *29*, 175–182. [CrossRef]
73. Jeon, Y.K.; Shin, M.J.; Kim, M.H.; Mok, J.H.; Kim, S.S.; Kim, B.H.; Kim, S.-J.; Kim, Y.K.; Chang, J.H.; Shin, Y.B.; et al. Low pulmonary function is related with a high risk of sarcopenia in community-dwelling older adults: The Korea National Health and Nutrition Examination Survey (KNHANES) 2008–2011. *Osteoporos. Int.* **2015**, *26*, 2423–2429. [CrossRef] [PubMed]
74. Borda, M.G.; Celis-Preciado, C.A.; Pérez-Zepeda, M.U.; Ríos-Zuluaga, J.D.; Cano-Gutiérrez, C.A. Sarcopenia en ancianos con antecedente de EPOC/asma: Resultados del estudio SABE—Bogotá. *Rev. Esp. Geriatr. Gerontol.* **2017**, *52*, 313–316. [CrossRef] [PubMed]
75. Lee, D.W.; Jin, H.J.; Shin, K.C.; Chung, J.H.; Lee, H.W.; Lee, K.H. Presence of sarcopenia in asthma–COPD overlap syndrome may be a risk factor for decreased bone-mineral density, unlike asthma: Korean national health and nutrition examination survey (KNHANES) IV and V (2008–2011). *Int. J. COPD* **2017**, *12*, 2355–2362. [CrossRef] [PubMed]
76. Hong, K.S.; Kim, M.C.; Ahn, J.H. Sarcopenia is an independent risk factor for NAFLD in COPD: A nationwide survey (KNHANES 2008–2011). *Int. J. COPD* **2020**, *15*, 1005–1014. [CrossRef] [PubMed]
77. Chung, J.H.; Hwang, H.J.; Han, C.H.; Son, B.S.; Kim, D.H.; Park, M.S. Association between sarcopenia and metabolic syndrome in chronic obstructive pulmonary disease: The Korea National Health and Nutrition Examination Survey (KNHANES) from 2008 to 2011. *COPD J. Chronic Obstr. Pulm. Dis.* **2015**, *12*, 82–89. [CrossRef]
78. Cruz-Jentoft, A.J.; Bahat, G.; Bauer, J.; Boirie, Y.; Bruyère, O.; Cederholm, T.; Cooper, C.; Landi, F.; Rolland, Y.; Sayer, A.A.; et al. Sarcopenia: Revised European consensus on definition and diagnosis. *Age Ageing* **2019**, *48*, 16–31. [CrossRef]

79. Nijholt, W.; ter Beek, L.; Hobbelen, J.S.M.; van der Vaart, H.; Wempe, J.B.; van der Schans, C.P.; Jager-Wittenaar, H. The added value of ultrasound muscle measurements in patients with COPD: An exploratory study. *Clin. Nutr. ESPEN* **2019**, *30*, 152–158. [CrossRef]
80. Neo, H.Y.; Xu, H.Y.; Wu, H.Y.; Hum, A. Prediction of Poor Short-Term Prognosis and Unmet Needs in Advanced Chronic Obstructive Pulmonary Disease: Use of the Two-Minute Walking Distance Extracted from a Six-Minute Walk Test. *J. Palliat. Med.* **2017**, *20*, 821–828. [CrossRef]
81. Wu, Z.Y.; Han, Y.X.; Niu, M.E.; Chen, Y.; Zhang, X.Q.; Qian, H.Y. Handgrip strength is associated with dyspnoea and functional exercise capacity in male patients with stable COPD. *Int. J. Tuberc. Lung Dis.* **2019**, *23*, 428–432. [CrossRef]
82. McDonald, M.L.N.; Diaz, A.A.; Ross, J.C.; Estepar, R.S.J.; Zhou, L.; Regan, E.A.; Eckbo, E.; Muralidhar, N.; Come, C.E.; Cho, M.H.; et al. Quantitative computed tomography measures of pectoralis muscle area and disease severity in chronic obstructive pulmonary disease: A cross-sectional study. *Ann. Am. Thorac. Soc.* **2014**, *11*, 326–334. [CrossRef]
83. Diaz, A.A.; Martinez, C.H.; Harmouche, R.; Young, T.P.; McDonald, M.L.; Ross, J.C.; Han, M.L.; Bowler, R.; Make, B.; Regan, E.A.; et al. Pectoralis muscle area and mortality in smokers without airflow obstruction. *Respir. Res.* **2018**, *19*, 6–13. [CrossRef] [PubMed]
84. Bak, S.H.; Kwon, S.O.; Han, S.S.; Kim, W.J. Computed tomography-derived area and density of pectoralis muscle associated disease severity and longitudinal changes in chronic obstructive pulmonary disease: A case control study. *Respir. Res.* **2019**, *20*, 226. [CrossRef] [PubMed]
85. Kao, C.C.; Hsu, J.W.-C.; Bandi, V.; Hanania, N.A.; Kheradmand, F.; Jahoor, F. Glucose and pyruvate metabolism in severe chronic obstructive pulmonary disease. *J. Appl. Physiol.* **2012**, *112*, 42–47. [CrossRef] [PubMed]
86. Rao, Z.Y.; Wu, X.T.; Wang, M.Y.; Hu, W. Comparison between measured and predicted resting energy expenditure in mechanically ventilated patients with COPD. *Asia Pac. J. Clin. Nutr.* **2012**, *21*, 338–346. [PubMed]
87. Kovarik, M.; Najpaverova, S.; Koblizek, V.; Zadak, Z.; Hronek, M. Association of resting energy expenditure and nutritional substrate oxidation with COPD stage and prediction indexes. *Respir. Med.* **2020**, *174*, 106174. [CrossRef] [PubMed]
88. Morikawa, K.; Tabira, K.; Takemura, H.; Inaba, S.; Kusuki, H.; Hashitsume, Y.; Suzuki, Y.; Tenpaku, Y.; Yasuma, T.; D'alessandro-Gabazza, C.N.; et al. A prediction equation to assess resting energy expenditure in Japanese patients with COPD. *J. Clin. Med.* **2020**, *9*, 3455. [CrossRef]
89. Bendavid, I.; Lobo, D.N.; Barazzoni, R.; Cederholm, T.; Coëffier, M.; de van der Schueren, M.; Fontaine, E.; Hiesmayr, M.; Laviano, A.; Pichard, C.; et al. The centenary of the Harris–Benedict equations: How to assess energy requirements best? Recommendations from the ESPEN expert group. *Clin. Nutr.* **2021**, *40*, 690–701. [CrossRef]
90. Jonker, R.; Deutz, N.E.P.; Ligthart-Melis, G.C.; Zachria, A.J.; Veley, E.A.; Harrykissoon, R.; Engelen, M.P.K.J. Preserved anabolic threshold and capacity as estimated by a novel stable tracer approach suggests no anabolic resistance or increased requirements in weight stable COPD patients. *Clin. Nutr.* **2019**, *38*, 1833–1843. [CrossRef]
91. Engelen, M.P.K.J.; Wouters, E.F.M.; Deutz, N.E.P.; Menheere, P.P.C.A.; Schols, A.M.W.J. Factors contributing to alterations in skeletal muscle and plasma amino acid profiles in patients with chronic obstructive pulmonary disease. *Am. J. Clin. Nutr.* **2000**, *72*, 1480–1487. [CrossRef]
92. Calder, P.C.; Laviano, A.; Lonnqvist, F.; Muscaritoli, M.; Öhlander, M.; Schols, A. Targeted medical nutrition for cachexia in chronic obstructive pulmonary disease: A randomized, controlled trial. *J. Cachexia. Sarcopenia Muscle* **2018**, *9*, 28–40. [CrossRef]
93. Deutz, N.E.; Ziegler, T.R.; Matheson, E.M.; Matarese, L.E.; Tappenden, K.A.; Baggs, G.E.; Nelson, J.L.; Luo, M.; Hegazi, R.; Jonnalagadda, S.S. Reduced mortality risk in malnourished hospitalized older adult patients with COPD treated with a specialized oral nutritional supplement: Sub-group analysis of the NOURISH study. *Clin. Nutr.* **2021**, *40*, 1388–1395. [CrossRef] [PubMed]
94. Jonker, R.; Deutz, N.E.P.; Schols, A.M.W.J.; Veley, E.A.; Harrykissoon, R.; Zachria, A.J.; Engelen, M.P.K.J. Whole body protein anabolism in COPD patients and healthy older adults is not enhanced by adding either carbohydrates or leucine to a serving of protein. *Clin. Nutr.* **2019**, *38*, 1684–1691. [CrossRef] [PubMed]
95. Jo, Y.S.; Choi, S.M.; Lee, J.; Park, Y.S.; Lee, S.M.; Yim, J.J.; Yoo, C.G.; Kim, Y.W.; Han, S.K.; Lee, C.H. The relationship between chronic obstructive pulmonary disease and comorbidities: A cross-sectional study using data from KNHANES 2010–2012. *Respir. Med.* **2015**, *109*, 96–104. [CrossRef] [PubMed]
96. Williams, M.T.; Effing, T.W.; Paquet, C.; Gibbs, C.A.; Lewthwaite, H.; Katrina Li, L.S.; Phillips, A.C.; Johnston, K.N. Counseling for health behavior change in people with COPD: Systematic review. *Int. J. COPD* **2017**, *12*, 2165–2178. [CrossRef]
97. Varraso, R.; Barr, R.G.; Willett, W.C.; Speizer, F.E.; Camargo, C.A. Fish intake and risk of chronic obstructive pulmonary disease in 2 large US cohorts. *Am. J. Clin. Nutr.* **2015**, *101*, 354–361. [CrossRef]
98. Kim, T.; Choi, H.; Kim, J. Association between Dietary Nutrient Intake and Chronic Obstructive Pulmonary Disease Severity: A Nationwide Population-Based Representative Sample. *COPD J. Chronic Obstr. Pulm. Dis.* **2020**, *17*, 49–58. [CrossRef]
99. Whyand, T.; Hurst, J.R.; Beckles, M.; Caplin, M.E. Pollution and respiratory disease: Can diet or supplements help? A review. *Respir. Res.* **2018**, *19*, 79. [CrossRef]
100. Hong, J.Y.; Lee, C.Y.; Lee, M.G.; Kim, Y.S. Effects of dietary antioxidant vitamins on lung functions according to gender and smoking status in Korea: A population-based cross-sectional study. *BMJ Open* **2018**, *8*, e020656. [CrossRef]
101. Park, H.J.; Byun, M.K.; Kim, H.J.; Kim, J.Y.; Kim, Y.I.; Yoo, K.H.; Chun, E.M.; Jung, J.Y.; Lee, S.H.; Ahn, C.M. Dietary vitamin C intake protects against COPD: The Korea National Health and Nutrition Examination Survey in 2012. *Int. J. COPD* **2016**, *11*, 2721–2728. [CrossRef]

102. Salari-Moghaddam, A.; Milajerdi, A.; Larijani, B.; Esmaillzadeh, A. Processed red meat intake and risk of COPD: A systematic review and dose-response meta-analysis of prospective cohort studies. *Clin. Nutr.* **2019**, *38*, 1109–1116. [CrossRef]
103. Min, J.E.; Huh, D.A.; Moon, K.W. The joint effects of some beverages intake and smoking on chronic obstructive pulmonary disease in Korean adults: Data analysis of the Korea national health and nutrition examination survey (KNHANES), 2008–2015. *Int. J. Environ. Res. Public Health* **2020**, *17*, 2611. [CrossRef] [PubMed]
104. Farooqi, N.; Nordström, L.; Lundgren, R.; Sandström, T.; Håglin, L. Changes in body weight and physical performance after receiving dietary advice in patients with chronic obstructive pulmonary disease (COPD): 1-year follow-up. *Arch. Gerontol. Geriatr.* **2011**, *53*, 70–75. [CrossRef] [PubMed]
105. Buys, D.R.; Campbell, A.D.; Godfryd, A.; Flood, K.; Kitchin, E.; Kilgore, M.L.; Allocca, S.; Locher, J.L. Meals Enhancing Nutrition After Discharge: Findings from a Pilot Randomized Controlled Trial. *J. Acad. Nutr. Diet.* **2017**, *117*, 599–608. [CrossRef] [PubMed]
106. Torre, G.L.A.; Cocchiara, R.A.; Sordo, E.L.O.; Chiarini, M.; Siliquini, R.; Firenze, A.; Maurici, M.; Agati, L.; Saulle, R.; Mannocci, A. Counseling intervention to improve quality of life in patients with pre-existing acute myocardial infarction (AMI) or chronic obstructive pulmonary disease (COPD): A pilot study. *J. Prev. Med. Hyg.* **2018**, *59*, E153–E158. [PubMed]
107. Ferreira, I.M.; Brooks, D.; White, J.; Goldstein, R. Nutritional supplementation for stable chronic obstructive pulmonary disease. *Cochrane Database Syst. Rev.* **2012**, *12*, CD000998. [CrossRef]
108. van Beers, M.; Rutten-van Mölken, M.P.M.H.; van de Bool, C.; Boland, M.; Kremers, S.P.J.; Franssen, F.M.E.; van Helvoort, A.; Gosker, H.R.; Wouters, E.F.; Schols, A.M.W.J. Clinical outcome and cost-effectiveness of a 1-year nutritional intervention programme in COPD patients with low muscle mass: The randomized controlled NUTRAIN trial. *Clin. Nutr.* **2020**, *39*, 405–413. [CrossRef]
109. Benito Martínez, M.d.P.; Guarro Riba, M.; La Serna Infantes, J.E.; Camere Colarossi, D.M.; Camere Torrealva, M.A.; Tort, G. Estado Nutricional y funcional en pacientes con enfermedad pulmonar obstructiva crónica: Efectos de la suplementación nutricional oral (Estudio OFOS). *Nutr. Hosp.* **2017**, *34*, 776–783.
110. Khan, N.A.; Kumar, N.; Daga, M.K. Effect of dietary supplementation on body composition, pulmonary function and health-related quality of life in patients with stable COPD. *Tanaffos* **2016**, *15*, 225–235.
111. van de Bool, C.; Rutten, E.P.A.; van Helvoort, A.; Franssen, F.M.E.; Wouters, E.F.M.; Schols, A.M.W.J. A randomized clinical trial investigating the efficacy of targeted nutrition as adjunct to exercise training in COPD. *J. Cachexia. Sarcopenia Muscle* **2017**, *8*, 748–758. [CrossRef]
112. Sugawara, K.; Takahashi, H.; Kashiwagura, T.; Yamada, K.; Yanagida, S.; Homma, M.; Dairiki, K.; Sasaki, H.; Kawagoshi, A.; Satake, M.; et al. Effect of anti-inflammatory supplementation with whey peptide and exercise therapy in patients with COPD. *Respir. Med.* **2012**, *106*, 1526–1534. [CrossRef]
113. Van De Bool, C.; Mattijssen-Verdonschot, C.; Van Melick, P.P.M.J.; Spruit, M.A.; Franssen, F.M.E.; Wouters, E.F.M.; Schols, A.M.W.J.; Rutten, E.P.A. Quality of dietary intake in relation to body composition in patients with chronic obstructive pulmonary disease eligible for pulmonary rehabilitation. *Eur. J. Clin. Nutr.* **2014**, *68*, 159–165. [CrossRef] [PubMed]
114. Payne, C.; Wiffen, P.; Martin, S. Interventions for fatigue and weight loss in adults with advanced progressive illness: A cochrane overview of systematic reviews. *Cochrane Database Syst. Rev.* **2017**, *2017*, CD008427.
115. Korkmaz, C.; Demirbas, S.; Vatansev, H.; Yildirim, E.; Teke, T.; Zamani, A. Effects of comprehensive and intensive pulmonary rehabilitation and nutritional support on quality of life and functional status in patients with chronic obstructive pulmonary disease. *J. Int. Med. Res.* **2020**, *48*, 1–14. [CrossRef] [PubMed]
116. Jonker, R.; Deutz, N.E.P.; Erbland, M.L.; Anderson, P.J.; Engelen, M.P.K.J. Hydrolyzed casein and whey protein meals comparably stimulate net whole-body protein synthesis in COPD patients with nutritional depletion without an additional effect of leucine co-ingestion. *Clin. Nutr.* **2014**, *33*, 211–220. [CrossRef] [PubMed]
117. Reeves, A.; White, H.; Sosnowski, K.; Tran, K.; Jones, M.; Palmer, M. Energy and protein intakes of hospitalised patients with acute respiratory failure receiving non-invasive ventilation. *Clin. Nutr.* **2014**, *33*, 1068–1073. [CrossRef] [PubMed]
118. Ogasawara, T.; Marui, S.; Miura, E.; Sugiura, M.; Matsuyama, W.; Aoshima, Y.; Kasamatsu, N.; Ogiku, M.; Ikematsu, Y. Effect of eicosapentaenoic acid on prevention of lean body mass depletion in patients with exacerbation of chronic obstructive pulmonary disease: A prospective randomized controlled trial. *Clin. Nutr. ESPEN* **2018**, *28*, 67–73. [CrossRef] [PubMed]
119. Wandrag, L.; Brett, S.J.; Frost, G.; Hickson, M. Impact of supplementation with amino acids or their metabolites on muscle wasting in patients with critical illness or other muscle wasting illness: A systematic review. *J. Hum. Nutr. Diet.* **2015**, *28*, 313–330. [CrossRef]
120. Jonker, R.; Ep Deutz, N.; Erbland, M.L.; Anderson, P.J.; Pkj Engelen, M. Effectiveness of essential amino acid supplementation in stimulating whole body net protein anabolism is comparable between COPD patients and healthy older adults HHS Public Access continuous IV infusion of L-[ring-2 H 5]-PHE and L-[ring-2 H2]-tyrosine. *Metabolism* **2017**, *69*, 120–129. [CrossRef]
121. Dal Negro, R.W.; Testa, A.; Aquilani, R.; Tognella, S.; Pasini, E.; Barbieri, A.; Boschi, F. Essential amino acid supplementation in patients with severe COPD: A step towards home rehabilitation. *Monaldi Arch. Chest Dis. Pulm. Ser.* **2012**, *77*, 67–75. [CrossRef]
122. Zhang, L.; Yuan, Q.Y. Vitamin D should be supplemented more actively in elderly patients with coronary heart disease combined with COPD. *Int. J. COPD* **2016**, *11*, 1359–1365. [CrossRef]
123. Hendryx, M.; Luo, J. A test of vitamin D benefits on respiratory health mediated through inflammatory markers. *Chron. Respir. Dis.* **2015**, *12*, 24–30. [CrossRef] [PubMed]

124. Gouzi, F.; Maury, J.; Héraud, N.; Molinari, N.; Bertet, H.; Ayoub, B.; Blaquière, M.; Bughin, F.; De Rigal, P.; Poulain, M.; et al. Additional effects of nutritional antioxidant supplementation on peripheral muscle during pulmonary rehabilitation in COPD patients: A randomized controlled trial. *Oxid. Med. Cell. Longev.* **2019**, *2019*, 5496346. [CrossRef] [PubMed]
125. Guertin, K.A.; Grant, R.K.; Arnold, K.B.; Burwell, L.; Hartline, J.; Goodman, P.J.; Minasian, L.M.; Lippman, S.M.; Klein, E.; Cassano, P.A. Effect of long-term vitamin E and selenium supplementation on urine F2-isoprostanes, a biomarker of oxidative stress. *Free Radic. Biol. Med.* **2016**, *95*, 349–356. [CrossRef] [PubMed]
126. Vogiatzis, I.; Zakynthinos, S. The physiological basis of rehabilitation in chronic heart and lung disease. *J. Appl. Physiol.* **2013**, *115*, 16–21. [CrossRef] [PubMed]
127. Constantin, D.; Menon, M.K.; Houchen-Wolloff, L.; Morgan, M.D.; Singh, S.J.; Greenhaff, P.; Steiner, M.C. Skeletal muscle molecular responses to resistance training and dietary supplementation in COPD. *Thorax* **2013**, *68*, 625–633. [CrossRef]
128. Meys, R.; Stoffels, A.A.F.; de Brandt, J.; van Hees, H.W.H.; Franssen, F.M.E.; Sillen, M.J.H.; Wouters, E.F.M.; Burtin, C.; Klijn, P.; Bij de Vaate, E.; et al. Beta-alanine supplementation in patients with COPD receiving non-linear periodised exercise training or neuromuscular electrical stimulation: Protocol of two randomised, double-blind, placebo-controlled trials. *BMJ Open* **2020**, *10*, e038836. [CrossRef]
129. Coppi, F.; Nasi, M.; Farinetti, A.; Manenti, A.; Gallina, S.; Mattioli, A.V. Physical activity, sedentary behaviour, and diet in menopausal women: Comparison between COVID19 "first wave" and "second wave" of pandemic in Italy. *Prog. Nutr.* **2021**, *23*, e2021194. [CrossRef]
130. Loprinzi, P.D.; Walker, J.F. Increased daily movement associates with reduced mortality among COPD patients having systemic inflammation. *Int. J. Clin. Pract.* **2016**, *70*, 286–291. [CrossRef]
131. Fekete, M.; Kerti, M.; Fazekas-Pongor, V.; Balazs, P.; Csizmadia, Z.; Nemeth, A.N.; Tarantini, S.; Varga, J.T. Effect of interval training with non-invasive ventilation in severe chronic obstructive pulmonary disease—A prospective cohort study with matched control group. *Ann. Palliat. Med.* **2021**, *10*, 5289–5298. [CrossRef]
132. Emtner, M.; Hallin, R.; Arnardottir, R.H.; Janson, C. Effect of physical training on fat-free mass in patients with chronic obstructive pulmonary disease (COPD). *Ups. J. Med. Sci.* **2015**, *120*, 52–58. [CrossRef]
133. Paulin, F.V.; Zagatto, A.M.; Chiappa, G.R.; Müller, P. de T. Addition of vitamin B12 to exercise training improves cycle ergometer endurance in advanced COPD patients: A randomized and controlled study. *Respir. Med.* **2017**, *122*, 23–29. [CrossRef] [PubMed]
134. Parker, D.R.; Liu, J.; Roberts, M.B.; Eaton, C.B. Is inflammatory chronic obstructive pulmonary disease a coronary heart disease risk equivalent? A longitudinal analysis of the third National Health and Nutrition Examination Survey (NHANES III), 1988–1994. *BMC Pulm. Med.* **2014**, *14*, 195. [CrossRef] [PubMed]
135. Park, S.K.; Larson, J.L. The relationship between physical activity and metabolic syndrome in people with chronic obstructive pulmonary disease. *J. Cardiovasc. Nurs.* **2014**, *29*, 499–507. [CrossRef] [PubMed]
136. Yentes, J.M.; Sayles, H.; Meza, J.; Mannino, D.M.; Rennard, S.I.; Stergiou, N. Walking abnormalities are associated with COPD: An investigation of the NHANES III dataset. *Respir. Med.* **2011**, *105*, 80–87. [CrossRef] [PubMed]
137. Lewthwaite, H.; Olds, T.; Williams, M.T.; Effing, T.W.; Dumuid, D. Use of time in chronic obstructive pulmonary disease: Longitudinal associations with symptoms and quality of life using a compositional analysis approach. *PLoS ONE* **2019**, *14*, e214058. [CrossRef]
138. Shah, A.M.; Shah, R.B.; Kachoria, S. Health-related quality of life and associated factors in patients with chronic obstructive pulmonary disease. *Drugs Ther. Perspect.* **2019**, *35*, 241–249. [CrossRef]
139. Loprinzi, P.D.; Walker, J.F.; Lee, H. Association between physical activity and inflammatory markers among U.S. Adults with chronic obstructive pulmonary disease. *Am. J. Health Promot.* **2014**, *29*, 81–88. [CrossRef]
140. WHO. *WHO Guidelines on Physical Activity and Sedentary Behaviour*; World Health Organization: Geneva, Switzerland, 2020. Available online: https://www.ncbi.nlm.nih.gov/books/NBK566045/ (accessed on 16 January 2023).
141. Susanthy, D.; Erna, K.; Rahayu, W.K.S. Effect of Ophiocephalus striatus Extract on the Levels of TNF-α, CRP, Leptin, Adiponectin, and COPD Assessment Test (CAT) Score in Stable COPD Patients with Muscle Wasting. *Turk. J. Immunol.* **2018**, *6*, 23–29. [CrossRef]
142. Ingadottir, A.R.; Beck, A.M.; Baldwin, C.; Weekes, C.E.; Geirsdottir, O.G.; Ramel, A.; Gislason, T.; Gunnarsdottir, I. Oral nutrition supplements and between-meal snacks for nutrition therapy in patients with COPD identified as at nutritional risk: A randomised feasibility trial. *BMJ Open Respir. Res.* **2019**, *6*, e000349. [CrossRef]
143. Lee, S.H.; Kim, S.J.; Han, Y.; Ryu, Y.J.; Lee, J.H.; Chang, J.H. Hand grip strength and chronic obstructive pulmonary disease in Korea: An analysis in KNHANES VI. *Int. J. COPD* **2017**, *12*, 2313–2321. [CrossRef]
144. Jeong, M.; Kang, H.K.; Song, P.; Park, H.K.; Jung, H.; Lee, S.-S.; Koo, H.-K. Hand grip strength in patients with chronic obstructive pulmonary disease. *Int. J. Chron. Obstruct. Pulmon. Dis.* **2017**, *12*, 2385–2390. [CrossRef] [PubMed]
145. Poot, C.C.; Meijer, E.; Kruis, A.L.; Smidt, N.; Chavannes, N.H.; Honkoop, P.J. Integrated disease management interventions for patients with chronic obstructive pulmonary disease. *Cochrane Database Syst. Rev.* **2021**, *2021*, CD009437. [CrossRef]
146. Valentijn, P.I.M.P.; Tymchenko, L.; Arends, R.Y. Effectiveness of Integrated Care for Diabetes Mellitus Type 2, Cardiovascular and Chronic Respiratory Diseases: A Systematic Review and Meta-Analysis. *Int. J. Integr. Care* **2024**, *24*, 16. [CrossRef] [PubMed]
147. Beijers, R.J.H.C.G.; Steiner, M.C.; Schols, A.M.W.J. The role of diet and nutrition in the management of COPD. *Eur. Respir. Rev.* **2023**, *32*, 230003. [CrossRef]

148. Allard, J.P.; Keller, H.; Gramlich, L.; Jeejeebhoy, K.N.; Laporte, M.; Duerksen, D.R. GLIM criteria has fair sensitivity and specificity for diagnosing malnutrition when using SGA as comparator. *Clin. Nutr.* **2020**, *39*, 2771–2777. [CrossRef]
149. Malmstrom, T.K.; Miller, D.K.; Simonsick, E.M.; Ferrucci, L.; Morley, J.E. SARC-F: A symptom score to predict persons with sarcopenia at risk for poor functional outcomes. *J. Cachexia Sarcopenia Muscle* **2016**, *7*, 28–36. [CrossRef] [PubMed] [PubMed Central]

nutrients

MDPI

Article

Impact of Elexacaftor–Tezacaftor–Ivacaftor Therapy on Body Composition, Dietary Intake, Biomarkers, and Quality of Life in People with Cystic Fibrosis: A Prospective Observational Study

Francisco Hevilla [1,2,3], Nuria Porras [2,3], María Victoria Girón [4], María García-Olivares [1,2,3], Marina Padial [1,2,3], Francisco José Sánchez-Torralvo [2,3], Casilda Olveira [1,2,4,*] and Gabriel Olveira [1,2,3,5,*]

1 Departamento de Medicina y Dermatología, Facultad de Medicina, University of Malaga, 29010 Malaga, Spain
2 Instituto de Investigación Biomédica de Málaga (IBIMA), Plataforma Bionand, 29010 Malaga, Spain
3 Unidad de Gestión Clínica de Endocrinología y Nutrición, Hospital Regional Universitario de Málaga, 29007 Malaga, Spain
4 Unidad de Gestión Clínica de Neumología, Hospital Regional Universitario de Málaga, 29010 Malaga, Spain
5 Centro de Investigación Biomédica en Red de Diabetes y Enfermedades Metabólicas Asociadas (CIBERDEM), Instituto de Salud Carlos III, 28029 Madrid, Spain
* Correspondence: casi1547@separ.es (C.O.); gabolvfus@uma.es (G.O.)

Abstract: Background: The combination of elexacaftor–tezacaftor–ivacaftor modulators (ETI) has improved clinical outcomes for people with cystic fibrosis (pwCF). **Objectives:** This study aimed to evaluate changes in nutritional and morphofunctional assessments, as well as anxiety, depression symptoms, and quality of life, in pwCF after starting ETI therapy. **Methods:** This was a prospective observational study. We measured body composition (fat mass [FM] and fat-free mass [FFM]) using bioelectrical impedance analysis (BIA) and skinfold thickness measurements (SMs). We also assessed hand grip strength, dietary intake via surveys, blood and stool biomarkers, symptoms of anxiety and depression using the Hospital Anxiety and Depression Scale [HADS], and quality of life through the Cystic Fibrosis Questionnaire—Revised (CFQR). **Results:** A total of 31 pwCF were evaluated. Significant improvements were observed in respiratory function and quality of life, alongside an average weight increase of approximately 5 kg (60% FM and 40% FFM). The prevalence of malnutrition, based on BMI and the FFM index, decreased significantly, while the rate of overweight/obesity increased. Biomarker analysis indicated better nutrient absorption and reduced intestinal inflammation, as evidenced by significant changes in faecal calprotectin, nitrogen, and fat levels, as well as blood lipid and vitamin profiles. **Conclusions:** Despite a reduction in caloric intake, an increase in weight was observed one year after initiating ETI. This increase was attributed to gains in both FM and FFM, suggesting improved metabolic efficiency and nutrient absorption. Both SM and BIA were found to be useful assessment tools. These findings indicate the need to modify the nutritional approach, focusing on the quality rather than the quantity of intake, and aiming for an appropriate body composition (FFM) rather than solely focusing on BMI.

Keywords: cystic fibrosis; elexacaftor–tezacaftor–ivacaftor (ETI); body composition; bioelectrical impedance analysis (BIA); skinfold thickness measurement; dietary surveys

1. Introduction

Cystic fibrosis (CF) is a disease caused by the alteration of a single gene, the CFTR gene (cystic fibrosis transmembrane conductance regulator). The protein encoded by the CFTR gene functions as a chloride channel, and mutations result in a defect in chloride transport in the epithelial cells of the respiratory, hepatobiliary, gastrointestinal, reproductive, pancreatic, and sweat gland systems. Due to the multitude of organs and systems it affects, CF is a complex and multisystemic disease that requires a multidisciplinary approach [1].

Currently, the triple combination of CFTR modulators, elexacaftor–tezacaftor–ivacaftor (ETI), has become the new standard of care for people with CF (pwCF) carrying at least one F508del CFTR variant [2,3]. Data from randomised clinical trials revealed improvements in respiratory outcomes (respiratory symptoms, lung function, exacerbations) and body mass index [2,4,5], which were largely confirmed in real-world studies [6–8].

CF-associated poor nutritional status is a multifactorial syndrome caused by nutrient malabsorption, inadequate nutrient intake, decreased appetite, and higher energy needs [9]. Poor nutritional status is linked to worse pulmonary function and increased mortality in pwCF. Improved nutritional CF care significantly reduced the rate of malnutrition before the generalisation of ETI modulator treatment; however, figures close to 25% continued to be reported in both children and adults [10,11].

The guidelines emphasise the need to conduct a longitudinal assessment of body composition to obtain estimates of fat mass (FM) and fat-free mass (FFM) [3,12] because their association with respiratory outcomes is stronger than for BMI alone, and because a normal or high BMI can mask low FFM [13–15]. This could be important in the context of CFTR modulator therapy [3,15]. The choice of body composition (BC) method should be guided based on availability, resources, technical factors, and clinical factors [12].

Weight improvements have been published in the vast majority of real-life studies after ETI treatment [6–8]. However, few have evaluated the change in BC [11,16–19], and the findings regarding which components—fat mass and/or fat-free mass—increase remain inconsistent. Additionally, no study has examined the use of anthropometric methods, such as skinfold thickness measurements (SMs), in patient follow-up. These could be particularly useful in settings where more advanced techniques like bioelectrical impedance analysis (BIA), dual-energy X-ray absorptiometry (DXA), ultrasonography, or computed tomography (CT) are unavailable. The mechanisms behind weight gain after ETI remain unclear and are likely multifactorial. Improvements in intestinal absorption [20] and changes in biomarkers such as lipids and vitamins have been observed [8,20]. Moreover, only one study has prospectively evaluated dietary intake [21]. It is important to note that dietary intake may be influenced by anxiety and depression symptoms, which are common in pwCF and may, in turn, affect their quality of life in all its dimensions [22]. To date, no study has holistically evaluated all these aspects.

With this background, the objective of this study was to prospectively and comprehensively assess mid-term changes in morphofunctional evaluation, including body composition (via BIA and SM), hand dynamometry, prospective dietary surveys, blood and stool biomarkers, as well as symptoms of anxiety and depression, and quality of life in adults with cystic fibrosis (pwCF) following the initiation of ETI therapy.

2. Materials and Methods

Design: Prospective observational study of routine clinical practice. Adult pwCF from the Cystic Fibrosis Adult Unit who began taking elexacaftor–tezacaftor–ivacaftor were eligible for inclusion and were studied at baseline and one year after starting ETI treatment.

2.1. Morphofunctional Assessment

2.1.1. Body Composition

Weight and BC (phase angle, fat-free mass, and fat mass) were assessed using a BIA scale (TANITA MC980MA, TANITA Corporation, Tokyo, Japan), and height was obtained using a stadiometer (Holtain Limited, Crymych, UK). The skinfolds measured were the triceps, biceps, subscapular, and supra-iliac, using a Holtain constant pressure caliper (Holtain Limited, Crymych, UK). The same investigator (N.P.) performed the measurements in triplicate for each of the skinfolds assessed, and the mean was calculated. FM and FFM were estimated according to the formulas of Siri and Durnin [23,24]. The FFM index (FFMI) was calculated using anthropometry and BIA. The prevalence of malnutrition was determined according to the criteria: <15 kg/m^2 for women or <17 kg/m^2 for men.

2.1.2. Muscle Strength

Muscle strength was assessed using a Jamar dynamometer (Asimow Engineering Co., Los Angeles, CA, USA) on the dominant hand. The measurement was repeated three times, and the mean was calculated.

2.1.3. Dietary Questionnaire

A 4-day prospective dietary questionnaire was completed. The data provided were analysed using a computer application designed by our group for this purpose (Dietstat®, FIMABIS, Málaga, Spain) [25] and the food composition tables of Jiménez and Mataix [26,27] and BEDCA [28] were used. In cases where patients were receiving medical nutritional therapy through oral nutritional supplements or enteral nutrition via a feeding tube, the composition was also included in the database of the DIETSTAT programme and accounted for.

2.1.4. Laboratory Measurements

A complete blood test was performed to assess haemogram, coagulation, and biochemical values, including albumin, prealbumin, C-reactive protein, immunoglobulins (with an autoanalyzer), glycated haemoglobin (following the international recommendations for standardisation of the HbA1c measurement [29]), and fat-soluble vitamins (A, D, and E). Vitamins A and E were measured using High-Performance Liquid Chromatography (HPLC, Agilent 1200, Bio-Rad, Hercules, CA, USA) and vitamin D was assessed through an electrochemiluminescent immunoassay (Modular E-170, Roche Diagnostics, Mannheim, Germany). A 72 h stool sample was collected for the quantitative measurement of faecal fat and nitrogen by means of a spectrophotometer technique (near-infrared reflectance analysis), as well as elastase 1 (ELISA ScheBo, Biotech AG, Gießen, Germany)) and calprotectin (ELISA Calprest® Eurospital, Trieste, Italy).

2.2. Quality of Life—CFQR14+ (Spain)

It consists of 50 items divided into twelve domains. Scores range from 0 to 100, with higher scores indicating better HRQoL [30].

2.3. Assessment of Respiratory Status

The exacerbations recorded during the annual examination were assessed, considering those occurring in the year prior to the evaluation. They were classified into mild/moderate or severe (suggestive symptoms that worsen and require hospitalisation and/or intravenous antibiotics on an outpatient basis). Chronic colonisation was defined as the presence of three or more consecutive positive cultures for the same pathogen over a period of at least twelve months, with samples taken at least one month apart. Moreover, patients underwent forced spirometry following the guidelines of the Spanish Society of Pulmonology and Thoracic Surgery (SEPAR), determining the values of forced vital capacity (FVC), forced expiratory volume in 1 s (FEV1), and the ratio between both (FEV1/FVC) [31]. The values were expressed in absolute terms in ml and as percentages according to a reference population. We also evaluated the E-FACED-Score [32].

2.4. Hospital Anxiety and Depression Scale

It is a 14-item instrument: 7 questions measure depression and 7 measure anxiety. Respondents indicated the severity of each symptom over the past week. The maximum score is 21. A score of less than 8 is considered a negative result in the screening [33].

2.5. Statistical Analysis

Quantitative variables were expressed as the mean ± standard deviation, and the distribution was assessed using the Shapiro–Wilk test. Differences between quantitative variables were analysed using the paired Student's *t*-test or Wilcoxon test. Comparisons between the three groups were performed using ANOVA with Bonferroni post hoc tests or Kruskal–Wallis tests. The associations of the variables were evaluated by estimating the Pearson or Spearman correlation coefficient according to normality. For the comparison of proportions of qualitative variables, such as the percentage of malnourished and obese individuals before and after ETI, McNemar's test was used. For calculations, significance was set at $p < 0.05$ for two-tailed tests. Data analysis was performed with the JAMOVI program (version 2.3.28).

2.6. Ethics

All subjects gave their informed consent to participate in the study. The study was conducted in accordance with the Declaration of Helsinki, and the protocol was approved by the Research Ethics Committee of Málaga on 30 March 2021.

3. Results

A total of 34 adults with CF who initiated ETI were recruited, among which three were excluded during follow-up (one for lack of compliance and two for voluntarily undertaking a low-calorie diet to lose weight during the follow-up period). The patients began treatment with ETI at a mean age of 30.7 ± 9 years, and the average follow-up time was 1 year and 1 month. F508del homozygotes made up 29% of the study cohort, F508del heterozygotes 58%, and four patients (13%) received treatment as compassionate use (without the F508del mutation). Twenty-seven (87%) had pancreatic insufficiency, eight (26%) had carbohydrate intolerance, and seven had CF-related diabetes (22.5%), among which six received insulin treatment (19%). All patients treated with insulin continued the treatment after one year, and one person with carbohydrate intolerance achieved a normal curve without changes in the rest. Seven subjects were receiving oral nutritional supplements (ONSs) before treatment, and one person was on enteral nutrition via gastrostomy. After one year, only two continued ONSs, and gastrostomy was removed 6 months after starting ETI. Seven patients had HADSa (Hospital Anxiety and Depression Scale anxiety subscale) scores above 8, and after one year, only five remained the same; two had HADSd (depression subscale) scores above 8, and these remained unchanged after one year.

Tables 1–5 summarise the changes before and after treatment with ETI. We observed significant differences in respiratory spirometric parameters, exacerbations, and chronic colonisation by Staphylococcus aureus (Table 1); weight and body composition (BMI, FM, FFM, FFM index, and the percentage of people with malnutrition, overweight/obesity, and FFM malnutrition), both measured by SM and BIA (Table 2); calories from dietary intake and grams of macronutrients (total and monounsaturated fats and carbohydrates) (Table 3); LDL cholesterol, HbA1C, immunoglobulin G, vitamin A, nitrogen, fat, and faecal calprotectin (Table 4); and quality of life dimensions: vitality, body, eating, treatment, health, weight, and respiratory (Table 5).

The weight gain was significantly greater ($p < 0.05$) in patients with CF with a BMI less than 18.5 kg/m^2 at the beginning ($n = 7$: 7.2 ± 5 kg) and also in those with overweight or obesity (OW/O) ($n = 5$: 9.7 ± 5.4 kg) compared to those with normal weight ($n = 19$: 2.7 ± 2.7 kg).

We observed significant negative correlations between the increase in weight ($p = 0.043$), FM ($p = 0.023$), and FFM ($p = 0.033$) measured by skinfolds and the baseline FEV1/FVC ratio, as well as positive correlations between the number of severe exacerbations in the year prior to starting ETI and the increase in FFM (BIA) ($p = 0.022$) and almost significant FFM by skinfolds ($p = 0.08$).

Table 1. General characteristics and respiratory status.

	Pre ETI (n = 31)	Post ETI (n = 31)	p-Value
Age	30.7 (±9)	31.9 (±9)	<0.001
Pancreatic insufficiency (n, %)	27 (87%)	27 (87%)	1
Endocrine pancreas			
Glucose intolerance	8 (26%)	7 (22.5%)	0.9
CF related diabetes	7 (22.5%)	7 (22.5%)	1
Insulin therapy	6 (19%)	6 (19%)	1
Mild exacerbations	1.1 (±1.2)	0.4 (±0.7)	0.004
Severe exacerbations	0.6 (±0.9)	0.1(±0.3)	0.021
FEV_1 (mL)	1849.0 (±977.3)	2105.1 (±1012.8)	0.001
% FEV_1	51.4 (±22.2)	58.5 (±23.3)	<0.001
FVC (mL)	2711.0 (±1095.6)	3043.6 (±1126.7)	<0.001
% FVC	61.3 (±19.0)	68.0 (±19.0)	<0.001
FEV_1/FVC	0.66 (±0.12)	0.67 (±0.11)	0.289
Chronic colonisation of the respiratory tract (n, %)			
Haemophilus influenzae	2 (6%)	2 (6%)	1
Pseudomonas aeruginosa	12 (35%)	8 (23.5%)	0.125
Staphylococcus aureus	18 (53%)	12 (35%)	0.031
E-FACED Score	3.6 (±20.1)	3.1 (±15.3)	0.100

Data are shown as mean (±standard deviation). Elexacaftor–tezacaftor–ivacaftor (ETI); FEV_1: forced expiratory volume in 1 s; FVC: forced vital capacity. E-FACED is a scoring system used to predict the risk of exacerbations in patients with bronchiectasis: (exacerbations, forced expiratory volume in 1 s (FEV1), age, colonisation with pseudomonas aeruginosa, radiological extent of the disease, and dyspnoea).

Table 2. Body composition and muscle strength.

	Pre ETI (n = 31)	Post ETI (n = 31)	p-Value
Weight (kg)	59.2 (±15.2)	64.1 (±17.1)	<0.001
BMI (kg/m^2)	21.5 (±3.8)	23.2 (±4.2)	<0.001
% low BMI	22.6	3.2	0.020
% overweight/obesity	16.1	25.8	0.020
% FM_{SM}	20.7 (±8.7)	23.3 (±9.5)	<0.001
FM_{SM} (kg)	12.3 (± 6.5)	14.9 (±7.6)	<0.001
% FM_{SM}	79.3 (±8.7)	76.7 (±9.5)	<0.001
FFM_{SM} (kg)	46.0 (±11.1)	48.0 (±12.0)	<0.001
$FFMI_{SM}$ (kg/m^2)	16.8 (±2.6)	17.4 (±2.7)	<0.001
% low $FFMI_{SM}$	35.5	16.7	0.030
% FM_{BIA}	22.9 (±11.4)	24.5 (±7.8)	0.326
FM_{BIA} (kg)	13.5 (±6.8)	16.8 (±8.3)	<0.001
%FFM_{BIA}	77.2 (±11.5)	75.3 (±8.0)	0.210
FFM (kg) $_{BIA}$	46.5 (±10.8)	48.6 (±11.5)	<0.001
$FFMI_{BIA}$	16.9 (±2.3)	17.6 (±2.4)	<0.001
% low $FFMI_{BIA}$	29	10.3	0.063
Phase angle (°)	5.3 (±0.8)	5.5 (±0.8)	0.099
Triceps ST (mm)	12.6 (±7.0)	15.1 (±7.8)	<0.001
Biceps ST (mm)	7.2 (±4.5)	8.9 (±5.5)	0.028
Subscapular ST (mm)	11.5 (±5.9)	13.7 (±6.8)	0.002
Abdominal ST (mm)	15.7 (±9.1)	17.7 (±9.3)	0.067
Suprailiac ST (mm)	10.6 (±7.5)	12.6 (±7.4)	0.029
MUAC (cm)	25.9 (±3.6)	27.2 (±4.1)	0.002
Max. dynamometry (kg)	34.1 (±12.7)	34.2 (±11.9)	0.884
Mean dynamometry (kg)	33.0 (±12.5)	33.3 (±11.7)	0.645

Data are shown as the mean (±standard deviation). Elexacaftor–tezacaftor–ivacaftor (ETI); BMI: body mass index; low BMI: BMI < 18.5 kg/m^2; overweight: BMI ≥ 25 and <30; obesity: BMI ≥ 30; FM: fat mass; $_{SM}$: estimated according to skinfold thickness measurements; FFM: fat-free mass; FFMI: fat-free mass index; low FFMI: <17 kg/m^2 in men and <15 kg/m^2 in women; $_{BIA}$: measured by bioelectrical impedance (BIA); ST: skinfold thickness; MUAC: mid-upper arm circumference; Max. dynamometry: maximum hand grip dynamometry.

Table 3. Dietary survey.

	Pre ETI (n = 31)	Post ETI (n = 31)	p-Value
Energy (kcal)	2621.0 (±456.3)	2355.9 (±369.7)	0.022
Protein (g)	109.6 (±29.4)	100.0 (±24.0)	0.064
Protein (% energy)	16.7 (±2.6)	16.9 (±2.6)	0.218
Total fat (g)	126.3 (±30.6)	107.6 (±22.7)	0.006
Total fat (% energy)	42 (±5.8)	39.0 (±4.2)	0.216
Saturated fat (g)	29.8 (±6.4)	26.9 (±6.1)	0.073
Saturated fat (% of fat)	28.0 (±5.4)	29.1 (±6.9)	0.616
Monounsaturated fat (g)	55.4 (±14.6)	47.2 (±11.2)	0.012
Monounsaturated fat (% of fat)	52.8 (±4.4)	51.7 (±6.1)	0.615
PUFAs (g)	19.9 (±10.4)	16.1 (±7.0)	0.112
PUFAs (% of fat)	18.6 (±7.2)	18.1 (±5.7)	0.834
PUFA-Omega 3 (g)	2.3 (±1.7)	2.3 (±1.3)	0.906
Carbohydrate (g)	261.1 (±48.8)	245.1 (±49.1)	0.035
Carbohydrate (% energy)	39.8 (±5.9)	41.1 (±5.1)	0.439
Fiber (g)	19.7 (±8.0)	19.0 (±8.7)	0.575
Medical nutritional therapy (n, %)			
Tube feeding	1 (2.9%)	0 (0%)	0.031
Oral nutritional supplements	7 (20%)	2 (5.8%)	

Data are shown as mean (±standard deviation. This refers to the average daily intake of energy and macronutrients. Elexacaftor–tezacaftor–ivacaftor (ETI); PUFAs: polyunsaturated fatty acids.

Table 4. Blood and stool test parameters.

	Pre ETI (n = 31)	Post ETI (n = 31)	p-Value
Neutrophils ($\times 10^3/\mu$L)	5.2 (±2.7)	4.4 (±3.0)	0.350
% Neutrophils	60.3 (±10.7)	56.2 (±11.0)	0.15
% Prothrombin time	93.1 (±14.3)	98.5 (±12.3)	0.172
Total cholesterol (mg/dL)	146.1 (± 34.9)	158.3 (±44.8)	0.098
HDL (mg/dL)	54.1 (±17.3)	52.8 (± 13.6)	0.639
LDL (mg/dL)	84.7 (±26.4)	101.7 (±34.5)	0.023
Triglycerides (mg/dL)	77.2 (±22.3)	89.9 (±33.1)	0.192
HbA1c (%)	5.9 (±0.8)	5.6 (±0.5)	0.017
Albumin (g/dL)	3.8 (±0.5)	3.9 (±0.3)	0.441
Prealbumin (mg/dL)	23.4 (±4.9)	26.4 (±7.7)	0.048
C-reactive protein (mg/dL)	11.7 (±16.7)	4.2 (±4.2)	0.130
Immunoglobulin G (mg/dL)	1606.8 (±393.5)	1392.5 (±324.1)	0.002
Vitamin A (µg/dL)	48. 1 (± 15.4)	55.7 (± 16.3)	0.048
Vitamin D3 (ng/mL)	36.1 (±16.2)	33.5 (±12.9)	0.570
Vitamin E (µg/dL)	1185.9 (± 354.0)	1277.6 (± 419.1)	0.389
Zinc (µg/dL)	77.3 (±18.1)	84.7 (±9.1)	0.153
Faecal nitrogen (g)	7.2 (±5.0)	3.7 (±2.6)	0.021
Faecal fat (g)	11.7 (±7.0)	8.3 (±4.6)	0.049
Faecal pancreatic elastase (µg/g)	107.6 (±183.3)	153.2 (±211.2)	0.369
Faecal calprotectin (µg/g)	623.1 (±835.1)	96.9 (±87.4)	0.048

Data are shown as mean (±standard deviation). Elexacaftor–tezacaftor–ivacaftor (ETI).

Table 5. Quality of life questionnaires (CFQ-R) and Hospital Anxiety and Depression Scale.

	Pre ETI (n = 31)	Post ETI (n = 31)	p-Value
$HADS_A$	4.9 (±3.5)	4.6 (±3.6)	0.640
$HADS_D$	2.9 (±2.2)	2.5 (±3.2)	0.520
CFQ-R role	87.0 (±15.0)	89.0 (±16.8)	0.606
CFQ-R vitality	67.3 (±19.1)	76.3 (±19.5)	0.032
CFQ-R emotion	84.5 (±13.7)	84.3 (±15.5)	0.943
CFQ-R social	76.9 (±13.6)	82.0 (±15.7)	0.082
CFQ-R physical	65.8 (±20.7)	70.2 (±27.3)	0.344
CFQ-R body	68.9 (±20.8)	77. 8 (±18.4)	0.041

Table 5. *Cont.*

	Pre ETI (n = 31)	Post ETI (n = 31)	p-Value
CFQ-R eatings	88.5 (±17.4)	94.2 (±11.2)	0.048
CFQ-R treatment	54.7 (±21.3)	67.1 (±20.2)	0.017
CFQ-R health	60.5 (±19.0)	75.1 (±20.1)	0.009
CFQ-R weights	66.7 (±37.3)	81.3 (±27.4)	0.046
CFQ-R respiratory	61.3 (±1.9)	85.3 (±1.4)	<0.001
CFQ-R digestion	76.5 (±17.4)	78.2 (±16.2)	0.621

Data are shown as mean (±standard deviation). Elexacaftor–tezacaftor–ivacaftor (ETI); CFQ-R: Cystic Fibrosis Questionnaire—Revised. Application; HADSA: Hospital Anxiety and Depression Scale, anxiety subscale; HADSD: Hospital Anxiety and Depression Scale, depression subscale.

4. Discussion

In our study, we observed an average weight increase of approximately 5 kg during the first year of follow-up, consisting of 60% fat mass and 40% fat-free mass. Both skinfold measurements and bioelectrical impedance analysis were useful, yielding very similar results. These changes were accompanied by improvements in pulmonary function, quality of life, a decrease in caloric intake, and enhancements in biomarkers related to absorption and intestinal inflammation.

4.1. Morphofunctional Assessment

The prevalence of malnutrition (according to BMI) in our series decreased from 22.6% to 3.2%, while the prevalence of overweight/obesity (OW/O) increased from 16% to 26%. Both bioelectrical impedance (BIA) and skinfold measurements (SMs) are non-invasive, safe, quick, and accessible methods at the point of care, providing immediate results [14,34]. Using these techniques, the percentage of pwCF with FFM malnutrition decreased significantly, from 35% to 16% (estimated by skinfolds) and from 29% to 10% (estimated by BIA). The slight differences may be due to BIA generally overestimating the FFM compared to skinfold measurements in individuals with CF and bronchiectasis [14,34]. Increased adiposity along with low FFM may be even more detrimental to pulmonary function in pwCF [35].

In a large series of 434 patients with CF after ETI initiation, the percentage of patients with malnutrition (body mass index <18.5 kg/m^2) decreased from 38.6% to 11.3% at 12 months (p = 0.0001). The weight increased during the first year and then stabilised [7]. In the Petersen series, decreases were observed in the rates of underweight (7.5% to 2.2%) with increases in rates of overweight (19.4% to 31.3%) and obesity (7.5% to 9.7%) [8]. Similarly, in our group, Proud et al. demonstrated an increase in both FFM and FM using BIA, with mean increases of 2.5 kg and 2.1 kg, respectively, seven months after initiating ETI [19].

However, not all studies have observed increases in FFM. Grancini et al., in a group of 24 patients with CF-related diabetes, demonstrated that, after six months of treatment, FM (measured by BIA) significantly increased by a median value of 1.6 kg, but without a significant increase in FFM [16].

Knott-Torcal et al., in 36 pwCF, also observed a significant increase in BMI after six months of treatment, as well as an increase in FM and visceral fat area, with a trend towards an increase in FFM (by approximately 600 g), though this did not reach statistical significance [17]. This same group published, in 26 adult subjects, changes in body composition using CT scans at the level of the 12th dorsal vertebra and observed an increase in total body area, driven by increases in total FM, subcutaneous fat, visceral fat, and intermuscular fat (all with significant differences). The only muscle compartment that showed an increase after treatment was very-low-density muscle, suggesting an increase in myosteatosis [18].

In a retrospective study, an automated analysis of body composition on the chest CT scans of 66 adult patients with CF was performed. They observed marked increases in all adipose tissue ratios, including the total adipose tissue ratio (+46.21%); conversely, only small (but statistically significant) increases in the muscle ratio (+1.63%). Study participants who were initially categorised as underweight experienced more pronounced effects on the total adipose tissue ratio, while gains in muscle ratio were equally distributed across BMI categories [11]. In our series, in contrast, both patients with CF with low BMI at initiation and those with overweight/obesity (OW/OB) gained more weight compared to those with normal BMI (who showed the least total weight gain).

Concomitant with the changes in body composition, we observed significant improvements in spirometric parameters, a reduction in both total and severe respiratory exacerbations, and a decrease in chronic bacterial colonisation. Having a higher number of severe exacerbations prior to ETI treatment was associated in our sample with an increase in FFM in the first year, as well as a lower FEV1/FVC ratio with greater weight gain in FM and FFM. Stewart et al. also observed in a series of young adults that younger age and more frequent prior pulmonary exacerbations had the strongest relationships to 6-month increases in BMI [36]. In the study by Navas-Moreno, higher levels of very low-density muscle prior to treatment were associated with lower final FEV1 and less improvement in FEV1 after therapy [18].

While all studies document weight and fat mass increases, discrepancies in FFM changes among studies may be due to various factors: differences in pwCF populations (with a varying severity of disease at baseline), measurement techniques of BC, and levels of physical exercise or training. In a series by Gruber et al., it was observed that, after ETI treatment, pwCF had a significant increase in steps/day (+25%) [37]. Increased physical activity could lead to improvements in FFM. In a Danish prospective study of 229 pwCF evaluating the impact of CFTR modulators on exercise capacity using the cardiopulmonary exercise test (CPET), a significant increase in oxygen uptake was observed; however, the change was not clinically relevant and considerable variability was observed in the sample. Changes in FEV1% and BMI were able to explain some of the differences [38]. In another series with long-term prospective follow-up evaluating exercise capacity in pwCF (measured by incremental cycle test), an improvement was only observed in pwCF using ETI, whereas pwCF not using ETI showed a small decrease; however, overall, the impact of ETI on all aspects of physical fitness was small [39]. It is likely that CFTR modulators alone are not sufficient for recovering physical deconditioning, but should be supplemented with physical activity and respiratory physiotherapy [40]. Unfortunately, we did not assess the changes in the physical activity levels of our patients, although indirectly, we observed a significant increase in the vitality dimension of the CFQR test. Conversely, we did not observe changes in strength as measured by hand grip dynamometry.

4.2. Serum and Faecal Biomarkers

The causes underlying weight increases following modulator therapies are not well understood but could be multiple, including a reduction in energy expenditure and systemic inflammation, improvement in glycaemic control, changes in dietary intake, and changes in fat absorption, gut inflammation, and microbiota modifications [7,8,16,20].

In our study, we observed significant decreases in faecal calprotectin levels, as well as nitrogen and fat in the stools, while LDL cholesterol and vitamin A levels increased significantly, with vitamin E, albumin, and total cholesterol levels nearing significance. Additionally, the dimensions of quality of life, body image, eating problems, and weight improved, indicating better nutrient absorption and reduced intestinal inflammation. Statna et al. also observed lower pancreatic enzyme replacement requirements and improved defecation in adult patients with CF on ETI, along with increased albumin and prealbumin levels [20]. In Burgel et al.'s series, significant increases in serum concentrations of vitamins A and E were noted [7], and Petersen et al. and Docherty et al. reported increases in total cholesterol and LDL [8,41].

Numerous studies have demonstrated improvements in metabolic control following ETI, with a reduction or even discontinuation of insulin therapy [7,8,16,42]. In our series, metabolic control also improved with significant decreases in HbA1c by 0.2%, although insulin was not discontinued in any patient. The underlying mechanism is still not completely understood and could be related to a decreased inflammatory state, improved insulin sensitivity, and better beta-cell function.

4.3. Dietary Intake

These changes occurred in our series despite observing a decrease in total caloric dietary intake and grams of macronutrients (except fibre), but not in their percentage. Of the seven patients taking oral nutritional supplements prior to ETI initiation, only two maintained their intake after one year, and the only person with a gastrostomy discontinued it within the first six months. These findings align with the series by Caley et al., in a group of 40 adult pwCF, where weight increased despite a reduction in caloric intake [21]. In Burgel et al.'s series, a 50% decrease in the number of patients using oral nutritional supplements and the discontinuation of the enteral tube feeding in most patients was observed over the first year following ETI initiation [7].

4.4. Psychological Symptoms

Depressive and/or anxious symptoms can also influence intake as they can worsen the perception of quality of life and adherence to treatment [22,43]. Although CFTR modulator therapies provide hope for improving clinical outcomes, worsening depression and anxiety occur in some patients when starting these novel agents [44]. We did not observe changes in depression and anxiety symptoms or the corresponding dimension of the CFQR. In a study of 100 pwCF, no changes in symptoms were observed; however, a quarter of patients did display a change in psychiatric medications [43].

4.5. Limitations

Although some results did not reach statistical significance, the observed changes in body composition, respiratory function, quality of life, blood and stool biomarkers, and dietary caloric intake provide meaningful clinical insights for healthcare professionals managing CF patients post-ETI therapy. These findings underscore the importance of adopting a holistic approach to care.

The strengths of this study include its prospective nature and the use of various techniques for a comprehensive assessment of morphofunctional changes (body composition by BIA and SM, hand grip dynamometry, prospective dietary survey, blood and stool biomarkers, quality of life) as well as anxiety and depression symptoms in adult pwCF. This study is limited by its single-centre observational design and relatively small sample size, which increases the risk of Type 1 and Type 2 errors and limits the generalisability of the results. Functionality was also assessed using only handgrip dynamometry.

5. Conclusions

Adults with CF one year after initiating ETI treatment increased weight at the expense of FM and FFM. Both SM and BIA were useful for the longitudinal monitoring of body composition. These changes were parallel to improvements in pulmonary function, quality of life, biomarkers related to absorption and intestinal inflammation, and a decrease in caloric intake and the need for oral nutritional supplements. These results emphasise the importance of monitoring patients with CF with a focus on the quality rather than quantity of intake, and on body composition and exercise rather than BMI. Future studies with larger cohorts are essential to validate these results and further elucidate the mechanisms underlying these changes.

Author Contributions: Conceptualisation, G.O. and F.H.; methodology, N.P., F.H. and G.O.; formal analysis, G.O.; investigation, F.H., N.P., M.V.G., M.G.-O., M.P., F.J.S.-T., C.O. and G.O.; resources, G.O.; data curation, N.P. and G.O.; writing—original draft preparation G.O. and F.H.; writing—review and editing, All authors; supervision, C.O. and G.O.; project administration G.O.; funding acquisition, G.O. All authors have read and agreed to the published version of the manuscript.

Funding: This study was partially funded by an unrestricted grant from VegenatHealthcare (Spain). Marina Padial holds an IPFIS (IFI20/00034) contract from the Carlos III National Health Institute, co-funded by European Social Fund Plus "The FSE invests in your future".

Institutional Review Board Statement: The study was conducted in accordance with the Declaration of Helsinki and approved by Research Ethics Committee of Malaga on 30 March 2021 (reference number #30032021).

Informed Consent Statement: Informed consent was obtained from all subjects involved in the study.

Data Availability Statement: The original contributions presented in the study are included in the article, and further inquiries can be directed to the corresponding author due to privacy reasons.

Acknowledgments: The authors would like to thank all the individuals who participated in this study for their willingness to collaborate.

Conflicts of Interest: The authors declare no conflicts of interest. The funders had no role in the design of the study; in the collection, analyses, or interpretation of data; in the writing of the manuscript; or in the decision to publish the results.

References

1. Olveira Fuster, G.; Olveira Fuster, C. Care of People with Cystic Fibrosis: What Is the Role of Specialists in Endocrinology and Nutrition? *Endocrinol. Diabetes Nutr.* **2021**, *68*, 215–217. [CrossRef] [PubMed]
2. Barry, P.J.; Mall, M.A.; Álvarez, A.; Colombo, C.; de Winter-de Groot, K.M.; Fajac, I.; McBennett, K.A.; McKone, E.F.; Ramsey, B.W.; Sutharsan, S.; et al. Triple Therapy for Cystic Fibrosis Phe508del-Gating and -Residual Function Genotypes. *N. Engl. J. Med.* **2021**, *385*, 815–825. [CrossRef] [PubMed]
3. Southern, K.W.; Addy, C.; Bell, S.C.; Bevan, A.; Borawska, U.; Brown, C.; Burgel, P.R.; Button, B.; Castellani, C.; Chansard, A.; et al. Standards for the Care of People with Cystic Fibrosis; Establishing and Maintaining Health. *J. Cyst. Fibros.* **2024**, *23*, 12–28. [CrossRef] [PubMed]
4. Middleton, P.G.; Mall, M.A.; Dřevínek, P.; Lands, L.C.; McKone, E.F.; Polineni, D.; Ramsey, B.W.; Taylor-Cousar, J.L.; Tullis, E.; Vermeulen, F.; et al. Elexacaftor–Tezacaftor–Ivacaftor for Cystic Fibrosis with a Single Phe508del Allele. *N. Engl. J. Med.* **2019**, *381*, 1809–1819. [CrossRef] [PubMed]
5. Heijerman, H.G.M.; McKone, E.F.; Downey, D.G.; Van Braeckel, E.; Rowe, S.M.; Tullis, E.; Mall, M.A.; Welter, J.J.; Ramsey, B.W.; McKee, C.M.; et al. Efficacy and Safety of the Elexacaftor plus Tezacaftor plus Ivacaftor Combination Regimen in People with Cystic Fibrosis Homozygous for the F508del Mutation: A Double-Blind, Randomised, Phase 3 Trial. *Lancet* **2019**, *394*, 1940–1948. [CrossRef] [PubMed]
6. Carrasco Hernández, L.; Girón Moreno, R.M.; Balaguer Cartagena, M.N.; Peláez, A.; Sole, A.; Álvarez Fernández, A.; Felipe Montiel, A.; Olveira, C.; Olveira, G.; Gómez Bonilla, A.; et al. Experience With Elexacaftor/Tezacaftor/Ivacaftor in Patients With Cystic Fibrosis and Advanced Disease. *Arch. Bronconeumol.* **2023**, *59*, 556–565. [CrossRef]
7. Burgel, P.-R.; Paillasseur, J.-L.; Durieu, I.; Reynaud-Gaubert, M.; Hamidfar, R.; Murris-Espin, M.; Danner-Boucher, I.; Chiron, R.; Leroy, S.; Douvry, B.; et al. Multisystemic Effects of Elexacaftor-Tezacaftor-Ivacaftor in Adults with Cystic Fibrosis and Advanced Lung Disease. *Ann. Am. Thorac. Soc.* **2024**, *21*, 1053–1064. [CrossRef]
8. Petersen, M.C.; Begnel, L.; Wallendorf, M.; Litvin, M. Effect of Elexacaftor-Tezacaftor-Ivacaftor on Body Weight and Metabolic Parameters in Adults with Cystic Fibrosis. *J. Cyst. Fibros.* **2022**, *21*, 265–271. [CrossRef]
9. Turck, D.; Braegger, C.P.; Colombo, C.; Declercq, D.; Morton, A.; Pancheva, R.; Robberecht, E.; Stern, M.; Strandvik, B.; Wolfe, S.; et al. ESPEN-ESPGHAN-ECFS Guidelines on Nutrition Care for Infants, Children, and Adults with Cystic Fibrosis. *Clin. Nutr.* **2016**, *35*, 557–577. [CrossRef] [PubMed]
10. Culhane, S.; George, C.; Pearo, B.; Spoede, E. Malnutrition in Cystic Fibrosis: A Review. *Nutr. Clin. Pract.* **2013**, *28*, 676–683. [CrossRef]
11. Westhölter, D.; Haubold, J.; Welsner, M.; Salhöfer, L.; Wienker, J.; Sutharsan, S.; Straßburg, S.; Taube, C.; Umutlu, L.; Schaarschmidt, B.M.; et al. Elexacaftor/Tezacaftor/Ivacaftor Influences Body Composition in Adults with Cystic Fibrosis: A Fully Automated CT-Based Analysis. *Sci. Rep.* **2024**, *14*, 9465. [CrossRef] [PubMed]
12. Wilschanski, M.; Munck, A.; Carrion, E.; Cipolli, M.; Collins, S.; Colombo, C.; Declercq, D.; Hatziagorou, E.; Hulst, J.; Kalnins, D.; et al. ESPEN-ESPGHAN-ECFS Guideline on Nutrition Care for Cystic Fibrosis. *Clin. Nutr.* **2024**, *43*, 413–445. [CrossRef] [PubMed]
13. Calella, P.; Valerio, G.; Brodlie, M.; Donini, L.M.; Siervo, M. Cystic Fibrosis, Body Composition, and Health Outcomes: A Systematic Review. *Nutrition* **2018**, *55–56*, 131–139. [CrossRef] [PubMed]
14. Contreras-Bolívar, V.; Olveira, C.; Porras, N.; García-Olivares, M.; Girón, M.V.; Sánchez-Torralvo, F.J.; Ruiz-García, I.; Alonso-Gallardo, S.P.; Olveira, G. Assessment of Body Composition in Cystic Fibrosis: Agreement between Skinfold Measurement and Densitometry. *Nutr. Hosp.* **2022**, *39*, 376–382. [CrossRef]

15. Stallings, V.A.; Stark, L.J.; Robinson, K.A.; Feranchak, A.P.; Quinton, H. Evidence-Based Practice Recommendations for Nutrition-Related Management of Children and Adults with Cystic Fibrosis and Pancreatic Insufficiency: Results of a Systematic Review. *J. Am. Diet. Assoc.* **2008**, *108*, 832–839. [CrossRef]
16. Grancini, V.; Gramegna, A.; Zazzeron, L.; Alicandro, G.; Porcaro, L.L.; Piedepalumbo, F.; Lanfranchi, C.; Daccò, V.; Orsi, E.; Blasi, F. Effects of Elexacaftor/Tezacaftor/Ivacaftor Triple Combination Therapy on Glycaemic Control and Body Composition in Patients with Cystic Fibrosis-Related Diabetes. *Diabetes Metab.* **2023**, *49*, 101466. [CrossRef]
17. Knott-Torcal, C.; Sebastián-Valles, F.; Girón Moreno, R.M.; Martín- Adán, J.C.; Jiménez-Díaz, J.; Marazuela, M.; Sánchez de la Blanca, N.; Fernández-Contreras, R.; Arranz-Martín, A. A Prospective Study to Assess the Impact of a Novel CFTR Therapy Combination on Body Composition in Patients with Cystic Fibrosis with F508del Mutation. *Clin. Nutr.* **2023**, *42*, 2468–2474. [CrossRef]
18. Navas-Moreno, V.; Sebastian-Valles, F.; Rodríguez-Laval, V.; Knott-Torcal, C.; Marazuela, M.; de la Blanca, N.S.; Arranz Martín, J.A.; Girón, R.M.; Sampedro-Núñez, M.A. Impact of CFTR Modulator Therapy on Body Composition as Assessed by Thoracic Computed Tomography: A Follow-up Study. *Nutrition* **2024**, *123*, 112425. [CrossRef]
19. Proud, D.; Duckers, J. Weight a Minute: Exploring the Effect on Weight and Body Composition after the Initiation of Elexacaftor/Tezacaftor/Ivacaftor in Adults with CF. *J. Cyst. Fibros.* **2023**, *22*, 847–850. [CrossRef]
20. Stastna, N.; Kunovsky, L.; Svoboda, M.; Pokojova, E.; Homola, L.; Mala, M.; Gracova, Z.; Jerabkova, B.; Skrickova, J.; Trna, J. Improved Nutritional Outcomes and Gastrointestinal Symptoms in Adult Cystic Fibrosis Patients Treated with Elexacaftor/Tezacaftor/Ivacaftor. *Dig. Dis.* **2024**, *42*, 361–368. [CrossRef]
21. Caley, L.R.; Jarosz-Griffiths, H.H.; Smith, L.; Gale, L.; Barrett, J.; Kinsey, L.; Davey, V.; Nash, M.; Jones, A.M.; Whitehouse, J.L.; et al. Body Mass Index and Nutritional Intake Following Elexacaftor/Tezacaftor/Ivacaftor Modulator Therapy in Adults with Cystic Fibrosis. *J. Cyst. Fibros.* **2023**, *22*, 1002–1009. [CrossRef] [PubMed]
22. Olveira, C.; Sole, A.; Girón, R.M.; Quintana-Gallego, E.; Mondejar, P.; Baranda, F.; Alvarez, A.; Prados, C.; Rodríguez-González, J.; Herrero-Labarga, I.; et al. Depression and Anxiety Symptoms in Spanish Adult Patients with Cystic Fibrosis: Associations with Health-Related Quality of Life. *Gen. Hosp. Psychiatry* **2016**, *40*, 39–46. [CrossRef] [PubMed]
23. Siri, W.E. Body Composition from Fluid Spaces and Density: Analysis of Methods. *Nutrition* **1993**, *9*, 480–491; discussion 480, 492. [PubMed]
24. Durnin, J.V.; Womersley, J. Body Fat Assessed from Total Body Density and Its Estimation from Skinfold Thickness: Measurements on 481 Men and Women Aged from 16 to 72 Years. *Br. J. Nutr.* **1974**, *32*, 77–97. [CrossRef] [PubMed]
25. Contreras-Bolívar, V.; Olveira, C.; Porras, N.; Abuín-Fernández, J.; García-Olivares, M.; Sánchez-Torralvo, F.J.; Girón, M.V.; Ruiz-García, I.; Olveira, G. Oral Nutritional Supplements in Adults with Cystic Fibrosis: Effects on Intake, Levels of Fat-Soluble Vitamins, and Bone Remodeling Biomarkers. *Nutrients* **2021**, *13*, 669. [CrossRef]
26. Jimenez, A.; Jiménez, A. *Tablas de Composición de Alimentos*; Novartis Consumer Health, S.A.: Barcelona, Spain, 2002.
27. Mataix, J. *Tablas de Composición de Alimentos Españoles*; Universidad de Granada: Granada, Spain, 2003.
28. Base de Datos BEDCA. Available online: https://www.bedca.net/bdpub/ (accessed on 25 September 2024).
29. Hanas, R.; John, G.; on behalf of the International HbA1c Consensus Committee. 2010 Consensus Statement on the Worldwide Standardization of the Hemoglobin A1C Measurement. *Diabetes Care* **2010**, *33*, 1903–1904. [CrossRef]
30. Quittner, A.L.; Buu, A.; Messer, M.A.; Modi, A.C.; Watrous, M. Development and Validation of The Cystic Fibrosis Questionnaire in the United States: A Health-Related Quality-of-Life Measure for Cystic Fibrosis. *Chest* **2005**, *128*, 2347–2354. [CrossRef] [PubMed]
31. Máiz Carro, L.; Baranda, F.; Coll, R.; Prados, C.; Vendrell, M.; Escribano, A.; Gartner, S.; De Gracia, S.; Martínez, M.; Salcedo, A.; et al. Normativa Del Diagnóstico y El Tratamiento de La Afección Respiratoria En La Fibrosis Quística. *Arch. Bronconeumol.* **2001**, *37*, 316–324. [CrossRef]
32. Martinez-Garcia, M.A.; Athanazio, R.A.; Girón, R.; Máiz-Carro, L.; de la Rosa, D.; Olveira, C.; de Gracia, J.; Vendrell, M.; Prados-Sánchez, C.; Gramblicka, G.; et al. Predicting High Risk of Exacerbations in Bronchiectasis: The E-FACED Score. *Int. J. COPD* **2017**, *12*, 275–284. [CrossRef]
33. Zigmond, A.S.; Snaith, R.P. The Hospital Anxiety and Depression Scale. *Acta Psychiatr. Scand.* **1983**, *67*, 361–370. [CrossRef]
34. Doña, E.; Olveira, C.; Palenque, F.J.F.J.; Porras, N.; Dorado, A.; Martín-Valero, R.; Godoy, A.M.A.M.; Espíldora, F.; Contreras, V.; Olveira, G.; et al. Body Composition Measurement in Bronchiectasis: Comparison between Bioelectrical Impedance Analysis, Skinfold Thickness Measurement, and Dual-Energy X-ray Absorptiometry before and after Pulmonary Rehabilitation. *J. Acad. Nutr. Diet.* **2018**, *118*, 1464–1473. [CrossRef]
35. Alvarez, J.A.; Ziegler, T.R.; Millson, E.C.; Stecenko, A.A. Body Composition and Lung Function in Cystic Fibrosis and Their Association with Adiposity and Normal-Weight Obesity. *Nutrition* **2016**, *32*, 447–452. [CrossRef] [PubMed]
36. Stewart, K.L.; Szczesniak, R.; Liou, T.G. Predicting Weight Gain in Patients with Cystic Fibrosis on Triple Combination Modulator. *Pediatr. Pulmonol.* **2024**, *59*, 1724–1730. [CrossRef] [PubMed]
37. Gruber, W.; Stehling, F.; Blosch, C.; Dillenhoefer, S.; Olivier, M.; Brinkmann, F.; Koerner-Rettberg, C.; Sutharsan, S.; Mellies, U.; Taube, C.; et al. Longitudinal Changes in Habitual Physical Activity in Adult People with Cystic Fibrosis in the Presence or Absence of Treatment with Elexacaftor/Tezacaftor/Ivacaftor. *Front. Sport. Act. Living* **2024**, *6*, 1284878. [CrossRef] [PubMed]

38. Philipsen, L.K.D.; Olesen, H.V.; Jensen, J.H.; Olsen, M.F.; Faurholt-Jepsen, D.; Buchvald, F.; Nielsen, K.G.; Skov, M.; Pressler, T. Changes in Exercise Capacity in People with Cystic Fibrosis after One Year of Elexacaftor/Tezacaftor/Ivacaftor Treatment—A Danish Prospective Cohort. *J. Cyst. Fibros.* **2024**, S1569-1993(24)00055-9. [CrossRef] [PubMed]
39. Welsner, M.; Gruber, W.; Blosch, C.; Koerner-Rettberg, C.; Brinkmann, F.; Dillenhoefer, S.; Sutharsan, S.; Taube, C.; Mellies, U.; Olivier, M.; et al. Longitudinal Evaluation of Physical Fitness in Adults with Cystic Fibrosis in the Era of CFTR-Modulating-Therapies. *Res. Q. Exerc. Sport* **2024**, 1–9. [CrossRef] [PubMed]
40. Stastna, N.; Hrabovska, L.; Homolka, P.; Homola, L.; Svoboda, M.; Brat, K.; Fila, L. The Long-Term Effect of Elexacaftor/Tezacaftor/Ivacaftor on Cardiorespiratory Fitness in Adolescent Patients with Cystic Fibrosis: A Pilot Observational Study. *BMC Pulm. Med.* **2024**, *24*, 260. [CrossRef]
41. Docherty, R.; Folganan, J.; Dempsey, O. Effect of Elexacaftor-Tezacaftor-Ivacaftor on Lipid Parameters in Adults with Cystic Fibrosis: A Single Centre Preliminary Report. *Respir. Med. Res.* **2024**, *86*, 101102. [CrossRef] [PubMed]
42. Granados, A.; Chan, C.L.; Moheet, A.; Vigers, T.; Arbeláez, A.M.; Larson Ode, K. The Impact of Elexacaftor/Tezacaftor/Ivacaftor on Body Composition in a Small Cohort of Youth with Cystic Fibrosis. *Pediatr. Pulmonol.* **2023**, *58*, 1805–1811. [CrossRef]
43. Zhang, L.; Albon, D.; Jones, M.; Bruschwein, H. Impact of Elexacaftor/Tezacaftor/Ivacaftor on Depression and Anxiety in Cystic Fibrosis. *Ther. Adv. Respir. Dis.* **2022**, *16*, 1–10. [CrossRef]
44. Arslan, M.; Chalmers, S.; Rentfrow, K.; Olson, J.M.; Dean, V.; Wylam, M.E.; Demirel, N. Suicide Attempts in Adolescents with Cystic Fibrosis on Elexacaftor/Tezacaftor/Ivacaftor Therapy. *J. Cyst. Fibros.* **2023**, *22*, 427–430. [CrossRef] [PubMed]

nutrients

MDPI

Article

Sarcopenia in the Oldest-Old Adults in the Capital of Brazil: Prevalence and Its Associated Risk Factors

Hudson Azevedo Pinheiro [1], Ruth Losada de Menezes [2], Camila Kellen de Souza Cardoso [3], Rômulo Roosevelt da Silva Filho [3], Farah Registre [3], César de Oliveira [4] and Erika Aparecida Silveira [3,*]

1 Health Department of the Federal District, Brasília 72010-120, Brazil; hudsonap@gmail.com
2 Study, Research, and Extension Group on Functional Health and Aging, Interdisciplinary Center on Aging, Postgraduate Program in Health Sciences, Institute of Tropical Pathology and Public Health, Federal University of Goiás, Goiania 74605-050, Brazil; ruthlosada@ufg.br
3 Postgraduate Health Science Program, Medicina Faculty, Federal University of Goiás, Goiania 74690-900, Brazil; camilacardoso_nut@hotmail.com (C.K.d.S.C.); romulordsf@gmail.com (R.R.d.S.F.); farah.registre@yahoo.fr (F.R.)
4 Department of Epidemiology & Public Health, Institute of Epidemiology & Health Care, University College London, London WC1E 6BT, UK; c.oliveira@ucl.ac.uk
* Correspondence: erikasil@terra.com.br; Tel.: +55-(62)99217-3302

Abstract: Background: In light of the demographic context in which the older adult population is prominent, sarcopenia emerges as a significant concern for the health of these individuals. Aim: To assess the frequency of sarcopenia and severe sarcopenia and the associated risk factors in the oldest adults living in the community. Methods: There were 399 participants aged 80 or older, of both sexes, using primary health care services in the metropolitan area of Brasília, Brazil. Sarcopenia was evaluated based on European Working Group on Sarcopenia in Older People 2 (EWGSOP2). Muscle mass was measured by calf circumference, muscle function by handgrip strength, and muscle performance by gait speed. Clinical and socioeconomic variables, comorbidities, falls, and urinary incontinence were collected. The prevalence of sarcopenia was calculated with a 95% (IC) prevalence. Multivariate Poisson regression analysis was performed in Stata, with $p < 5\%$. Results: Among participants, 78.2% were women. Prevalence of pre-sarcopenia was 31.8%, sarcopenia 3.3%, and severe sarcopenia 25.1%. After multivariate regression, sarcopenia was associated with the female sex, low weight, and a dependency for activities of daily living (ADLs). Similarly, severe sarcopenia remained associated with female sex, low weight, and an ADLs dependency. Sarcopenia and severe sarcopenia were not associated with the level of education, marital status, income, physical activity, medications, falls, nor comorbidities. Conclusions: A quarter of older adults had severe sarcopenia. Sarcopenia and severe sarcopenia were associated with being a woman, being low weight, and have an ADLs dependence.

Keywords: sarcopenia; thinness; risk factors; activities of daily living; prevalence; aged 80 and over

1. Introduction

As life expectancy continues to rise globally, the proportion of older adults is also increasing. This demographic trend is observed in many countries including Brazil, where the population aged 80 and over is growing fast [1,2].

According to the United Nations Organization (ONU) (2022), Brazil's population aged 65 or older may increase by approximately 20% over the next five decades [3]. The demographic shift towards an older population presents significant challenges for health systems, social care services, and the scientific community. This underscores the critical need to understand and address the economic, health, social, and psychological needs in later life [4–6].

In light of the demographic context in which the older adult population is prominent, sarcopenia emerges as a significant concern for the health of these individuals. With increasing age, the decline in muscle mass and function becomes inevitable, gradual, and continuous. This decline results in limitations in daily activities, an increased risk of falls and fractures, and a poorer prognosis for several chronic diseases [7–9].

There are still few studies of community-dwelling that have included people aged 80 years or older which investigate severe sarcopenia, sarcopenia and pre-sarcopenia and its associated factors, especially in Latin American countries, including Brazil. Sarcopenia is a geriatric syndrome, the impact of which on disabilities and mortality, however, needs to be investigated further in older adults at or exceeding 80 years old [10–12]. The few Brazilian studies mostly investigate this population in Sao Paulo [13].

Our study is the first with this specific population (80+) to be conducted in Brasilia, the capital of Brazil, the third largest metropolitan region. To investigate these outcomes in oldest or older adults brings relevant clinical and public health information. In Brazil, a study found that 16.1% of women and 14.4% of men aged 60 and over in São Paulo were affected by sarcopenia; the most significant risk factors for sarcopenia are age, cognitive decline, and the risk of malnutrition [13]. The present study chose not to explore cognitive declines because it understands that neurological problems and dementia syndromes in themselves are determining factors for functional dependence and to demystify that not every person over 80 years of age has cognitive deficits or even dementia senile.

In Fortaleza, Ceará, Brazil, the prevalence of probable sarcopenia was 25.52%, with 11.98% cases of sarcopenia and 9.90% of severe sarcopenia in individuals aged 60 years or older. The results indicated that probable sarcopenia was more prevalent in males and in patients receiving multiple medications, while calf circumference below 31 cm was more frequent in patients with sarcopenia and severe sarcopenia. Furthermore, the presence of osteoporosis was more common in cases of severe sarcopenia [14].

Despite numerous studies on sarcopenia, no specific research has been identified that addresses the prevalence and risk factors of sarcopenia and severe sarcopenia in older adults over the age of 80 in Brazil; with the progressive aging of the population, especially in more vulnerable regions (socially, economically, and environmentally), the identification of the sarcopenia phenotype becomes necessary as a public policy within the Unified Health System (UHS), the Brazilian program that finances government actions relating to health policies aiming to minimize impacts such as exacerbation of chronic diseases, dependence on carrying out activities of daily life (ADLs), caregiver burden, and high costs for services [15,16].

This paper aims to contribute to a more comprehensive understanding of this condition in Brazil and improve the quality of life in later life. Additionally, the findings will inform the development of more effective public health policies and clinical practices.

2. Materials and Methods

2.1. Study Design and Populations

This is a cross-sectional study carried out between September 2015 and December 2018 with community-dwelling older adults assisted by the UHS in the southwest region of Brasilia (the third largest Brazilian metropolis), from eight basic health units (BHU) and a family clinic, Federal District, Brazil, with an estimated population of 828,703 inhabitants. We know that individuals from 80 years and older in a country with a high rate of violence do not accept unfamiliar strangers into their homes. To minimize the recuses in our study and reduce bias, we include individuals who use the BHU. A Brazilian study reveals that 46.2% of the population over 60 years in age uses the health services [17]. Approximately 20% of that population is 80 or older, and their per capita income is around USD 315.04 [18].

The inclusion criterion adopted was older adults referred by BHU to the reference clinic in geriatrics and gerontology, located in Taguatinga, Brasilia/Federal District, Brazil. These patients were in conditions of vulnerability diagnosed by a doctor or a family health strategy team according to the criteria established by The Elderly Person's Health Booklet in the context of Primary Care [19] or in consultation by an interdisciplinary team composed of a nurse, a physiotherapist, and a nutritionist who was duly trained for this purpose and who recorded the medications in use, the socioeconomic characteristics, and the clinical comorbidities previously diagnosed. They also recorded in the electronic medical record, in addition to specifically related complaints of vulnerability such as the number of falls in the previous year, if any regular physical activity was performed (i.e., at least 150 min of weekly practice of any modality), urinary incontinence, dependence in ADLs, and sarcopenia status.

The exclusion criteria for this research were those older adults who presented sequelae of neurological diseases (cerebrovascular disease, Parkinson's disease, among others) or a cognitive deficit assessed by the mini-mental state (MMS) [20], in addition to amputees, since such injuries are related to the increased risk of dependence for ADLs and the increased risk of immobility.

During the interdisciplinary consultation, the following steps were completed sequentially, with the participation of family members and/or caregivers of these elderly individuals. Initially, an interview was conducted to survey a profile with issues related to income, marital status, and education, in addition to the ratification of information contained in the reason for referral, such as the presence of urinary incontinence, one or more falls in the last six months, or number of medications in use.

The study was approved by the Ethics and Research Committee of the Health Education and Research Foundation under opinion number 1,128,355/2015. All participants and their family members or caregivers have provided a signed and informed consent form.

2.2. *Measurements*

2.2.1. Anthropometric Variables

Anthropometric variables were measured by height (cm) and weight (kg) using a scale with a stadiometer brand Filizola® (São Paulo, Brazil) to subsequently calculate the body mass index (BMI), using the Lipschitzl recommendation; this classified the older adults with values less than 22 kg/cm^2 as low weight, the older adults with values between 22 and 27 kg/cm^2 as eutrophic subjects, and the older adults with a BMI greater than 27 kg/cm^2 as excess weight, these measures being more sensitive for public health [21].

2.2.2. Sarcopenia

To classify whether the older adults were sarcopenic, the criteria recommended by the EWGSOP2 were used, where subjects who presented reduced muscle strength and reduced quality of muscle mass were classified as sarcopenic. To be defined as severe sarcopenic, older adults should also present reduced physical performance, and pre-sarcopenia adults present only reduced muscle mass or only reduced muscle quality [22].

To measure muscle strength, the handgrip strength test was measured with a hydraulic dynamometer JAMAR® (São Paulo, Brazil). Three measurements with an interval were performed in the dominant hand. One minute between them is considered sarcopenic if they present values lower than 27 kg/F for men and 16 kg/F for women [23].

The quality of muscle mass was measured by the circumference of the calf with the participant sitting on a chair, with legs relaxed, feet flat on the floor, and knees bent at 90°. After identifying the most protruding region of the legs through an inelastic measuring tape, the perimetry was gauged, and individuals with values equal to or less than 33 cm for women and 34 cm for men were considered at risk for sarcopenia [24,25].

Finally, the physical performance was measured by the usual gait speed test performed in a corridor, where participants were instructed to walk at their usual speed, being able to use an auxiliary device for locomotion. The time taken to move three meters was measured, after the acceleration and deceleration time were disregarded; a speed slower than 0.8 m/s was considered a risk. All functional capacity tests were conducted by a qualified examiner [26].

2.2.3. The Activity of Daily Living Assessment

The Barthel index was applied to assess the degree of functional independence, using the version validated and cross-culturally adapted for the Brazilian population, whose cutoff point greater than or equal to 60 suggests the subjects are independent for ADLs [27].

2.3. Statistical Analyses

The statistical analyses were performed in the software Stata 12.0. The outcomes of this study were sarcopenia and severe sarcopenia. We estimated the prevalence ratio with their 95% confidence intervals and associated risk factors according to all sociodemographic and clinical variables.

All variables with p-value $\leq$ 0.20 in bivariate Poisson regression were included in the multivariable Poisson regression to control for potential confounders. The criteria to maintain variables on the final regression model as p-value $\leq$ 0.05 denominated as the adjusted model on the tables.

3. Results

Our analytical sample included 399 older adults aged 80 to 104 years. The mean age was 87.34 years (SD = 5.22), the mean BMI was 25.71 kg/m^2 (SD = 5.32), the mean calf circumference was 31.77 cm (SD = 4.11), and the mean hand grip strength was 17.73 kg/F (SD = 6.23).

The prevalence of pre-sarcopenia was 31.8% (95% CI = 26.9–36.1), sarcopenia was 3.3% (CI 95%= 1.5–5.1), and severe sarcopenia 25.1% (95% CI = 20.8–29.6), represented in Figure 1. The prevalence of pre-sarcopenia and severe sarcopenia were statistically different between the sexes. The prevalence of pre-sarcopenia was significantly higher in men than in women (p-value = 0.013). Severe sarcopenia was more prevalent in women (28.5%) than in men (12.6%) (p-value = 0.03).

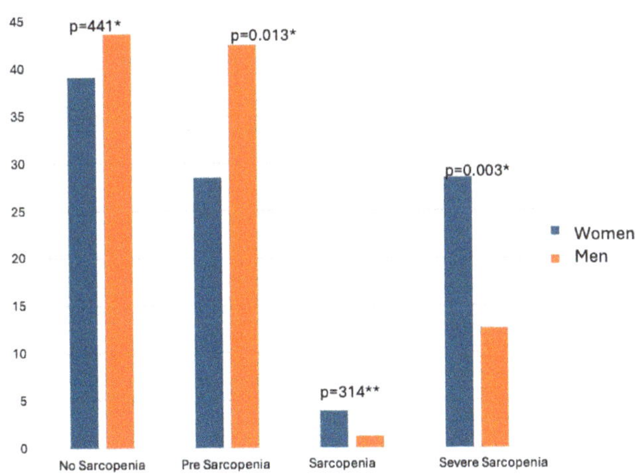

Figure 1. Prevalence of pre-sarcopenia, sarcopenia, and severe sarcopenia by sex in community-dwelling older adults (n = 399). Notes: * Chi-square test; ** Fisher's exact test.

The prevalence of non-sarcopenia, pre-sarcopenia, sarcopenia, and severe sarcopenia according to sociodemographic characteristics and physical activity were statistically different by sex, marital status, monthly income, and activities of daily living (ADLs) dependence. The data are available in Table 1.

Table 1. Prevalence of pre-sarcopenia, sarcopenia, and severe sarcopenia and their associations with sociodemographic variables and physical activity in community-dwelling older adults (n = 399).

Variables	n (%)	No Sarcopenia (%)	Pre-Sarcopenia (%)	Sarcopenia (%)	Severe Sarcopenia (%)	p
Sex						
Female	312 (78.2)	122 (39.1)	89 (28.5)	12 (3.8)	89 (28.5)	0.004 *
Male	87 (21.8)	38 (43.7)	37 (42.2)	1 (1.2)	11 (12.6)	
Level of education						
Illiterate	106 (26.6)	38 (35.8)	31 (29.3)	1 (0.9)	36 (33.9)	0.113 *
≤6 years	212 (53.1)	86 (40.6)	70 (33.0)	11 (5.2)	45 (21.2)	
>7 years	81 (20.3))	36 (44.4)	25 (30.9)	1 (1.2)	19 (23.5)	
Marital status						
Not married/divorced	50 (12.6)	22 (44.0)	15 (30)	0 (0.0)	13 (26.0)	0.022 *
Married	111 (27.9)	49 (44.1)	42 (37.8)	5 (4.5)	15 (13.5)	
Widower	237 (59.5)	89 (37.5)	68 (28.7)	8 (3.4)	72 (30.4)	
Monthly income per person						
≤U$200	106 (26.6)	48 (45.3)	30 (28.3)	0 (0.0)	28 (26.4)	0.036 *
U$200–400	227 (57.0)	81 (35.7)	82 (36.1)	11 (4.9)	53 (23.3)	
≥400	65 (16.3)	30 (46.2)	14 (21.5)	2 (3.1)	19 (29.2)	
Physical Activity Status (>150 min/week)						
No	216 (54.1)	80 (37.0)	75 (34.7)	6 (2.8)	55 (25.5)	0.401 **
Yes	183 (45.9)	80 (43.7)	51 (27.8)	7 (3.8)	45 (24.6)	

Note: * Fisher's exact test; ** Chi-square test.

The prevalence of pre-sarcopenia, sarcopenia, and severe sarcopenia and their association with health variables in community-dwelling older adults were statistically different in individuals with low weight, ADLs independence, and COPD. The data are available in Table 2.

Table 2. Prevalence of pre-sarcopenia, sarcopenia, and severe sarcopenia and their associations with health variables in community-dwelling older adults (n = 399).

Variables	n (%)	No Sarcopenia (%)	Pre-Sarcopenia (%)	Sarcopenia (%)	Severe Sarcopenia (%)	p
Low weight						
No	297 (74.4)	153 (51.5)	78 (26.7)	8 (2.6)	58 (19.5)	$p < 0.001$ *
Yes	102 (25.6)	7 (6.9)	48 (47.1)	5 (4.9)	42 (41.2)	
Falls						
No	224 (56.3)	92 (41.1)	75 (33.5)	8 (3.6)	49 (21.9)	0.377 *
Yes	174 (43.7)	68 (39.1)	50 (28.7)	5 (2.9)	51 (29.3)	
Femur fractures						
No	386 (96.7)	157 (40.7)	121 (31.3)	13 (3.4)	95 (24.6)	0.465 *
Yes	13 (3.3)	3 (23.1)	5 (38.5)	0 (0.0)	5 (38.5)	
Independence for ADLs						
No	25 (6.3)	7 (28.0)	4 (16.0)	0 (0.0)	14 (56.0)	0.008 *
Yes	374 (93.7)	153 (40.9)	122 (32.6)	13 (3.5)	86 (23.1)	
Arterial hypertension						
No	62 (15.6)	18 (29.0)	26 (41.9)	3 (4.8)	15 (24.2)	0.127 *
Yes	336 (84.4)	141 (41.9)	100 (29.8)	10 (3.0)	85 (25.3)	
Cardiopathy						
No	297 (74.4)	124 (41.7)	92 (31.0)	11 (3.7)	70 (23.6)	0.478 *
Yes	102 (25.6)	36 (35.3)	34 (33.3)	2 (2.0)	30 (29.4)	
Diabetes						
No	253 (63.4)	102 (40.3)	81 (32.0)	8 (3.2)	62 (24.5)	0.980 *
Yes	146 (36.6)	58 (39.7)	45 (30.8)	5 (3.4)	38 (26.0)	

Table 2. *Cont.*

Variables	*n* (%)	No Sarcopenia (%)	Pre-Sarcopenia (%)	Sarcopenia (%)	Severe Sarcopenia (%)	*p*
Depression						
No	220 (55.3)	89 (40.5)	72 (32.7)	5 (2.3)	54 (24.5)	0.732 *
Yes	178 (44.7)	70 (39.3)	54 (30.3)	8 (4.5)	46 (25.8)	
Arthrosis						
No	210 (52.6)	77 (36.7)	73 (34.8)	6 (2.9)	55 (25.7)	0.389 **
Yes	189 (47.4)	83 (43.9)	53 (28.0)	7 (3.7)	46 (24.3)	
Hypothyroidism						
No	341 (85.5)	137 (40.2)	107 (32.4)	10 (2.9)	87 (25.5)	0.739 *
Yes	58 (14.5)	23 (39.7)	19 (32.8)	3 (5.2)	13 (22.4)	
Chronic obstructive pulmonary disease (COPD)						
No	391 (98.0)	160 (40.9)	122 (31.2)	13 (3.3)	96 (24.5)	0.048 *
Yes	8 (2.0)	0 (0.0)	4 (50.0)	0 (0.0)	4 (50.0)	
Urinary incontinence						
No	166 (41.6)	66 (39.8)	59 (35.5)	6 (3.6)	35 (21.2)	0.344 **
Yes	233 (58.4)	94 (40.3)	67 (28.8)	7 (3.0)	65 (27.9)	
Medications (number)						
† 0–4	158 (39.6)	60 (37.9)	52 (32.9)	7 (4.4)	39 (24.7)	0.668 **
5 or more	241 (60.4)	100 (41.5)	74 (30.7)	6 (2.5)	61 (25.3)	

Note: * Fisher's exact test. ** Chi-square test; † 10 older adults did not use medication.

Sex, marital status, low weight, ADLs dependency, and depression were statistically associated with sarcopenia in the unadjusted regression analysis. However, multivariate regression analyses included additional factors such as level of education, COPD, urinary incontinence, and falls. After the multivariate analysis, sarcopenia showed statistically significant associations with the female sex (PR 2.34, 95% CI 1.35–4.07), a low weight status (PR 1.93, 95% CI 1.45–2.59), and an ADLs dependence (PR 1.94, 95% CI 1.35–2.79). The data are available in Table 3.

Table 3. Association of sarcopenia in community-dwelling older adults, simple and multivariate Poison regression ($n = 399$).

Variables	Simple Regression		Multivariate Regression	
	RP (CI 95%)	***p*-Value (Wald)**	**RP (CI 95%)**	***p*-Value**
Sex		0.0024		
Female	2.35 (1.35–4.07)		2.34	0.002
Male	1		1	
Level of education		0.1930	-	
Illiterate	1.41 (0.89–2.24)		-	-
≤6 years	1.07 (0.69–1.66)		-	-
>7 years	1			
Marital status		0.0153		
Not married/divorced	1.44 (0.78–2.67)		-	-
Married	1		-	-
Widower	1.87 (1.21–2.89)			
Monthly income per person		0.6991		
≤U$200	1		-	-
U$200–400	1.07 (0.73–1.56)		-	-
≥400	1.22 (0.76–1.97)		-	-
Physical Activity status		0.9693	-	-
No	1		-	-
Yes	1.00 (0.73–1.38)			
Medications (number)		0.7758	-	-
0–4	1		-	-
5 or more	0.95 (0.69–1.31)			-

Table 3. *Cont.*

Variables	Simple Regression RP (CI 95%)	p-Value (Wald)	Multivariate Regression RP (CI 95%)	p-Value
Low weight		0.0000		
No	1		1	
Yes	2.07 (1.54–2.79)		1.93 (1.45–2.59)	0.000
Falls		0.1394	-	
No	1			
Yes	1.26 (0.93–1.73)			
Femur fractures		0.3776		
No	1			
Yes	1.37 (0.68–2.79)			
Independence for ADLs		0.0001	-	0.000
No	2.1 (1.44–3.11)		1.94 (1.35–2.79)	
Yes	1		1	
Arterial hypertension		0.9029		
No	1.03 (0.67–1.57)		-	-
Yes	1		-	-
Cardiopathy		0.4226		
No	1		-	-
Yes	1.15 (0.82–1.62)		-	-
Diabetes		0.7027		
No	1		-	-
Yes	1.06 (0.77–1.47)		-	-
Depression		0.0000		
No	1		-	-
Yes	1.13 (0.83–1.54)		-	-
Arthrosis		0.9069		
No	1.02 (0.74–1.39)		-	-
Yes	1		-	-
Hypothyroidism		0.8937		
No	1.03 (0.66–1.62)		-	-
Yes	1		-	-
Chronic obstructive pulmonary disease (COPD)		0.1078		
No	1		-	-
Yes	1.79 (0.88–3.65)		-	-
Urinary incontinence		0.1809		
No	1		-	-
Yes	1.25 (0.90–1.74)		-	-

Concerning severe sarcopenia, the associated variables were the female sex, marital status, underweight, ADLs dependency, and depression in the simple regression analysis. Level of education, falls, COPD and urinary incontinence have also been included in the multivariate Poisson regression. After the multivariable analysis, the associated variables with severe sarcopenia were female sex PR 2.32 (IC 95% 1.29–4.14), underweight PR 2.00 (IC 95% 1.46–2.75), and ADLs dependency PR 2.13 (IC 95% 1.47–3.10). The data are available in Table 4.

Table 4. Association of severe sarcopenia in community-dwelling older adults, simple and multivariate Poison regression (n = 399).

Variables	Simple Regression		Multivariate Regression	
	RP (CI 95%)	p-Value (Wald)	RP (CI 95%)	p-Value
Sex		0.0044		0.004
Female	2.32 (1.30–4.14)		2.32 (1.29–4.14)	
Male	1		1	

Table 4. *Cont.*

Variables	Simple Regression		Multivariate Regression	
	RP (CI 95%)	*p*-Value (Wald)	RP (CI 95%)	*p*-Value
Level of education		0.0624		
Illiterate	1.53 (1.06–2.22)		-	-
≤6 years	1		-	-
>7 years	1.06 (0.66–1.69)		-	-
Marital status		0.0082		
Not married/divorced	1.84 (0.95–3.56)		-	-
Married	1		-	-
Widower	2.22 (1.34–3.69)			
Monthly income per person		0.6572		
≤U$200	1.08 (0.72–1.60)		-	-
U$200–400	1		-	-
≥400	1.23 (0.79–1.91)		-	-
Physical Activity status		0.890		
No	0.97 (0.69–1.37)		-	-
Yes	1		-	-
Medications (number)		0.9774		
0–4	1		-	-
5 or more	1.00 (0.71–1.42)		-	-
Low weight		0.0000		
No	1		1	
Yes	2.16 (1.56–2.98)		2.00 (1.46–2.75)	0.000
Falls		0.0969		
No	1		-	-
Yes	1.33 (0.95–1.86)		-	-
Femur fractures		0.2552		
No	1			
Yes	1.51 (0.74–3.07)			
Independence for ADLs		0.0000		
No	2.35 (1.58–3.48)		2.13 (1.47–3.10)	0.000
Yes	1		1	
Arterial hypertension		0.9169	-	-
No	1		-	-
Yes	0.97 (0.61–1.57)			
Cardiopathy		0.2712		
No	1		-	-
Yes	1.22 (0.85–1.76)		-	-
Diabetes		0.7222		
No	1		-	-
Yes	1.06 (0.75–1.51)		-	-
Depression		0.0000		
No	1		-	-
Yes	1.08 (1.02–1.51)		-	-
Arthrosis		0.789		
No	1.05 (0.75–1.47)		-	-
Yes	1		-	-
Hypothyroidism		0.683		
No	1.11 (0.67–1.85)		-	-
Yes	1		-	-
Chronic obstructive pulmonary disease (COPD)		0.063		
No	0		-	-
Yes	1.97 (0.96–4.02)		-	-
Urinary incontinence		0.134		
No	1		-	-
Yes	1.31 (0.92–1.88)		-	-

4. Discussion

This study not only represents the first comprehensive investigation into the prevalence of sarcopenia and severe sarcopenia in older Brazilians aged 80 and older but also sheds light on the associated risk factors, paving the way for targeted interventions and improved public health strategies for this population.

The results showed a prevalence of possible sarcopenia, sarcopenia, and severe sarcopenia in older adults aged 80 or older at rates of 31.8%, 3.3%, and 25.1%, respectively. When compared with international studies, the rates vary.

In China, 38.5% of older adults over 80 years of age had possible sarcopenia, 18.6% had sarcopenia, and 8.0% had severe sarcopenia [10]. In Chile, the prevalence among people aged 80 years and older was 38.5% [28]. In contrast, in Finland, older adult men had lower rates: 4.8% probable sarcopenia and 2.7% confirmed sarcopenia [14].

The differences in prevalence rates may be due to population characteristics, highlighting the importance of addressing this issue in healthcare and promoting strategies to maintain muscle health as older adults.

In Brazilian studies, the prevalence of sarcopenia in primary care showed that males were more likely to develop pre-sarcopenia, and the female sex was a risk factor for sarcopenia, since, due to hormonal changes beginning from the age of 50, there is an accelerated loss of strength in women; there is also increased risk for individuals aged over 76 years [29,30].

The study found a higher prevalence of pre-sarcopenia in men and severe sarcopenia in women (28.5% vs. 12.6%). This is consistent with the findings from Sousa et al., [29] showing that probable sarcopenia is more prevalent in men. In contrast, Wu et al. [10] reported higher possible sarcopenia in women (40.7% vs. 36.3%), while Lera et al. [28] found equal sarcopenia prevalence (19.1%) in both sexes in Chile. These variations could be attributed to age, lifestyle, and genetic factors.

Our study has assessed the prevalence of different stages of sarcopenia, analysing sociodemographic data and physical activity levels. Significant differences were observed concerning gender, marital status, monthly income, and dependence to perform ADLs.

A systematic review focusing on community-dwelling older adults aged 60 and over identified the following factors associated with sarcopenia: advanced age, marital status, ADLs, and low weight. Nevertheless, no significant associations were found between sarcopenia and either male or female sex in this study [6]. Concerning monthly income, no significant differences were observed between groups of older adults with varying degrees of sarcopenia [13].

Our findings revealed statistically significant differences in the prevalence of pre-sarcopenia, sarcopenia, and severe sarcopenia, as well as their relationships with health variables, especially related to low weight, independence for ADLs, and COPD. Santos et al. [31] noted a higher prevalence of sarcopenia in underweight older adults aged 80 to 84 years. On the other hand, Jones et al. [32] linked increased sarcopenia prevalence with COPD progression in older adults with an average age of 70.4 years.

According to Wu X et al., [10] having a history of chronic lung diseases was associated with a higher risk of possible sarcopenia. However, no identified association was found between the severity of COPD and the prevalence of sarcopenia in the study by Jones et al. [32]. These results highlight the importance of considering various health variables when evaluating sarcopenia in older adults.

The results of the multivariate analysis indicated that female sex, low weight, and ADLs remained statistically significant after controlling for other variables. These factors demonstrated associations with sarcopenia and severe sarcopenia, indicating their importance even after consideration of additional factors such as education, COPD, urinary incontinence, and falls.

Previous studies, such as Yen et al., [33] also identified female gender as a risk factor for severe sarcopenia. Additionally, Oliveira et al. [34] found that female sex is associated with sarcopenia in institutionalized older individuals. These findings underscore the significance of gender in the risk profile for sarcopenia and suggest that targeted interventions for women may be necessary.

Our findings align with Sri-On et al. [35] who showed that low weight is linked to sarcopenia and severe sarcopenia in individuals aged 70 and above. Another study indicated that malnutrition is associated with an approximately four times greater risk of developing sarcopenia or severe sarcopenia with advancing age due to a poorly balanced diet and a reduction in micro- and macronutrients [36].

Conversely, in individuals with severe obesity, the complexity of identifying negative variables for muscle health is compounded by factors such as chronic inflammation, insulin resistance, dysphagia, and low physical activity [37,38]. These elements are crucial for muscle mass loss and reduced strength, which can give rise to further complications.

Regarding sedentary lifestyle, Brazilian studies found that those elderly people who had higher income regularly practiced some physical activity while low-income subjects considered occupational activity as physical activity. In addition, subjects with low income tend to adopt other less healthy habits, such as smoking and alcohol consumption, due to a lack of information, contributing to the development of comorbidities or chronic diseases regardless of sex [13,39].

Concerning ADLs, a survey of older adults indicated that sarcopenia was directly linked to greater disability in ADLs and lower physical functionality. Older individuals with sarcopenia were twice as likely to face limitations in ADLs compared to those without this condition. Furthermore, sarcopenia was associated with weakness in the lower limbs, which caused difficulties such as bending, kneeling, lifting loads above 5 kg, and walking 400 m [8,40,41].

The association between sarcopenia and dependence on ADLs results in increased care costs, greater caregiver burden, and a greater risk of hospitalization [42–45]. Therefore, it is essential to identify sarcopenia early and implement effective interventions to enhance muscle strength and function in older adults, mainly in primary care which is responsible for ensuring access to basic healthcare and preventing diseases such as sarcopenia through physical, nutritional, and clinical health education actions throughout the course of life and close to one's home [46].

This study has limitations that should be acknowledged. The lack of data on lifestyle such as smoking status, alcohol consumption, leisure activities, ethnicity, religion, and biochemical markers could be a potential limitation. These factors may potentially impact the development of sarcopenia and should be considered in future research involving older individuals. By including these variables, we can better understand their impact on the sarcopenia process.

Additionally, our study excluded individuals with pre-existing physical or mental limitations, assuming they already had reduced mobility and increased dependence on ADLs. However, investigating sarcopenia in these populations can provide valuable insights into how such conditions influence sedentary behaviours and lifestyles.

It is essential to note that the prevalence and associated factors of sarcopenia may change over the lifespan. Recent evidence indicates that the risk factors commonly associated with sarcopenia in later life may not apply to the oldest elderly individuals living in the community. For instance, the correlation between physical activity levels and daily functioning with sarcopenia may not be as straightforward as previously thought. Indeed, being overweight may even offer protection against this condition, contrary to trends observed in older adults more broadly. Nevertheless, further research is required to investigate the risk factors for sarcopenia and severe sarcopenia, particularly in long-lived elderly populations, to inform the development of more effective preventive strategies and interventions.

5. Conclusions

The high prevalence of severe sarcopenia affects approximately a quarter of the oldest seniors. Several factors have been associated with sarcopenia and severe sarcopenia risk, including being female, low weight, and ADLs dependency. This research highlights the pressing requirement for public health policies and strategies to reduce the effects of sarcopenia and encourage a healthy and active ageing process.

Author Contributions: Conceptualization, H.A.P. and R.L.d.M.; methodology, H.A.P. and R.L.d.M.; software, C.K.d.S.C.; validation, F.R. and R.R.d.S.F.; formal analysis, C.K.d.S.C. and E.A.S.; investigation, H.A.P. and R.L.d.M.; resources, F.R., R.R.d.S.F.; data curation, H.A.P.; writing—original draft preparation, F.R., R.R.d.S.F. and C.d.O.; writing—review and editing, C.d.O., E.A.S. and H.A.P.; visualization, E.A.S.; supervision, E.A.S.; project administration, E.A.S. and C.d.O.; funding acquisition, E.A.S. All authors have read and agreed to the published version of the manuscript.

Funding: This work was developed with support from the Research Support Program of the Escola Superior de Ciências da Saúde (ESCS), with resources from the Foundation for Teaching and Research in Health Sciences (FEPECS) TOA05/2023 and Postgraduate Program in Health Sciences, Faculty of Medicine, Federal University of Goiás.

Institutional Review Board Statement: The study was conducted in accordance with the Declaration of Helsinki and approved by the Ethics and Research Committee of the Health Education and Research Foundation under opinion number 1,128,355/2015 on 29 June 2015.

Informed Consent Statement: Informed consent was obtained from all subjects involved in the study.

Data Availability Statement: The Excel file with the database can be made available by the authors upon request.

Acknowledgments: The Health Department of the Federal District (Brasília, Brazil) and all patients and their families who participated in the present study.

Conflicts of Interest: The authors declare no conflicts of interest.

References

1. Vanella, P.; Deschermeier, P.; Wilke, C.B. An overview of population projections—Methodological concepts, international data availability, and use cases. *Forecasting* **2020**, *2*, 346–363. [CrossRef]
2. Kuliński, W.; Brawer, I. Physical therapy in disability prevention in long-lived persons. indexed in pubmed/medline, scopus, embase, ebsco, index copernicus, polish ministry of education and science, polish medical bibliography. *Wiad Lek.* **2023**, *76*, 1517–1526. [CrossRef] [PubMed]
3. Pérez, R.A.; Tejada, C.A.O.; Triaca, L.M.; Bertoldi, A.D.; Dos Santos, A.M.A. Socioeconomic inequality in health in older adults in Brazil. *Dialogues Health* **2022**, *1*, 100009. [CrossRef] [PubMed]
4. World Health Organization. *Integrated Care for Older People (ICOPE): Guidance for Person-Centred Assessment and Pathways in Primary Care*; World Health Organization: Geneva, Switzerland, 2019.
5. Xu, W.; Chen, T.; Cai, Y.; Hu, Y.; Fan, L.; Wu, C. Sarcopenia in community-dwelling oldest old is associated with disability and poor physical function. *J. Nutr. Health Aging* **2020**, *24*, 339–345. [CrossRef] [PubMed]
6. Gao, Q.; Hu, K.; Yan, C.; Zhao, B.; Mei, F.; Chen, F.; Zhao, L.; Shang, Y.; Ma, Y.; Ma, B. Associated Factors of Sarcopenia in Community-Dwelling Older Adults: A Systematic Review and Meta-Analysis. *Nutrients* **2021**, *13*, 4291. [CrossRef]
7. Cruz-Jentoft, A.J.; Baeyens, J.P.; Bauer, J.M.; Boirie, Y.; Cederholm, T.; Landi, F.; Martin, F.C.; Michel, J.P.; Rolland, Y.; Schneider, S.M.; et al. Sarcopenia: European consensus on definition and diagnosis: Report of the European Working Group on Sarcopenia in Older People. *Age Ageing* **2010**, *39*, 412–423. [CrossRef]
8. Sato, P.H.R.; Ferreira, A.A.; Rosado, E.L. The prevalence and risk factors for sarcopenia in older adults and long-living older adults. *Arch Gerontol. Geriatr.* **2020**, *89*, 104089. [CrossRef]
9. Kim, H.; Hirano, H.; Edahiro, A.; Ohara, Y.; Watanabe, Y.; Kojima, N.; Kim, M.; Hosoi, E.; Yoshida, Y.; Yoshida, H.; et al. Sarcopenia: Prevalence and associated factors based on different suggested definitions in community-dwelling older adults. *Geriatr. Gerontol. Int.* **2016**, *16*, 110–122. [CrossRef]
10. Wu, X.; Li, X.; Xu, M.; Zhang, Z.; He, L.; Li, Y. Sarcopenia prevalence and associated factors among older Chinese population: Findings from the China Health and Retirement Longitudinal Study. *PLoS ONE* **2021**, *16*, e0247617. [CrossRef]
11. Kaufman, H.; Howell, S.; Stolow, J.; Andrinopoulos, K.; Anglewicz, P.; Burt, M.; Castro, A. Self-perceived health of older adults in Latin America and the Caribbean: A scoping review. *Rev. Panam. Salud Pública* **2023**, *47*, e105. [CrossRef]
12. Tsekoura, M.; Billis, E.; Matzaroglou, C.; Tsepis, E.; Gliatis, J. Prevalence of probable sarcopenia in community-dwelling older Greek people. *J. Frailty Sarcopenia Falls* **2021**, *6*, 204. [CrossRef] [PubMed]
13. Alexandre, T.; Wong, R. Prevalence and Associated Factors of Sarcopenia among Elderly in Brazil: Findings from the SABE Study. *J. Nutr. Health Aging* **2014**, *18*, 284–290. [CrossRef] [PubMed]

14. Sousa, C.R.D.; Coutinho, J.F.V.; Marques, M.B.; Barbosa, R.G.B.; Roriz Filho, J.D.S.; Soares, E.S.; Nogueira, C.B.; Souza, R.L.D.P. Prevalence of characteristics associated with sarcopenia in elders: A cross-sectional study. *Rev. Bras. Enferm.* **2023**, *76*, e20220209. [CrossRef] [PubMed]
15. Freitas, J.L.D.S.; Silva, J.M.; Nóbrega, J.C.L.; Simões, R.F.; Medeiros, J.B.; Alves, R.O.; Santos, J.L.; Duarte, Y.A.O.; Zatz, M.; Matheson, D.; et al. Health-related quality of life and associated factors: Regional differences among oldest-old in Brazil. *INQUIRY J. Health Care Organ. Provis. Financ.* **2022**, *59*, 00469580221086922. [CrossRef] [PubMed]
16. Nunes, B.P.; Thumé, E.; Facchini, L.A. Multimorbidity in older adults: Magnitude and challenges for the Brazilian health system. *BMC Public Health* **2015**, *15*, 1–11. [CrossRef]
17. Cesário, V.A.C.; Santos, M.M.; Mendes, T.C.O.; Souza-Júnior, P.R.B.; Lima, K.C. Trends in the access and use of health services in PHC among Brazilian older adults in the years 2008, 2013 and 2019. *Ciência Saúde Coletiva* **2021**, *26*, 4033–4044. [CrossRef]
18. CODEPLAN-COMPANHIA DEPDOD. FEDERAL. Pesquisa Distrital por Amostra de Domicílios do Distrito Federal-PDAD-DF-2015. Published online 2015.
19. Gomes, N.M.C.; da Cunha, A.M.S.; de Almeida, A.B. *A CADERNETA DE SAÚDE DA PESSOA IDOSA NO CONTEXTO DA ATENÇÃO BÁSICA*; Universidade Federal de Alagoas: Maceió, Brazil, 2018.
20. Wajman, J.R.; Oliveira FF de Schultz, R.R.; de Marin, S.M.C.; Bertolucci, P.H.F. Educational bias in the assessment of severe dementia: Brazilian cutoffs for severe Mini-Mental State Examination. *Arq. Neuropsiquiatr.* **2014**, *72*, 273–277. [CrossRef]
21. Silveira, E.A.; Barbosa, L.S.; Noll, M.; Pinheiro, H.A.; de Oliveira, C. Body fat percentage prediction in older adults: Agreement between anthropometric equations and DXA. *Clin. Nutr.* **2021**, *40*, 2091–2099. [CrossRef]
22. Cruz-Jentoft, A.J.; Bahat, G.; Bauer, J.; Boirie, Y.; Bruyère, O.; Cederholm, T.; Cooper, C.; Landi, F.; Rolland, Y.; Sayer, A.A.; et al. Sarcopenia: Revised European consensus on definition and diagnosis. *Age Ageing* **2019**, *48*, 16–31. [CrossRef]
23. Lino, V.T.S.; Rodrigues, N.C.P.; O'Dwyer, G.; de Andrade, M.K.N.; Mattos, I.E.; Portela, M.C. Handgrip strength and factors associated in poor elderly assisted at a primary care unit in Rio de Janeiro, Brazil. *PLoS ONE* **2016**, *11*, e0166373. [CrossRef]
24. Pagotto, V.; Santos, K.F.; dos Malaquias, S.G.; Bachion, M.M.; Silveira, E.A. Calf circumference: Clinical validation for evaluation of muscle mass in the elderly. *Rev. Bras. Enferm.* **2018**, *71*, 322–328. [CrossRef] [PubMed]
25. Buccheri, E.; Dell'Aquila, D.; Russo, M.; Chiaramonte, R.; Musumeci, G.; Vecchio, M. Can artificial intelligence simplify the screening of muscle mass loss? *Heliyon* **2023**, *9*, e16323. [CrossRef] [PubMed]
26. Karpman, C.; LeBrasseur, N.K.; DePew, Z.S.; Novotny, P.J.; Benzo, R.P. Measuring gait speed in the out-patient clinic: Methodology and feasibility. *Respir. Care* **2014**, *59*, 531–537. [CrossRef] [PubMed]
27. Minosso, J.S.M.; Amendola, F.; Alvarenga, M.R.M.; De Campos Oliveira, M.A. Validação, no Brasil, do Índice de Barthel em idosos atendidos em ambulatórios. *ACTA Paul. Enferm.* **2010**, *23*, 218–223. [CrossRef]
28. Lera, L.; Albala, C.; Sánchez, H.; Angel, B.; Hormazabal, M.J.; Márquez, C.; Arroyo, P. Prevalence of sarcopenia in community-dwelling Chilean elders according to an adapted version of the European Working Group on Sarcopenia in Older People (EWGSOP) criteria. *J. Frailty Aging* **2017**, *6*, 12–17.
29. Jyväkorpi, S.K.; Urtamo, A.; Kivimäki, M.; Strandberg, T.E. Macronutrient composition and sarcopenia in the oldest-old men: The Helsinki Businessmen Study (HBS). *Clin. Nutr.* **2020**, *39*, 3839–3841. [CrossRef]
30. Souza, L.F.D.; Fontanela, L.C.; Leopoldino, A.A.O.; Mendonça, V.A.; Danielewicz, A.L.; Lacerda, A.C.R.; Avelar, N.C.P.D. Are sociodemographic and anthropometric variables effective in screening probable and confirmed sarcopenia in community-dwelling older adults? A cross-sectional study. *Sao Paulo Med. J.* **2022**, *141*, e2022141. [CrossRef]
31. dos Santos, V.R.; Christofaro, D.G.D.; Gomes, I.C.; Agostinete, R.R.; Freitas Júnior, I.F.; Gobbo, L.A. Factors associated with sarcopenia in subjects aged 80 years and over. *Rev. Nutr.* **2015**, *28*, 319–326. [CrossRef]
32. Jones, S.E.; Maddocks, M.; Kon, S.S.; Canavan, J.L.; Nolan, C.M.; Clark, A.L.; Polkey, M.I.; Man, W.D. Sarcopenia in COPD: Prevalence, clinical correlates and response to pulmonary rehabilitation. *Thorax* **2015**, *70*, 213–218. [CrossRef]
33. Yen, H.; Lee, S.; Lin, C.; Lai, H.; Yamaguchi, Y.; Lee, P. Prevalence of sarcopenia and its association with diet and physical activity in older adults with type 2 diabetes: A cross-sectional study. *Nurs. Health Sci.* **2023**, *25*, 628–635. [CrossRef]
34. de Oliveira Neto, L.; de Oliveira, L.P.; Agrícola, P.M.D.; de Oliveira Tavares, V.D.; Gomes, I.C.; Sales, M.C.; Lima, K.C. Factors associated with sarcopenia in institutionalized elderly. *J. Public Health* **2021**, *43*, 806–813. [CrossRef] [PubMed]
35. Sri-On, J.; Fusakul, Y.; Kredarunsooksree, T.; Paksopis, T.; Ruangsiri, R. The prevalence and risk factors of sarcopenia among Thai community-dwelling older adults as defined by the Asian Working Group for Sarcopenia (AWGS-2019) criteria: A cross-sectional study. *BMC Geriatr.* **2022**, *22*, 786. [CrossRef] [PubMed]
36. Beaudart, C.; Sanchez-Rodriguez, D.; Locquet, M.; Reginster, J.Y.; Lengelé, L.; Bruyère, O. Malnutrition as a strong predictor of the onset of sarcopenia. *Nutrients* **2019**, *11*, 2883. [CrossRef] [PubMed]
37. da Costa Teixeira, L.A.; Avelar, N.C.P.; Peixoto, M.F.D.; Parentoni, A.N.; Santos, J.M.D.; Pereira, F.S.M.; Danielewicz, A.L.; Leopoldino, A.A.O.; Costa, S.P.; Arrieiro, A.N.; et al. Inflammatory biomarkers at different stages of Sarcopenia in older women. *Sci. Rep.* **2023**, *13*, 10367. [CrossRef] [PubMed]
38. Cerceau, V.R.; Pinheiro, H.A.; da Silva Boaventura, E.D.; de Matos, N.M.; de Araújo Lima, Z.R.A.; Stival, M.M. Prevalência e fatores associados ao risco de disfagia em pessoas idosas da comunidade. *Estud. Interdiscip. Sobre Envelhec.* **2024**. [CrossRef]
39. Zaitune, M.P.D.A.; Barros, M.B.D.A.; César, C.L.G.; Carandina, L.; Goldbaum, M. Fatores associados ao sedentarismo no lazer em idosos, Campinas, São Paulo, Brasil. *Cad. Saúde Pública* **2007**, *23*, 1329–1338. [CrossRef]

40. Pinheiro, H.A.; Cerceau, V.R.; Pereira, L.C.; Funghetto, S.S. Effects of the Home-based Older People's Exercise (HOPE) protocol on body composition and functional capacity of older Brazilians with sarcopenia: A randomized clinical trial. *Int. J. Dev. Res.* **2021**, *11*, 44824–44828.
41. Drummond, A.; Pimentel, W.R.T.; Pagotto, V.; Menezes, R.L. Disability on performing daily living activities in the elderly and history of falls: An analysis of the National Health Survey, 2013. *Rev. Bras. Epidemiol.* **2020**, *23*, e200055. [CrossRef]
42. Darvishi, A.; Hemami, M.R.; Shafiee, G.; Daroudi, R.; Mohseni, M.; Shekarabi, F.H.; Heshmat, R. Sarcopenia screening strategies in older people: A cost effectiveness analysis in Iran. *BMC Public Health* **2021**, *21*, 1–13. [CrossRef]
43. Silveira, E.A.; Souza, J.D.D.; Santos, A.S.E.A.D.C.; Canheta, A.B.D.S.; Pagotto, V.; Noll, M. What are the factors associated with sarcopenia-related variables in adult women with severe obesity? *Arch. Public Health* **2020**, *78*, 71. [CrossRef]
44. Martinez, B.P.; Batista, A.K.M.S.; Gomes, I.B.; Olivieri, F.M.; Camelier, F.W.R.; Camelier, A.A. Frequency of sarcopenia and associated factors among hospitalized elderly patients. *BMC Musculoskelet. Disord.* **2015**, *16*, 108. [CrossRef] [PubMed]
45. Cerri, A.P.; Bellelli, G.; Mazzone, A.; Pittella, F.; Landi, F.; Zambon, A.; Annoni, G. Sarcopenia and malnutrition in acutely ill hospitalized elderly: Prevalence and outcomes. *Clin. Nutr.* **2015**, *34*, 745–751. [CrossRef] [PubMed]
46. Bispo-Júnior, J.P.; Almeida, E.R. Equipes multiprofissionais (eMulti): Potencialidades e desafios para a ampliação da atenção primária à saúde no Brasil. *Cad. Saúde Pública* **2023**, *39*, e00120123. [CrossRef] [PubMed]

nutrients

MDPI

Article

Determinants of Malnourishment in the Institutionalized Older Population: The FRAGILESS Study

Julia Leira †, Ana Maseda *,†, Rocío López-López, Laura Lorenzo-López, Nuria Cibeira, Leire Lodeiro-Fernández and José C. Millán-Calenti

Universidade da Coruña, Gerontology and Geriatrics Research Group, Instituto de Investigación Biomédica de A Coruña (INIBIC), Complexo Hospitalario Universitario de A Coruña (CHUAC), SERGAS, 15071 A Coruña, Spain; julia.leira.morano@udc.es (J.L.); rocio.lopez.lopez@udc.es (R.L.-L.); laura.lorenzo.lopez@udc.es (L.L.-L.); nuria.cibeira@udc.es (N.C.); leire.lodeiro@udc.es (L.L.-F.); jcmillan@udc.es (J.C.M.-C.)

* Correspondence: amaseda@udc.es; Tel.: +34-881-015-983

† These authors contributed equally to this work.

Abstract: Background/Objectives: Malnutrition is a very common condition among older people and strongly affects their quality of life. The current literature relates the presence of nutritional deficiencies to several health-related factors that usually emerge at advanced stages of life. This study aimed to assess the associations between malnutrition and its determinants in a group of institutionalized older people via the Mini Nutritional Assessment–Short Form (MNA-SF) and the full MNA. Methods: The MNA-SF was compared with the full MNA to evaluate the nutritional status of 207 older people. A multinomial logistic regression analysis was performed. Results: The data revealed that institutionalized older people with cognitive impairment, frailty syndrome, dysphagia, a low BMI, a high duration of institutionalization, and a low educational level are more likely to be malnourished or at risk of malnutrition. Conclusions: The results reveal that the MNA or MNA-SF may not identify common determinants of malnutrition or nutritional risk. The identified determinants depend on the test. Therefore, the data obtained determine the need to use adequate nutritional screening tools to control the presence of malnutrition. Nutritional screening is essential to decrease public costs, hospitalizations, rates of disability, dependence, morbidity, and even mortality among institutionalized older people.

Keywords: malnutrition; undernutrition; Mini Nutritional Assessment; elderly

1. Introduction

According to the World Health Organization (WHO), malnutrition refers to "deficiencies or excesses in nutrient intake, imbalance of essential nutrients or impaired nutrient utilization" [1]. Malnutrition is a global public health problem and very prevalent in developed countries. Current evidence affirms that the risk of malnutrition is much greater among older individuals [2,3]. The WHO clarifies that malnutrition includes malnutrition, vitamin or mineral imbalance, overweight, obesity, and diseases that compromise nutrition. The percentage of older adults with problems of overweight and obesity is approximately 45%, whereas 462 million older adults experience moderate or severe malnutrition [1]. Malnutrition percentages are approximately 12–50%, specifically in hospitalized people, and 23–60% in institutionalized older people [4].

As mentioned, malnutrition is very common among older adults. The presence of this condition may be partly due to the physiological decline that humans suffer at this stage of life, the appearance of certain degenerative diseases, or the decrease in intake of food and essential nutrients [2]. Malnutrition deteriorates the quality of life and significantly increases public spending for its treatment, progressively increases hospitalization and increases the mortality rate [2,5–8]. The results of a systematic review of six longitudinal studies demonstrated that age was a risk factor for the development of malnutrition [9]. Specifically, malnutrition is also very common in older people with a good state of health [10].

The percentage of malnutrition considerably increases in older people in situations of isolation, dependence, and depression [4]. In cases of malnutrition, older people may experience an increased risk of falls, a substantial reduction in autonomy, gait disorders, and problems with healing wounds [11]. In addition, other very common pathologies or conditions at advanced ages represent risk factors for malnutrition, such as frailty in institutionalized people, polypharmacy, cognitive impairment, deterioration in general health, Parkinson's disease, institutionalization, and the presence of dysphagia or swallowing abnormalities [9,12]. A study revealed that dementia and Alzheimer's disease (AD) were less common in older people with a correct nutritional status [13]. In this sense, malnutrition can be linked to emotional factors such as the presence of depression [14,15]. Low food and nutrient intake may be more specifically due to the feeling of loss of an active social role, deprivation of affection, or depression, which may be caused by institutionalization. In other words, emotional problems largely stem from feelings of uselessness, a sedentary lifestyle or the passive role of older people [15,16].

Meanwhile, malnutrition is also linked to functional and physical factors such as sarcopenia and frailty [17]. Cognitive impairment has been shown to correlate to an incorrect nutritional status among older people [12,18]. Socio-environmental factors must be considered. The percentage of malnutrition often increases if there are physical barriers, great distances between homes and places where food is supplied, etc. An older person may not be able to access fresh products for proper nourishment for many reasons [19].

The current literature emphasizes the importance of early attention to malnutrition in older people. The aforementioned risk factors should be considered for early detection. Additionally, they can offer strategies for individualized and specific identification and treatment. In addition, they can lead to the creation of prevention techniques and instruments [2,9].

Currently, the methods used to evaluate the nutritional status of older adults are complicated and time-consuming [20]. Specifically, the Mini Nutritional Assessment (MNA) and its short version (MNA-SF) are excellent instruments to assess the nutritional status of older people. It is a very complete, standardized, and validated instrument that also predicts the risk of hospitalization and even mortality [20,21]. However, the use of malnutrition detection instruments, the correct application of diagnostic criteria, quantification of protein deficiencies and potential causes of malnutrition, and the assessment of individual resources are necessary throughout this process [22]. Nevertheless, the MNA contains questions to self-evaluate nutritional and health status, which may reduce its applicability in patients with dementia or impaired speech capacity [23,24]. Questions that address food choices, portion size, and mode of feeding may also not be appropriate for patients who are nutritionally stable. Thus, MNA cannot be used in patients who receive enteral nutrition [24]. MNA and MNA-SF are useful tools to detect the likelihood of undernutrition in frail older adults and malnutrition in the early stages with good reliability and sensitivity [25].

Early treatment can improve the quality of life for older people [3,11]. Eating a balanced diet, consuming the right amount of foods rich in proteins, vitamins, and minerals, and adequate intake of water constitute a good basis to treat and prevent eating problems [11]. Therefore, the hypothesis is that nutritional status can be linked to the development of health-related parameters in older adults. A high percentage of older people report this type of problem, so the need to promote new lines of research that address these types of risk factors, which are linked to the evolution and development of nutritional problems, is becoming increasingly evident. The identification of all of these factors will be beneficial for the creation of action protocols to improve the quality of life of this group and reduce the health costs, dependence, disability, and mortality rates [26].

Thus, the main objective of this study was to examine the relationship of a series of multi-dimensional risk factors related to the health and nutritional status in institutionalized older people and to compare the prevalence of malnutrition and the identification of its determinants using MNA-SF with that using the full MNA.

2. Materials and Methods

2.1. Design

A comparative, descriptive, and cross-sectional study was performed on a sample of older people aged $\geq$ 65 years, who were recruited from a gerontological complex in Galicia (Spain). All participants, or their relatives in the case of inability, gave their written informed consent. The research protocol was reviewed and approved by the Autonomous Research Ethics Committee of Galicia (Spain). The study was conducted following the ethical standards in the Declaration of Helsinki.

2.2. Participants

The study participants were recruited from a gerontological center, where different qualified professionals are in charge of the care for older people, most of whom have frailty or dependence problems. The center has several places for daytime stays and other places for permanent stays.

In total, 207 older adults participated in the study. The participants were selected based on the following inclusion criteria: (a) aged 65 years or older and (b) agreed to and signed the informed consent form. Participants who were unable to complete the assessment measures were excluded.

2.3. Instruments and Outcome Measures

All participants underwent a Comprehensive Gerontological Assessment (VGI). The objective was to globally assess the nutritional, physical functioning, psychological, and social status of each individual. The assessments were performed by a multi-disciplinary team composed of nutritionists, occupational and speech therapists, psychologists, and nurses. Information on the gender, age, educational level, length of institutionalization (months), or use of chewing aids was reported.

To perform the nutritional assessment, the Mini Nutritional Assessment (MNA) [27] and Mini Nutritional Assessment Short Form (MNA-SF) [28] scales were used. These tools reveal the current nutritional status of each participant. In addition, they classify each individual in a state of malnutrition, risk of malnutrition, or well-nourished according to the score obtained from the test, and the cutoff points are different in the long version and short version (For MNA, scores < 17 of 30 indicate "undernutrition", scores 17–23.5 indicate "at risk of malnutrition" and scores > 23.5 indicate "normal/well nourished". For MNA-SF, scores of 0–7 indicate "malnourishment", scores 8–11 indicate "at risk of malnutrition" and scores 12–14 indicate "normal"). It is especially designed for older people and widely used in care settings. Currently, it is available in several languages and is a good predictor of mortality and hospital costs due to malnutrition [29].

Weight and height measurements were obtained by a trained nurse. The BMI was estimated by dividing the weight (kilograms) by the square of the height (in meters). A clothing adjustment of approximately 0.8 kg for women and 1.2 kg for men was made [30]. The degree of comorbid illness was measured at the baseline using the Charlson Comorbidity Index (CCI) [31]. The age-adjusted CCI was computed.

The Spanish versions of the Mini-Mental State Examination (MMSE) [32] and severe MMSE (sMMSE) [33] were used as screening tools for dementia and cognitive impairment. MMSE scores of 0–30 were adjusted for the age and level of education considering cognitive impairment with scores $\leq$ 24. This tool enables rapid detection of mild or moderate cognitive impairment in clinical, community, and research contexts. Currently, it is the best-known and most commonly used method [34]. The sMMSE score range is also 0–30, where lower scores indicate greater impairment, and sMMSE is used when patients score 10 or less on the MMSE.

In addition, the Geriatric Depression Scale-Short Form (GDS-15) [35] was used to check for depressive symptomatology among the study participants, and a cutoff of 5 or higher was used to consider the existence of probable clinical depression. This scale, which was designed specifically for the geriatric population, explores the presence of depressive symptoms through 15 easy-to-understand questions with a dichotomous response pattern to facilitate its completion by the person being evaluated. The Cornell Scale for Depression in Dementia (CSDD) [36,37] was used to evaluate symptoms of major depression in patients with dementia by interviewing the patients and their formal caregivers. A cutoff point below 6 was considered the absence of significant depressive symptoms. Analysis of prescribed medications was based on the medical register. The Anatomical Therapeutic Chemical (ATC) classification was used to categorize the medications [38].

The study participants were classified as frail and pre-frail (non-frail or robust participants were not identified in our sample) according to Fried's frailty criteria [39]. These criteria assess the unintentional weight loss, self-reported exhaustion, slow walking speed, weakness (grip strength), and low physical activity of each individual. If 3 or more different domains are met, individuals are classified as frail; if 1 or 2 frailty domains are met, they are classified as pre-frail.

The Swallowing Performance Scale (SPS) [40] was used to detect dysphagia. The scale quantifies dysphagia with a score of 1–7 according to the criteria of oral impairment, pharyngeal impairment, aspiration, and diet. A higher score indicates more severe dysphagia [41]. In this study, a score of 3 or higher was considered dysphagia.

2.4. Statistical Analysis

The baseline characteristics of the sample were analyzed using descriptive statistics to compare the distributions of participant characteristics for each variable. Chi-square tests and one-way analysis of variance (ANOVA) were used to detect possible differences according to the nutritional status (normal/well-nourished, at risk of malnutrition or malnutrition) after the administration of the Mini Nutritional Assessment (MNA) or MNA-SF. Column proportions were used for the pairwise comparisons of categorical variables. In addition, Spearman's correlation coefficients were calculated between the independent variables and the total scores of the MNA and MNA-SF.

To determine the associations between the characteristics of the participants and their nutritional status (normal/well-nourished, at risk of malnutrition or malnutrition), which was determined by the administration of the MNA or MNA-SF, a multinomial logistic regression analysis was performed. Additionally, odds ratios (ORs) were estimated, and 95% confidence intervals (CIs) were calculated after adjustment for covariates. All statistical analyses were performed with IBM SPSS Statistics v.27.0 and R statistical software v.3.6.1 (using the R packages Rcmdr, MASS, and nparLD).

3. Results

3.1. Total Sample Characteristics

In total, 207 people were included in this study, 149 of whom were women, i.e., 72% of the sample. The mean age was 84.5 ± 7.8 years. The percentage of people who had received 8 or fewer years of education was 46.3%, 41.1% had 9–17 years of education, and only 12.6% had 18 or more years of education. The average length of institutionalization in the gerontological complex until the moment of data collection was 20.9 ± 24.1 months.

The MNA or MNA-SF was used to assess the nutritional status. After applying the MNA, a mean score of 20.3 ± 4.3 was obtained, and after applying the MNA-SF, a mean score of 9.7 ± 2.6 was obtained, which indicates that the majority of the sample was at risk of malnutrition according to both tests (no significant differences were found between the nutritional categories classified by MNA and MNA-SF, $p = 0.376$). Normal-status or well-nourished patients were present in only 25% of the sample, 60% were at risk of malnutrition, and approximately 15–20% presented malnourishment.

The mean BMI was 26.2 ± 5.7, and the age-adjusted CCI score was 6.2 ± 1.6. In total, 160 participants (78.8% of the sample) presented cognitive impairment, and, depression was observed in 44.2% of all participants. The mean number of drugs ingested per day was 8.4 ± 3.7. Frailty and pre-frailty criteria were observed in 68.6% and 31.4% of the sample, respectively. Furthermore, 65.7% used a type of chewing aid, and 33.2% suffered from swallowing problems.

3.2. Differences Between Multi-Dimensional Factors (Nutritional Status and MNA Score vs. MNA-SF Score)

The extended version of the MNA (Table 1) showed significant differences ($p = 0.008$) in the nutritional status by gender. The column proportions showed significant differences between normal individuals and those at risk of malnutrition, and women were at higher risk than men (79.3% vs. 20.7%). However, when the MNA-SF was used (Table 2), no significant differences ($p = 0.312$) were observed. The worst data in terms of nutrition were obtained from the examined women, but they were not significantly relevant. No significant differences were observed between the different nutritional statuses and the MNA versions in terms of age, level of education, age-adjusted CCI score, or use of chewing aids.

The length of institutionalization and number of drugs consumed significantly differed among the categories established by the MNA-SF. Patients who lived for more months in the nursing home were at risk of malnutrition ($p < 0.001$), and the number of drugs consumed decreased when the nutritional status worsened (9.0, 8.3, and 7.4, respectively, $p = 0.039$).

With respect to cognitive deficits, the tendency was similar between the MNA versions. Cognitive deficits were observed in 52–58.2% of cases with normal nutrition, 82.5–84.7% of cases at risk of malnutrition and 97.1–100% in malnutrition cases ($p < 0.001$). These percentages are not significantly different between those at risk of malnutrition and the malnourished.

Depressive symptoms occurred in 50.9% of cases at risk of malnutrition assessed by MNA, whereas they occurred in 26.5% of individuals with a normal nutritional status ($p = 0.015$). No significant differences were found in the presence of undernutrition assessment by the MNA-SF ($p = 0.161$).

Regarding the frailty phenotype, the trend was similar between both MNA versions: 81.8–91.2% of participants with malnutrition presented some criteria of frailty, as did 73.3–75.2% of those who presented an established risk of malnutrition and 42.0–46.3% of those who maintained a normal nutritional status ($p < 0.001$). The differences were not significant between risk of malnutrition and malnourishment.

Finally, the presence of dysphagia was similar between the two test versions, and there were significant differences between the groups. Dysphagia was detected in 60–69.4% of people with malnutrition, 30.6–32.8% of people at nutritional risk, and 12.5–16.7% of those with a normal nutritional status ($p < 0.001$).

Table 3 shows Spearman's correlations between the studied variables and the MNA and MNA-SF scores. The correlations between cognitive impairment, frailty phenotype, and swallowing performance were negative and ranged from −0.258 to −0.439. In other words, worse cognitive and frailty status and the presence of swallowing problems were associated with lower MNA and MNA-SF scores. A positive correlation was found with BMI: better nutritional status appeared at higher BMIs. In addition, a lower number of drugs consumed ($r = 0.154$) and the use of chewing aids ($r = -0.193$) were associated with better MNA-SF scores.

The logistic regression analysis identified important determinants of malnourishment or the risk of malnutrition. Older people with cognitive impairment, frailty, and dysphagia were more than 30 times more likely to be malnourished or at risk of malnourishment (Tables 4 and 5, with only significant variables included), although frailty was only identified using the full MNA analysis. In addition, as expected, low BMI is also a determinant of the risk of malnutrition or undernutrition. Finally, a longer duration of institutionalization and a lower educational level are determinants of malnutrition based on MNA-SF.

Table 1. One-way ANOVA and chi-square tests were used to compare older people according to their nutritional status (Mini Nutrition Assessment (MNA)), normal/well-nourished (24–30 points), at risk of malnutrition (17–23.5 points), and undernutrition (less than 17 points).

	Normal/Well-Nourished (n = 50)		At risk of Malnutrition (n = 121)		Undernutrition (n = 36)			Total (n = 207)	
	N or Mean	% or SD	N or Mean	% or SD	N or Mean	% or SD	*p* Value	N or Mean	% or SD
Gender (n, %) (1)							0.008 **		
Men	22	44.0	25	20.7	11	30.6		58	28.0
Women	28	56.0	96	79.3	25	69.4		149	72.0
Age (years; mean, SD)	83.8	8.1	84.7	7.6	84.6	7.9	0.785	84,5	7.8
Education (years; n, %)							0.444		
≤8	28	56.0	51	42.1	17	47.2		96	46.3
9–17	18	36.0	54	44.7	13	36.1		85	41.1
≥18	4	8.0	16	13.2	6	16.7		26	12.6
Months institutionalized (mean, SD)	20.5	19.4	22.6	28.0	15.9	12.8	0,347	20.9	24.1
Total MNA score (mean, SD)	25.5	1.4	20.3	1.9	13.3	2.4	<0.001 ***	20.3	4.3
Total MNA-SF (mean, SD)	12.2	1.3	9.8	1.7	6.0	2.3	<0.001 ***	9.7	2.6
BMI (kg/m2; mean, SD)	28.4	4.7	26.8	5.8	21.6	3.7	<0.001 ***	26.2	5.7
Age-adjusted CCI score (mean, SD)	5.7	1.4	6.3	1.6	6.3	1.8	0.070	6.2	1.6
Cognitive impairment (MMSE or sMMSE; n, %) (2)							<0.001 ***		
Yes	26	52.0	100	84.7	34	97.1		160	78.8
No	24	48.0	18	15.3	1	2.9		43	21.2
Presence of depressive symptoms by GDS-SF or Cornell (n, %) (3)							0.015 *		
Yes	13	26.5	59	50.9	16	47.1		88	44.2
No	36	73.5	57	49.1	18	52.9		111	55.8
Number of drugs (mean, SD)	8.2	4.4	8.7	3.6	7.8	2.9	0.412	8.4	3.7
Frailty phenotype (n, %) (4)							<0.001 ***		
Prefrailty	29	58.0	32	26.7	3	8.8		64	31.4
Frailty	21	42.0	88	73.3	31	91.2		140	68.6
Chewing aids (n, %)							0.363		
Yes	37	74.0	76	62.8	23	63.9		136	65.7
No	13	26.0	45	37.2	13	36.1		71	34.3
Dysphagia (Swallowing Performance Scale; n, %) (5)							<0.001 ***		
Yes	6	12.5	37	30.6	25	69.4		68	33.2
No	42	87.5	84	69.4	11	30.6		137	66.8

BMI: body mass index; CCI: Charlson Comorbidity Index; GDS-SF: Geriatric Depression Scale–Short Form; MMSE: Mini-Mental State Examination; sMMSE: Severe Mini-Mental State Examination. * Significant (*p* value) < 0.05; ** significant (*p* value) < 0.01; *** significant (*p* value) < 0.001.

Table 2. One-way ANOVA and chi-square tests were used to compare older people according to their nutritional status (Mini Nutrition Assessment–Short Form, MNA-SF), normal status (12–14 points), risk of malnutrition (8–11 points) and malnourishment status (less than 7 points).

	Normal (n = 55)		At risk of Malnutrition (n = 117)		Malnourishment (n = 35)		
	N or Mean	**% or SD**	**N or Mean**	**% or SD**	**N or Mean**	**% or SD**	***p* Value**
Gender (n, %)							0.312
Men	19	34.5	28	23.9	11	31.4	
Women	36	65.5	89	76.1	24	68.6	
Age (years; mean, SD)	83.8	7.7	84.8	7.9	84.2	7.1	0.749
Education (years; n, %)							0.179
≤8	32	58.2	50	42.7	14	40.0	
9–17	17	30.9	54	46.2	14	40.0	
≥18	6	10.9	13	11.1	7	20.0	
Months institutionalized (mean, SD)	18.9	17.9	23.7	28.6	13.7	10.9	<0.001 ***
Total MNA score (mean, SD)	24.6	2.3	20.3	2.5	13.8	3.1	0.043 *
Total MNA-SF (mean, SD)	12.7	0.8	9.6	1.0	5.4	1.7	<0.001 ***
BMI (kg/m^2; mean, SD)	28.9	4.7	26.7	6.1	21.7	5.2	0.315
Age-adjusted CCI score (mean, SD)	5.9	1.4	6.2	1.6	6.4	1.8	0.533
Cognitive impairment (MMSE or sMMSE; n, %) (1)							<0.001 ***
Yes	32	58.2	94	82.5	34	100.0	
No	23	41.8	20	17.5	0	0.0	
Presence of depressive symptoms by GDS-SF or Cornell (n, %)							0.161
Yes	19	34.5	52	46.0	17	54.8	
No	36	65.5	61	54.0	14	45.2	
Number of drugs (mean, SD)	9.0	4.4	8.3	3.5	7.4	3.3	0.039 *
Frailty phenotype (n, %) (2)							<0.001 ***
Prefrailty	29	53.7	29	24.8	6	18.2	
Frailty	25	46.3	88	75.2	27	81.8	
Chewing aids (n, %)							0.079
Yes	41	74.5	77	65.8	18	51.4	
No	14	25.5	40	34.2	17	48.6	
Dysphagia (Swallowing Performance Scale; n, %) (3)							<0.001 ***
Yes	9	16.7	38	32.8	21	60.0	
No	45	83.3	78	67.2	14	40.0	

BMI: body mass index; CCI: Charlson Comorbidity Index; GDS-SF: Geriatric Depression Scale–Short Form; MMSE: Mini-Mental State Examination; sMMSE: Severe Mini-Mental State Examination. * Significant (p value) < 0.05; *** significant (p value) < 0.001.

Table 3. Spearman's correlation coefficients among independent variables and Mini Nutritional Assessment (MNA) and MNA–Short Form (MNA-SF) total scores.

	MNA Total Score (max. 30 Points)	MNA-SF Score (max. 14 Points)
Gender	−0.082	−0.095
Age (years)	0.007	0.007
Education (years)	−0.084	−0.123
Months institutionalized	0.048	0.046
Total MNA Score		0.831 ***
Total MNA-SF score	0.831 ***	
BMI (kg/m^2)	0.447 ***	0.494 ***
Age-adjusted CCI score	−0.079	−0.042
Cognitive impairment	−0.375 ***	−0.306 ***
Presence of depressive symptoms	−0.127	−0.117
Number of drugs	0.039	0.154 *
Frailty phenotype	−0.354 ***	−0.272 ***
Dysphagia	−0.439 ***	−0.258 ***
Chewing aids	0.122	−0.193 **

BMI: body mass index; CCI: Charlson Comorbidity Index. * Significant (p value) < 0.05; ** significant (p value) < 0.01; *** significant (p value) < 0.001.

Table 4. Results of the multinomial logistic regression analysis for factors associated with normal/well-nourished status or risk of malnutrition relative to undernutrition (Mini Nutritional Assessment, MNA) ($\chi 2 = 112.268$, $p < 0.001$; −2 log likelihood 198.19, $p < 0.001$; Cox and Snell R2 0.487; Nagelkerke R2 0.579; 76.8% of cases precisely predicted). Only variables that indicate significant effects are included.

	Normal/Well-Nourished vs. Undernutrition			At Risk of Malnutrition vs. Undernutrition		
	OR	95% CI	p Value	OR	95% CI	p Value
BMI	1.607	1.1312–1.967	<0.001 ***	1.473	1.220–1.779	<0.001 ***
Presence of cognitive impairment	83.958	2.105–3348.642	0.018 *			
Presence of frailty	32.886	3.957–273.278	0.001 **	8.308	1.179–58.555	0.034 *
Presence of swallowing difficulties	33.995	4.995–231.376	<0.001 ***	11.166	2.436–51.171	0.002 **

BMI: Body mass index. * Significant (p value) < 0.05; ** significant (p value) < 0.01; *** significant (p value) < 0.001.

Table 5. Results of the multinomial logistic regression analysis for factors associated with normal or risk of malnutrition relative to malnourishment (Mini Nutritional Assessment, MNA-SF) ($\chi2 = 107.964$, $p < 0.001$; −2 log likelihood 215.64, $p < 0.001$; Cox and Snell R2 0.472; Nagelkerke R2 0.554; 72.8% of cases precisely predicted). Only variables that indicate significant effects are included.

	Normal vs. Malnourishment			At risk of Malnutrition vs. Malnourishment		
	OR	**95% CI**	***p* Value**	**OR**	**95% CI**	***p* Value**
BMI	1.731	1.374–2.181	<0.001 ***	1.586	1.271–1.980	<0.001 ***
Months institutionalized				1.074	1.013–1.139	0.017 *
Presence of cognitive impairment	9.2410	3.93510–2.25911	<0.001 ***			
Presence of swallowing difficulties	31.645	4.654–215.159	<0.001 ***	10.156	1.926–53.539	0.006 **
Low education (≤8 years)	0.025	0.002–0.317	0.004 **	0.059	0.006–0.583	0.015 *

BMI: Body mass index. * Significant (p value) < 0.05; ** significant (p value) < 0.01; *** significant (p value) < 0.001.

4. Discussion

To perform this study, the Mini Nutritional Assessment (MNA) and Mini Nutritional Assessment Short Form (MNA-SF) were used. The MNA is an excellent instrument for assessing the nutritional status of older adults [20,21], and the MNA-SF has greater sensitivity but lower specificity for patients aged over 65 years [42]. It is a validated and standardized screening tool that also helps to predict the hospitalization and mortality rates. However, Guyonnet et al. [3] reported that there were no standardized instruments to accurately detect malnutrition in this group; therefore, the malnutrition rate currently cannot be correctly estimated. Nevertheless, the MNA is a highly useful screening tool for detecting both nutritional risk and malnutrition, particularly in frail older people [43]. It is also ideal for routine use in health care and hospital settings [29]. The Short Nutritional Assessment Questionnaire (SNAQ), which is a screening tool used to predict the risk of malnutrition, can identify individuals who will lose weight earlier than MNA, but this scale is still rarely used. Currently, these scales are not used to detect nutritional problems in older adults because they require much time. The development of short versions aims to overcome this time limitation in professionals [3]. The Malnutrition Universal Screening Tool (MUST) was also identified as the most accurate nutritional screening tool for hospitalized patients in many clinical settings [42].

The percentage of malnutrition is the object of interest in this study. Hazzard et al. [4] reported a greater risk of malnutrition among older people who resided in a community. The reason may be situations of social isolation, self-imposed and environmental barriers and limitations. The barriers experienced by older people living in the community limit their access to food, which directly results in nutritional decline. Furthermore, the authors concluded that institutionalized people were subject to continuous medical care, unlike adults who live in the community. However, the rates reported by Kieswetter [6] of malnutrition among users of nursing homes and gerontological centers were very high (23–60%). Faravo-Moreira et al. [9] also noted that a person living in an institutional setting and in a situation of frailty was at high risk of malnutrition. Moreira et al. [44] affirmed that malnutrition was independently associated with residing in an institutionalized environment. Moreover, malnutrition is independent from the environment where a person is located and can occur in any scenario, except for those who live in the community [45]. In contrast, Donini et al. [16] explained that malnutrition in a community was frequent and continued to frequently occur in the most delicate and under-resourced groups of the population, e.g., older adults. Thus, they also stated that the malnutrition rate was higher among users of residences and institutional complexes. The reported data are as follows: 42.5% of women living in nursing homes suffer from malnutrition, whereas the percentage of older women with malnutrition living in a community is 14.5%. In the case of men, 30.8% of those living in nursing homes suffer from malnutrition, and only 2% of men living in a community are malnourished, which represents a great contrast between areas.

A study performed in residences for older people in Spain showed that malnutrition increased with age until 90 years of age, where the trend tends to stagnate. This rate has also been reported to be higher among older people institutionalized in residences in peripheral towns than among those in residences in the main cities [46]. Isenring et al. [47] reported that the nutritional risk of older adults living in a community was very low. Bell et al. [48] reported that approximately 20% of people who resided in nursing homes suffered from malnutrition. However, depending on the study, these rates are usually 1.5–66.5% of the total number of residents, so there is a wide range of variation between centers. Another study on public and private nursing homes in the city of Ankara [49] reported that 28.6% of residents suffered from malnutrition, and 44.5% were at risk of malnutrition. These alarming figures highlight a greater nutritional risk for nursing home users. However, another study with institutionalized older people in nursing homes in a rural area of Portugal [44] showed much lower percentages of malnutrition than expected in this context.

We observed a significant correlation between nutritional status and gender of the participants in the evaluation performed with the full MNA, but this correlation was not found in the regression model. The MNA-SF did not show this result because a study revealed that women were notably more likely to suffer from malnutrition than men, and this common difference is not understood today [50]. Therefore, although significant differences were found between several variables (such as gender or the presence of depressive symptoms) and nutritional status measured by MNA and/or MNA-SF, no evidence was found as determinants of malnutrition in the regression analysis.

A systematic review by O'Keeffe et al. [51] established conflicting evidence that depression was a determinant of malnutrition among older people, and it remains unclear whether depressive symptomatology is a cause or a consequence of malnutrition [52]. Yoshimura et al. [53] reported that depression and malnutrition tended to be closely related among young people but not among older people. Similarly, another study in China [54] reported that older people with malnutrition were 31% more likely to suffer from depression than older people who had a correct nutritional status. Our data revealed a significant difference only in the subjects evaluated by the full MNA and not in those assessed by MNA-SF.

In our study, no significant differences were detected between nutritional status and age or the use of chewing aids. Nevertheless, increased age can increase the risk of malnutrition due to physiological changes such as impaired taste, decreased gastric flexibility, and reduced appetite, which can exacerbate nutritional issues [52,55]. In addition, Moyihan et al. [56] reported that the use of specific aids such as dental prostheses could positively impact the nutritional status and cause greater enjoyment when eating. Hence, greater differences were observed in the data of people who use these aids and those who do not.

Low educational level and length of institutionalization were identified as determinants of malnourishment or risk of malnutrition only according to the MNA-SF. A meta-analysis revealed a significant relationship between low educational level and malnutrition or malnutrition risk, since individuals with higher education levels tend to have healthier and more diverse diets, which result in better nutritional status [57].

Our results identified important health-related parameters as determinants for malnutrition: frailty, cognitive impairment, and swallowing disorders. However, Bartali et al. [58] noted that low food intake was not related to the development of frailty among older people, and an association between malnutrition and/or the risk of malnutrition and frailty was found in a systematic review [59]. Favaro-Moreira et al. [9] established a decline in physical function as a very important risk factor for the development of malnutrition. Kieswetter [6] explained that if malnutrition was not correctly treated, the subject may be exposed to consequences at a physical functioning level. Another study reported that malnutrition detected by the MNA was significantly associated with functional measures based on the performance questionnaire [22]. Isenring et al. [47] reported that a higher rate of falls due to functional impairment was independently associated with nutritional risk. A study conducted in nursing homes in a Portuguese city [60] revealed that having cognitive decline and recurrent falls with associated injuries were not associated with poor nutritional status or risk of suffering from it. Our study revealed that cognitive impairment was also significantly associated with the poor nutritional status based on the full and short versions of the MNA. Kimura et al. [61] supported these data in their study and affirmed that the presence of malnutrition was very common among older adults with deterioration. In severe cognitive impairment, malnutrition may develop due to behavioral psychiatric symptoms of dementia (BPSD). A recent systematic review [12] mentioned possible causes of poor nutritional status and cognitive decline, since poor or deficient micronutrient intake plays key roles in the development and maintenance of brain structure and functions such as neurotransmitter activity, degeneration of nervous tissues and changes in brain functions. Another recent meta-analysis [62] revealed that older adults with cognitive frailty had a 3.77 times higher risk of malnutrition than those without cognitive frailty.

Swallowing disorders were also significantly associated with malnutrition status, as previously reported [63]. The consequences of the dysphagia–malnutrition relationship include weight loss, dehydration, muscle breakdown, fatigue, aspiration pneumonia, and a general decline in functional status [64]. Finally, our study did not suggest an association between the number of drugs consumed and malnutrition. Nevertheless, excessive polypharmacy was identified as a risk factor for malnutrition [9].

In summary, future studies should include the MNA and MNA-SF as ideal screening tools as part of a comprehensive assessment to identify multi-dimensional health factors that affect malnutrition. The nutritional status is an essential component to consider in long-term residential settings to establish an effective nutritional intervention, avoid increased morbidity and mortality and improve the quality of life of older people.

The main strength of this research is the large sample size, where data from institutionalized older people were comprehensively assessed. In addition, the analysis included potential health and social determinants. However, there are limitations, such as the cross-sectional nature of the study and the inability to determine the direction of the associations between the determinants and malnutrition or the risk of malnutrition. Furthermore, the limitations imposed by the descriptive nature of the study may hinder the generalization of the results. The Global Leadership Initiative on Malnutrition (GLIM) criteria were not published during the data collection; thus, they were not considered for diagnosing malnutrition [65].

5. Conclusions

In conclusion, this study analyzed the nutritional status and other health-related factors in a group of older people who resided in a gerontological center in a city in Spain. The results reveal that the MNA or MNA-SF can assess the nutritional status but do not identify the common determinants of malnutrition or nutritional risk. The relevant associated factors are cognitive impairment, frailty syndrome, dysphagia, low BMI, high length of institutionalization, and low educational level, depending on the test. Consequently, the findings highlight the need to use adequate nutritional screening tools to control the presence of malnutrition. This approach is crucial to reduce public costs, hospitalizations, rates of disability, dependence, morbidity, and mortality among institutionalized older people.

Author Contributions: Conceptualization, A.M. and J.C.M.-C.; data curation, J.L., A.M., R.L.-L., L.L.-L., N.C. and L.L.-F.; formal analysis, J.L. and A.M.; funding acquisition, L.L.-L.; investigation, J.L., A.M., R.L.-L., L.L.-L., N.C. and L.L.-F.; methodology, A.M. and J.C.M.-C.; resources, R.L.-L. and J.C.M.-C.; supervision, A.M. and J.C.M.-C.; writing—original draft, J.L. and A.M.; writing—review and editing, J.L., A.M., R.L.-L., L.L.-L., N.C., L.L.-F. and J.C.M.-C. All authors have read and agreed to the published version of the manuscript.

Funding: This research was funded by the Spanish Ministry of Science and Innovation: MCIN/AEI/ https://doi.org/10.13039/501100011033 [Grant PID2020-113788RB-I00].

Institutional Review Board Statement: The study was conducted in accordance with the Declaration of Helsinki, and approved by the Autonomous Research Ethics Committee of Galicia (Spain) (protocol code 08/2016 Institutional Review Board (or Ethics Committee), 15 April 2016).

Informed Consent Statement: Informed consent was obtained from all subjects involved in the study.

Data Availability Statement: The original contributions presented in the study are included in the article, further inquiries can be directed to the corresponding author.

Acknowledgments: We wish to thank all the patients and their relatives for their cooperation in the research. The authors are grateful to the staff at both the daycare center and the nursing home at the Gerontological Complex La Milagrosa, who took part in the management of the patients and provided administrative support during the study.

Conflicts of Interest: The authors declare no conflicts of interest. The funders had no role in the design of the study; in the collection, analyses, or interpretation of data; in the writing of the manuscript; or in the decision to publish the results.

References

1. World Health Organization. *Malnutrition*; World Health Organization: Geneva, Switzerland, 2020; Available online: https://www.who.int/health-topics/malnutrition#tab=tab_1 (accessed on 4 September 2024).
2. Dent, E.; Wright, O.R.L.; Woo, J.; Hoogendijk, E.O. Malnutrition in older adults. *Lancet* **2023**, *401*, 951–966. [CrossRef] [PubMed]
3. Guyonnet, S.; Rolland, Y. Screening for Malnutrition in Older People. *Clin. Geriatr. Med.* **2015**, *31*, 429–437. [CrossRef] [PubMed]
4. Hazzard, W.R.; Blass, J.P.; Ettinger, W.H., Jr.; Halter, J.B.; Ouslander, J.G. *Principles of Geriatric Medicine and Gerontology*, 4th ed.; McGraw-Hill: New York, NY, USA, 1999.
5. Mangels, A.R. CE: Malnutrition in older adults. *Am. J. Nurs.* **2018**, *118*, 34–41. [CrossRef] [PubMed]
6. Kiesswetter, E. Malnutrition in older people–Screening and assessment. *Dtsch. Med. Wochenschr.* **2020**, *145*, 1299–1305. [PubMed]
7. Donini, L.M.; Savina, C.; Piredda, M.; Cucinotta, D.; Fiorito, A.; Inelmen, E.M.; Sergi, G.; Domiguez, L.J.; Barbagallo, M.; Cannella, C. Senile anorexia in acute-ward and rehabilitation settings. *J. Nutr. Health Aging* **2008**, *12*, 511–517. [CrossRef] [PubMed]
8. De Lorenzo, A.; Deurenberg, P.; Pietrantuono, M.; Di Daniele, N.; Cervelli, V.; Andreoli, A. How fat is obese? *Acta Diabetol.* **2003**, *40*, S254–S257. [CrossRef]
9. Fávaro-Moreira, N.C.; Krausch-Hofmann, S.; Matthys, C.; Vereecken, C.; Vanhauwaert, E.; Declercq, A.; Bekkering, G.E.; Duyck, J. Risk factors for malnutrition in older adults: A systematic review of the literature based on longitudinal data. *Adv. Nutr.* **2016**, *7*, 507–522. [CrossRef]
10. Iizaka, S.; Tadaka, E.; Sanada, H. Comprehensive assessment of nutritional status and associated factors in the healthy, community-dwelling elderly. *Geriatr. Gerontol. Int.* **2008**, *8*, 24–31. [CrossRef]
11. Kalan, U.; Arik, F.; Pinar, S. Malnutrition in older people. In *Encyclopedia of Biomedical Gerontology*, 1st ed.; Rattan, S.I.S., Ed.; Academic Press: Cambridge, MA, USA, 2020; pp. 372–384.
12. Carey, S.; Deng, J.; Ferrie, S. The impact of malnutrition on cognition in older adults: A systematic review. *Clin. Nutr. ESPEN* **2024**, *63*, 177–183. [CrossRef]
13. O'Shea, E.; Trawley, S.; Manning, E.; Barrett, A.; Browne, V.; Timmons, S. Malnutrition in hospitalised older adults: A multicentre observational study of prevalence, associations and outcomes. *J. Nutr. Health Aging* **2017**, *21*, 830–836. [CrossRef] [PubMed]
14. Ramic, E.; Pranjic, N.; Batic-Mujanovic, O.; Karic, E.; Alibasic, E.; Alic, A. The effect of loneliness on malnutrition in elderly population. *Med. Arch.* **2011**, *65*, 92–95.
15. German, L.; Kahana, C.; Rosenfeld, V.; Zabrowsky, I.; Wiezer, Z.; Fraser, D.; Shahar, D.R. Depressive symptoms are associated with food insufficiency and nutritional deficiencies in poor community-dwelling elderly people. *J. Nutr. Health Aging* **2011**, *15*, 3–8. [CrossRef] [PubMed]
16. Donini, L.M.; Scardella, P.; Piombo, L.; Neri, B.; Asprino, R.; Proietti, A.R.; Carcaterra, S.; Cava, E.; Cataldi, S.; Cucinotta, D.; et al. Malnutrition in elderly: Social and economic determinants. *J. Nutr. Health Aging* **2013**, *17*, 9–15. [CrossRef] [PubMed]
17. Coelho, M.A.S.C.; Pereira, R.S.; Coelho, K.S.C. Antropometria e Composição Corporal em Idosos. In *Nutrição no Envelhecer*, 1st ed.; Frank, A.A., Soares, E.A., Eds.; Atheneu: Rio de Janeiro, Brazil, 2001; pp. 13–41.
18. Droogsma, E.; van Asselt, D.Z.; Schölzel-Dorenbos, C.J.; van Steijn, J.H.; van Walderveen, P.E.; van der Hooft, C.S. Nutritional status of community-dwelling elderly with newly diagnosed Alzheimer's disease: Prevalence of malnutrition and the relation of various factors to nutritional status. *J. Nutr. Health Aging* **2013**, *17*, 606–610. [CrossRef] [PubMed]
19. Rivière, S.; Gillette-Guyonnet, S.; Voisin, T.; Reynish, E.; Andrieu, S.; Lauque, S.; Salva, A.; Frisoni, G.; Nourhashemi, F.; Micas, M.; et al. A nutritional education program could prevent weight loss and slow cognitive decline in Alzheimer's disease. *J. Nutr. Health Aging* **2001**, *5*, 295–299.
20. Kagansky, N.; Berner, Y.; Koren-Morag, N.; Perelman, L.; Knobler, H.; Levy, S. Poor nutritional habits are predictors of poor outcome in very old hospitalized patients. *Am. J. Clin. Nutr.* **2005**, *82*, 784–791; quiz 913–914. [CrossRef]
21. Cereda, E. Mini nutritional assessment. *Curr. Opin. Clin. Nutr. Metab. Care* **2012**, *15*, 29–41. [CrossRef]
22. Kiesswetter, E.; Pohlhausen, S.; Uhlig, K.; Diekmann, R.; Lesser, S.; Heseker, H.; Stehle, P.; Sieber, C.C.; Volkert, D. Malnutrition is related to functional impairment in older adults receiving home care. *J. Nutr. Health Aging* **2013**, *17*, 345–350. [CrossRef]
23. Skates, J.; Anthony, P. The Mini Nutritional Assessment- An integral part of geriatric assessment. *Nutr. Today* **2009**, *44*, 21–28. [CrossRef]
24. Sieber, C.C. Nutritional screening tools—How does the MNA compare? Proceedings of the session held in Chicago May 2–3, 2006 (15 Years of Mini Nutritional Assessment). *J. Nutr. Health Aging* **2006**, *10*, 488–492; discussion 492–494.
25. Perry, E.; Walton, K.; Lambert, K. Prevalence of Malnutrition in People with Dementia in Long-Term Care: A Systematic Review and Meta-Analysis. *Nutrients* **2023**, *15*, 2927. [CrossRef] [PubMed]
26. Serón-Arbeloa, C.; Labarta-Monzón, L.; Puzo-Foncillas, J.; Mallor-Bonet, T.; Lafita-López, A.; Bueno-Vidales, N.; Montoro-Huguet, M. Malnutrition Screening and Assessment. *Nutrients* **2022**, *14*, 2392. [CrossRef] [PubMed]
27. Guigoz, Y.; Vellas, B.J.; Garry, P.J. Mini Nutritional Assessment: A practical assessment tool for grading the nutritional state of elderly patients. In *The Mini Nutritional Assessment (MNA)*; Vellas, B., Ed.; Serdi Publisher: Paris, France, 1994; Supplement No 2; pp. 15–59.
28. Kaiser, M.J.; Bauer, J.M.; Ramsch, C.; Uter, W.; Guigoz, Y.; Cederholm, T.; Thomas, D.R.; Anthony, P.; Charlton, K.E.; Maggio, M.; et al. Validation of the Mini Nutritional Assessment short-form (MNA-SF): A practical tool for identification of nutritional status. *J. Nutr. Health Aging* **2009**, *13*, 782–788. [CrossRef] [PubMed]

29. Vellas, B.; Guigoz, Y.; Nourhashemi, F.; Lauque, S.; Albarede, J.L. The Mini Nutritional Assessment (MNA) and its use in grading the nutritional state of elderly patients. *Nutrition* **1999**, *15*, 116–122. [CrossRef] [PubMed]
30. Whigham, L.D.; Schoeller, D.A.; Johnson, L.K.; Atkinson, R.L. Effect of clothing weight on body weight. *Int. J. Obes.* **2013**, *37*, 160–161. [CrossRef] [PubMed]
31. Charlson, M.E.; Pompei, P.; Ales, K.L.; MacKenzie, C.R. A new method of classifying prognostic comorbidity in longitudinal studies: Development and validation. *J. Chronic Dis.* **1987**, *40*, 373–383. [CrossRef] [PubMed]
32. Blesa, R.; Pujol, M.; Aguilar, M.; Santacruz, P.; Bertran-Serra, G.; Hernández, G.; Sol, J.M.; Peña-Casanova, J.; NORMACODEM Group. Clinical validity of the 'mini-mental state' for Spanish speaking communities. *Neuropsychologia* **2001**, *39*, 1150–1157. [CrossRef] [PubMed]
33. Buiza, C.; Navarro, A.; Díaz-Orueta, U.; González, M.F.; Alaba, J.; Arriola, E.; Hernández, C.; Zulaica, A.; Yanguas, J.J. Evaluación breve del estado cognitivo de la demencia en estadios avanzados: Resultados preliminares de la validación española del Severe Mini-Mental State Examination. *Rev. Esp. Geriatr. Gerontol.* **2011**, *46*, 131–138. [CrossRef]
34. Cockrell, J.R.; Folstein, M.F. Mini-Mental state examination (MMSE). *Psychopharmacol. Bull.* **1988**, *24*, 689–692.
35. Yesavage, J.A.; Sheikh, J.I. Geriatric Depression Scale (GDS). *Clin. Gerontol.* **1986**, *5*, 165–173. [CrossRef]
36. Alexopoulos, G.S.; Abrams, R.C.; Young, R.C.; Shamoian, C.A. Cornell scale for depression in dementia. *Biol. Psychiatry* **1988**, *23*, 271–284. [CrossRef] [PubMed]
37. Pujol-Doménech, J.; de Azpiazu, P.; Salamero, M.; Cuevas, R. Sintomatología depresiva de la demencia. Escala de Cornell: Validación de la versión en castellano. *Rev. Neurol.* **2001**, *33*, 397–398. [CrossRef]
38. WHO Collaborating Center for Drug Statistics Methodology. *Guidelines for ATC Classification and DDD Assignment 2013*; WHO Collaborating Centre for Drug Statistics Methodology: Oslo, Norway, 2013.
39. Fried, L.P.; Tangen, C.M.; Walston, J.; Newman, A.B.; Hirsch, C.; Gottdiener, J.; Seeman, T.; Tracy, R.; Kop, W.J.; Burke, G.; et al. Frailty in older adults: Evidence for a phenotype. *J. Gerontol. Med. Sci.* **2001**, *56*, M146–M156. [CrossRef] [PubMed]
40. Karnell, M.P.; MacCracken, E. A database information storage and reporting system for videofluorographic oropharyngeal motility (OPM) swallowing evaluations. *Am. J. Speech-Lang. Pathol.* **1994**, *3*, 54–60. [CrossRef]
41. Salama, J.K.; Stenson, K.M.; List, M.A.; Mell, L.K.; MacCracken, E.; Cohen, E.E.; Blair, E.; Vokes, E.E.; Haraf, D.J. Characteristics Associated with Swallowing Changes After Concurrent Chemotherapy and Radiotherapy in Patients with Head and Neck Cancer. *Arch. Otolaryngol. Head Neck Surg.* **2008**, *134*, 1060–1065. [CrossRef]
42. Cortes, R.; Yañez, A.M.; Capitán-Moyano, L.; Millán-Pons, A.; Bennasar-Veny, M. Evaluation of different screening tools for detection of malnutrition in hospitalised patients. *J. Clin. Nurs.* **2024**, *33*, 4759–4771. [CrossRef]
43. Pereira, M.L.; de Almeida Moreira, P.; Cunha de Oliveira, C.; Carneiro Roriz, A.K.; Teresópolis Reis Amaral, M.; Lima Mello, A.; Barbosa Ramos, L. Nutritional status of institutionalized elderly Brazilians: A study with the Mini Nutritional Assessment. *Nutr. Hosp.* **2014**, *31*, 1198–1204.
44. Moreira, A.L.; de Serpa, T.M.; García, N.P. Undernutrition and associated factors in Portuguese older adult community. *Rev. Nutr.* **2015**, *28*, 231–240.
45. Kaiser, M.J.; Bauer, J.M.; Rämsch, C.; Uter, W.; Guigoz, Y.; Cederholm, T.; Thomas, D.R.; Anthony, P.S.; Charlton, K.E.; Maggio, M.; et al. Frequency of malnutrition in older adults: A multinational perspective using the mini nutritional assessment. *J. Am. Geriatr. Soc.* **2010**, *58*, 1734–1738. [CrossRef]
46. Serrano-Urrea, R.; Garcia-Meseguer, M.J. Malnutrition in an elderly population without cognitive impairment living in nursing homes in Spain: Study of prevalence using the Mini Nutritional Assessment test. *Gerontology* **2013**, *59*, 490–498. [CrossRef] [PubMed]
47. Isenring, E.; Baker, J.; Kerr, G. Malnutrition and falls risk in community-dwelling older adults. *J. Nutr. Health Aging* **2013**, *17*, 277–279. [CrossRef] [PubMed]
48. Bell, C.L.; Lee, A.S.; Tamura, B.K. Malnutrition in the nursing home. *Curr. Opin. Clin. Nutr. Metab. Care* **2015**, *18*, 17–23. [CrossRef] [PubMed]
49. Kucuk, E.O.; Kapucu, S. Malnutrition in elderly staying in nursing homes. *Konuralp Tıp Derg.* **2017**, *9*, 46–51. [CrossRef]
50. Castel, H.; Shahar, D.; Harman-Boehm, I. Gender differences in factors associated with nutritional status of older medical patients. *J. Am. Coll. Nutr.* **2006**, *25*, 128–134. [CrossRef] [PubMed]
51. O'Keeffe, M.; Kelly, M.; O'Herlihy, E.; O'Toole, P.W.; Kearney, P.M.; Timmons, S.; O'Shea, E.; Stanton, C.; Hickson, M.; Rolland, Y.; et al. Potentially modifiable determinants of malnutrition in older adults: A systematic review. *Clin. Nutr.* **2019**, *38*, 2477–2498. [CrossRef] [PubMed]
52. Donini, L.M.; Stephan, B.C.M.; Rosano, A.; Molfino, A.; Poggiogalle, E.; Lenzi, A.; Siervo, M.; Muscaritoli, M. What Are the Risk Factors for Malnutrition in Older-Aged Institutionalized Adults? *Nutrients* **2020**, *12*, 2857. [CrossRef]
53. Yoshimura, K.; Yamada, M.; Kajiwara, Y.; Nishiguchi, S.; Aoyama, T. Relationship between depression and risk of malnutrition among community-dwelling young-old and old-old elderly people. *Aging Ment. Health* **2013**, *17*, 456–460. [CrossRef]
54. Wei, J.; Fan, L.; Zhang, Y.; Li, S.; Partridge, J.; Claytor, L.; Sulo, S. Association Between Malnutrition and Depression Among Community-Dwelling Older Chinese Adults. *Asia Pac. J. Public Health* **2018**, *30*, 107–117. [CrossRef]
55. Norman, K.; Haß, U.; Pirlich, M. Malnutrition in Older Adults-Recent Advances and Remaining Challenges. *Nutrients* **2021**, *13*, 2764. [CrossRef]

56. Moynihan, P.; Varghese, R. Impact of Wearing Dentures on Dietary Intake, Nutritional Status, and Eating: A Systematic Review. *JDR Clin. Trans. Res.* **2022**, *7*, 334–351. [CrossRef] [PubMed]
57. Besora-Moreno, M.; Llauradó, E.; Tarro, L.; Solà, R. Social and Economic Factors and Malnutrition or the Risk of Malnutrition in the Elderly: A Systematic Review and Meta-Analysis of Observational Studies. *Nutrients* **2020**, *12*, 737. [CrossRef] [PubMed]
58. Bartali, B.; Frongillo, E.A.; Bandinelli, S.; Lauretani, F.; Semba, R.D.; Fried, L.P.; Ferrucci, L. Low nutrient intake is an essential component of frailty in older persons. *J. Gerontol. A Biol. Sci. Med. Sci.* **2006**, *61*, 589–593. [CrossRef] [PubMed]
59. Lorenzo-López, L.; Maseda, A.; de Labra, C.; Regueiro-Folgueira, L.; Rodríguez-Villamil, J.L.; Millán-Calenti, J.C. Nutritional determinants of frailty in older adults: A systematic review. *BMC Geriatr.* **2017**, *17*, 108. [CrossRef] [PubMed]
60. Carrasco, C.; Reis, G.; Sim-Sim, M.; Parraca, J.A.; Fernandes, O.; Tomas-Carus, P. Sex, cognitive state and falls as factors associated with malnutrition: A cross-sectional study of institutionalized older adults living in a rural area of Portugal. *BMC Public Health* **2023**, *21* (Suppl. S2), 2337. [CrossRef] [PubMed]
61. Kimura, A.; Sugimoto, T.; Kitamori, K.; Saji, N.; Niida, S.; Toba, K.; Sakurai, T. Malnutrition is Associated with Behavioral and Psychiatric Symptoms of Dementia in Older Women with Mild Cognitive Impairment and Early-Stage Alzheimer's Disease. *Nutrients* **2019**, *11*, 1951. [CrossRef] [PubMed]
62. Feng, W.; Wang, J.; Zhang, H.; Wang, Y.; Sun, Z.; Chen, Y. Association between malnutrition and cognitive frailty in older adults: A systematic review and meta-analysis. *Geriatr. Nurs.* **2024**, *58*, 488–497. [CrossRef]
63. Nishioka, S.; Wakabayashi, H. Interaction between malnutrition and physical disability in older adults: Is there a malnutrition-disability cycle? *Nutr. Rev.* **2023**, *81*, 191–205. [CrossRef]
64. Ney, D.M.; Weiss, J.M.; Kind, A.J.; Robbins, J. Senescent swallowing: Impact, strategies, and interventions. *Nutr. Clin. Pract.* **2009**, *24*, 395–413. [CrossRef] [PubMed]
65. Cederholm, T.; Jensen, G.L.; Correia, M.I.T.D.; Gonzalez, M.C.; Fukushima, R.; Higashiguchi, T.; Baptista, G.; Barazzoni, R.; Blaauw, R.; Coats, A.; et al. GLIM criteria for the diagnosis of malnutrition-A consensus report from the global clinical nutrition community. *Clin. Nutr.* **2019**, *38*, 1–9. [CrossRef]

nutrients

Article

Muscle Biomarkers in Colorectal Cancer Outpatients: Agreement Between Computed Tomography, Bioelectrical Impedance Analysis, and Nutritional Ultrasound

Andrés Jiménez-Sánchez [1,*], María Elisa Soriano-Redondo [2], María del Carmen Roque-Cuéllar [1], Silvia García-Rey [1], Manuel Valladares-Ayerbes [3], José Luis Pereira-Cunill [1] and Pedro Pablo García-Luna [1]

1 Unidad de Gestión Clínica de Endocrinología y Nutrición, Instituto de Biomedicina de Sevilla, IBiS/Hospital Universitario Virgen del Rocío/CSIC/Universidad de Sevilla, Avda. Manuel Siurot s/n, 41013 Seville, Spain; mariac.roque@juntadeandalucia.es (M.d.C.R.-C.); silviam.garcia@juntadeandalucia.es (S.G.-R.); jpereira2@us.es (J.L.P.-C.)

2 Unidad de Gestión Clínica de Radiodiagnóstico, Hospital Universitario Virgen del Rocío, Avda. Manuel Siurot s/n, 41013 Seville, Spain

3 Unidad de Gestión Clínica de Oncología Médica, Instituto de Biomedicina de Sevilla, IBiS/Hospital Universitario Virgen del Rocío/CSIC/Universidad de Sevilla, Avda. Manuel Siurot s/n, 41013 Seville, Spain; mvalaye@icloud.com

* Correspondence: andres.jimenez.sanchez.sspa@juntadeandalucia.es

Abstract: Background: Muscle quality and mass in cancer patients have prognostic and diagnostic importance. Objectives: The objectives are to analyze agreement between gold-standard and bedside techniques for morphofunctional assessment. Methods: This cross-sectional study included 156 consecutive colorectal cancer outpatients that underwent computed tomography (CT) scanning at lumbar level 3 (L3), whole-body bioelectrical impedance analysis (BIA), point-of-care nutritional ultrasound® (US), anthropometry, and handgrip strength in the same day. Measured muscle biomarkers were stratified by sex, age, BMI-defined obesity, and malnutrition using Global Leadership in Malnutrition (GLIM) criteria. Whole-body estimations for muscle mass (MM) and fat-free mass were calculated using two different equations in CT (i.e., Shen, and Mourtzakis) and four different equations for BIA (i.e., Janssen, Talluri, Kanellakis, and Kotler). Muscle cross-sectional area at L3 was estimated using the USVALID equation in US. Different cut-off points for muscle atrophy and myosteatosis were applied. Sarcopenia was defined as muscle atrophy plus dynapenia. Intra-technique and inter-technique agreement were analyzed with Pearson, Lin (ρ), and Cohen (k) coefficients, Bland–Altman analyses, and hypothesis tests for measures of central tendency. Results: Intra-technique agreements on muscular atrophy (CT $k = 0.134$, BIA $k = -0.037$, US $k = 0.127$) and myosteatosis (CT $k = 0.122$) were low, but intra-technique agreement on sarcopenia in CT was fair ($k = 0.394$). Inter-technique agreement on muscular atrophy and sarcopenia were low. Neither CT and BIA ($\rho = 0.468$ to 0.772 depending on equation), nor CT and US ($\rho = 0.642$), were interchangeable. Amongst the BIA equations, MM by Janssen proved the best, with a 1.5 (3.6) kg bias, (−5.6, 8.6) kg LoA, and 9/156 (5.7%) measurements outside the LoA. Muscle biomarkers in all techniques were worse in aged, female, or malnourished participants. Obesity was associated with higher muscle mass or surface biomarkers in all techniques. Conclusions: Bedside techniques adequately detected patterns in skeletal muscle biomarkers, but lacked agreement with a reference technique in the study sample using the current methodology.

Keywords: muscle mass; validation study; computed tomography; bioelectrical impedance analysis; nutritional ultrasound®; obesity; GLIM; sarcopenia; colorectal cancer

1. Introduction

Computed tomography is a gold-standard body composition technique [1]. Software-based skeletal muscle segmentation at lumbar level 3 allows for the measurement of skeletal muscle area (L3-SMA) and density (L3-SMD). SMA can be used directly, indexed by height to produce the Skeletal Muscle Index (SMI), or used in different regression equations to obtain whole-body muscle mass (MM) [2] or fat-free mass (FFM) [3] estimates to diagnose low muscle mass (muscle atrophy). Muscle atrophy is part of the Global Leadership Initiative on Malnutrition (GLIM) [4] diagnostic criteria for malnutrition. As sarcopenia is a combination of muscle atrophy plus low strength (dynapenia), muscle atrophy is also part of the European Working Group on Sarcopenia in Older People (EWGSOP) diagnostic criteria [5]. In colorectal cancer patients, CT-determined muscle atrophy works as an independent predictor of survival and postoperative complications [6], functionality [7,8], and quality of life [9], amongst others. SMD acts as a surrogate measure for fatty infiltration (myosteatosis), a condition that associates worse prognosis and functionality in colorectal cancer [8,10]. Although it is an ionizing technique with limited accessibility, CT allows for opportunistic or retrospective measurements in routine studies requested in medical or surgical services for diagnostic–therapeutic purposes.

Bedside body composition analysis techniques, such as bioelectrical impedance analysis (BIA) and nutritional ultrasound® (US), are innocuous, relatively fast, portable, and cheaper. BIA is a doubly indirect technique that measures the following pure or raw bioelectrical parameters: Z (impedance), R_z (resistance), X_c (capacitive reactance), and phase angle (θ). These parameters may be introduced alongside age, sex, and basic anthropometric data in regression equations that estimate MM or FFM as measured by a reference technique [11,12]. US is an indirect technique that can evaluate muscular and adipose structures both in quantitative (thickness and area) and qualitative (echogenicity) terms. Using the nutritional ultrasound® methodology, muscle measurements take place in the distal third of the imaginary segment that joins the anterior superior iliac spine and the upper border of the patella, evaluating both the rectus femoris and vastus intermedius muscles [13]. US remains stable in fluid overload situations [14,15] and may predict muscle functionality [16]. Although it can diagnose myosteatosis based on echo-intensity levels, measurements from different devices may not coincide [17].

As previously stated, "The global clinical nutrition community needs to work together to come to consensus on the optimal tool(s) to use to assess nutrition status at the bedside" [18], and further studies that analyze agreement between CT and bedside body composition techniques are still needed [19]. To our knowledge, a simultaneous cross-sectional evaluation of the quantitative and qualitative agreement between a reference technique and two bedside techniques (BIA and US) in a colorectal cancer population has not yet been carried out. Performing all techniques on the same day avoids changes in body composition due to treatment or clinical evolution in an inter-technique time interval. If these techniques were directly interchangeable under the currently state of methodology and procedures, this could allow for more diagnostic efficiency and better continuity of care: US and BIA could be performed in the scheduled follow-up by Nutrition units, while CT scans requested for diagnostic or staging reasons could be analyzed opportunistically in between, thus having a closer follow-up of the subject's muscle status. Since CT scans can be analyzed retrospectively and with telemedicine, this closer monitoring would go unnoticed and without inconvenience for the patient. The aim of the present study is to analyze the degree of agreement in a simultaneous body composition analysis using CT, BIA, US, and anthropometry in a real-life sample of outpatients under follow-up for colorectal cancer, regardless of their treatment modality.

Our research questions were the following:

- Can all techniques detect similar patterns in body composition in the study sample?
- Are a reference (CT) and bedside techniques (BIA, US) interchangeable using current regression equations for MM or FFM in the study sample?
- How do current operational definitions of muscle atrophy, myosteatosis, and sarcopenia agree in the study sample?

Our hypothesis was that all techniques may detect similar patterns in the study sample, but direct interchangeability may not exist neither intra-technique nor inter-technique.

2. Materials and Methods

2.1. Study Design

This cross-sectional validation study was carried out in a single center (Hospital Universitario Virgen del Rocío, Seville, Spain). Consecutive sampling was used, and measurements took place from July 2022 to June 2023. This study protocol was designed following STROBE [19] and QUADAS-2 [20] recommendations.

The inclusion criteria were:

- Colorectal cancer outpatients over 50 years of age;
- Under active surveillance by the Oncology Department;
- With a programmed abdominal CT scan;
- Eastern Cooperative Oncology Group (ECOG) performance status of 0 to 3.

The exclusion criteria were

- ECOG 4-5;
- Terminal illness;
- Presence of a pacemaker, implantable cardioverter defibrillator, or intrathecal pain pump;
- Skin lesions or severe adhesive dermatitis that contraindicated electrode placement in the required areas for BIA;
- Severe cognitive impairment;
- Medical conditions that may artifact measurements at the discretion of the researcher (stroke with right residual hemiplegia, amyotrophic lateral sclerosis, or muscular dystrophy that may affect BIA and US; symptomatic rheumatoid arthritis or gouty arthritis of hand and wrist that may affect HGS);
- Unable to perform an informed consent or no desire for participation.

All measurements took place in the same day and order in a room with centrally-controlled temperature and devoid of strong electromagnetic fields. Liquid and solid intake was prohibited in the last two and eight hours, respectively. No patients received enteral or intravenous fluids during the fasting or measurement period, and no diuretic treatment was allowed during the fasting period. After emptying the bladder in a contiguous WC, participants undressed. Their clothing, smartphone, wearables, and jewelry were stored away. After a brief physical exploration looking for possible artifacts (central catheter, edema, or ostomy), participants rested in a supine position in an electrically isolated stretcher, covered by a hospital blanket. US was performed, with BIA measurements taking place immediately afterwards. Next, height, weight, and abdominal circumference were measured and annotated. Then, participants got dressed and handgrip strength was measured with a handheld dynamometer. Finally, patients were sent to Radiology so they could undergo their corresponding abdominal CT scan following normal procedures.

This study was conducted in accordance with the Declaration of Helsinki and approved by the Ethics Committee "CEI de los Hospitales Universitarios Virgen Macarena y Virgen del Rocío" (protocol code: 1006-N-22; date of approval: 23 May 2022). All patients participating in this study gave informed consent. "Written informed consent was conducted in person by A.J.-S. Each participant was provided with a written document detailing why they were contacted, what the participation consisted of, its possible risks and benefits, and pseudonymization of data. Only A.J-S. accessed the two separate password-encrypted databases of this study (one for patient identification, and one for data), which have been kept in custody in accordance with current European and Spanish legislation".

2.2. Procedures

2.2.1. Computed Tomography (CT) Scan Segmentation

Abdominal CT scans were requested by the Oncology Department of our center due to diagnostic–therapeutic reasons. Both the General Electric Revolution EVO (GE HealthCare Technologies Inc., Chicago, IL, USA) and Toshiba Aquilion (Toshiba, Minato, Japan) scanners were used. Portovenous phase scans with a slice thickness of either 1.00 or 1.25 mm were obtained after intravenous administration of a contrast medium following a standardized acquisition protocol. The images were retrospectively downloaded in Digital Imaging and Communication in Medicine (DICOM). DICOM files were then anonymized using DICOM Anonymizer v2.4.2 (https://www.dicomanonymizer.com/index.html, accessed on 1 November 2024).

Tissue segmentation was performed with Horos (Annapolis, MD, USA). Its 4.0.0RC4 version was used for this study (https://github.com/horosproject/horos/releases, accessed on 1 November 2024). The rationale behind its use has been previously explained [21].

All segmentations were performed on a Mac Mini M1 with 16 GB of RAM (Apple Inc., Cupertino, CA, USA) and an LG 32UN500P-W 31.5-inch screen with 4K resolution (LG Electronics, Seoul, Republic of Korea). The identification of the L3 vertebra and skeletal muscle segmentation using a −29 to +150 Hounsfield units (HU) threshold in a selected axial slice were performed following the Alberta protocol (TomoVision, Magog, QC, Canada, https://tomovision.com/Sarcopenia_Help/index.htm, accessed on 1 November 2024). Both the skeletal muscle cross-sectional area (L3-SMA) in square centimeters (cm^2) and skeletal muscle density (L3-SMD) in Hounsfield units (HU) were recorded.

2.2.2. Bioelectrical Impedance Analysis (BIA)

Bioelectrical impedance was measured with a phase-sensitive touch screen impedance device (Nutrilab™, Akern SRL; Pontassieve, Florence, Italy), working with an alternating sinusoidal electric current of 230 μA at an operating frequency of 50 kHz (±1%). The device was calibrated every morning using the standard control circuit supplied by the manufacturer with a known impedance resistance (R_Z) = 380 Ω; reactance (X_c) = 45 Ω. Impedance data are shown directly in a LCD touchscreen and stored into an internal memory. Accuracy: R_Z: ±0.1 Ω; X_c: ±0.1 Ω; CV% <1%. The pure bioelectric parameters obtained were: Z (in Ω), R_Z (in Ω), X_c (in Ω) and θ ($\theta = \tan^{-1}(X_c/R_Z)$, in °). The measurement technique was conducted according to ASPEN and ESPEN recommendations [18,22], with arms separated at 30° and legs at 45°. The electrode placement area was cleaned with 70° alcohol. Once dry, two sets of adhesive Ag/AgCl low impedance electrode (Bivatrodes™, Akern Srl; Pontassieve, Florence, Italy), designed for accurate and sensitive bioimpedance measurements, were placed proximal to the phalangeal–metacarpal joint on the dorsal surface of the right hand and distal to the transverse arch on the superior surface of the right foot. Sensor electrodes were placed at the midpoint between the distal prominence of the radius and ulna of the right wrist, and between the medial and lateral malleoli of the right ankle. The clamps of the measuring cable were then attached, avoiding the occurrence of loops. After an approximate time of five minutes in the supine position, participants underwent three consecutive measurements and each R, X_c, and θ were registered. Its respective means were used as input in Bodygram HBO version 3.1.6 (Akern SRL, Pontassieve, Florence, Italy) to calculate Talluri equations for both MM and FFM, or RStudio version 2023.06.1 + 524 to calculate other MM and FFM equations (Janssen, Kanellakis, and Kotler).

2.2.3. Nutritional Ultrasound® (US)

US was performed using a Butterly iQ+™ (Butterfly Network Inc., Burlington, MA, USA), a point-of-care (POC) handheld device with a 1–10 MHz range and a built-in battery that was connected via cable to a Samsung Galaxy S9 smartphone (Samsung Group, Suwon, Republic of Korea). Images were recorded using the "Musculoskeletal/Soft Tissue" presets, and the depth was adjusted as needed to visualize all structures of interest following previous recommendations [13]. All recorded images were stored in the Butterfly Network in a pseudo-anonymized manner. Images where then downloaded as .PNG files and measured in ImageJ in the same computer where CT scan segmentation took place. After calibrating each image measuring two centimeters in its built-in scale with the "Straight" tool and the Shift command to ensure a straight line, the "Set Scale" tool was then used to set the scale for that given image. Both Quad-MT (the whole depth of the vastus intermedius plus the rectus femoris of the quadriceps muscle in millimeters) and RF-MT (the depth of the rectus femoris of the quadriceps muscle in millimeters) were measured using the "Straight" tool. RF-CSA (the rectus femoris cross-sectional area in square centimeters) was measured using a manual "Polygon" tool.

2.2.4. Anthropometry Protocol

Height and weight measurements were performed according to ASPEN recommendations [18]. Height was measured with a SECA wall-mounted measuring rod (seca GmbH & Co. KG, Hamburg, Germany), installed at 200 mm. Weight was measured using a new and calibrated portable weight CAS-PB-150 (CAS Corporation, Seoul, Republic of Korea), with a capacity of up to 150 kg and two ranges of measuring sensitivity (20-g differences up to 60 kg; 50-g differences between 60 and 150 kg).

2.2.5. Handgrip Strength (HGS) Measurements

Handgrip strength was measured in kilograms (kg) using a JAMAR Plus handheld dynamometer (Performance Health Sammons Preston, Warrenville, IL, USA) in the dominant side following the Southampton protocol [23], and the best of three attempts was used for this study. Further details are discussed elsewhere [24].

2.2.6. Clinical Variables and Cancer Staging

The following clinical variables were obtained from digitized health records ("DIRAYA Clinical Station"): date of birth and age, ECOG Performance Status [25], type of baseline disease, tumor staging (according to AJCC-TNM 8th edition) [26], type and date of treatment, previous weight, active treatment, and presence of metallic artifacts. Different systemic anticancer therapies were applied following standard schemes according to Oncology guidelines [27].

2.2.7. Operative Definitions of Muscle Atrophy, Myosteatosis, Dynapenia, Sarcopenia, Malnutrition, and Obesity

Muscle atrophy in CT and BIA was defined on multiple muscle biomarkers using different cut-off points, applying EWGSOP-II [5] and GLIM [4] recommendations whenever possible (Table 1). Myosteatosis was defined by applying different cut-off points on SMD (Table 1). BIA equations were compared with CT biomarkers, including whole-body prediction equations for MM (Shen et al. [2]) and FFM (Mourtzakis et al. [3]). In US, muscle atrophy was based on the "confirmed sarcopenia" cut-off points from the DRECO study in Spanish inpatients with a simultaneous US, BIA and physical performance evaluation [28].

Table 1. Muscle biomarkers, definitions of muscle atrophy, and myosteatosis.

Technique	Muscle Biomarker	European Cut-Off Points
CT	SMI-CT (cm^2/m^2) = L3-SMA/H^2	Van Vugt et al. [29]: See Table A1 Dolan et al. [30]: <45 cm^2/m^2 if BMI < 25 kg/m^2 ♂, <53 cm^2/m^2 if BMI ≥ 25 kg/m^2 ♂, <39 cm^2/m^2 if BMI < 25 kg/m^2 ♀, <41 cm^2/m^2 if BMI ≥ 25 kg/m^2 ♀
	SMD (HU)	Van Vugt et al. [29]: See Table A1 Dolan et al. [30]: <34 HU if BMI < 25.0 kg/m^2 in both sexes, <32 HU if BMI ≥ 25 kg/m^2 in both sexes
	SMG (AU) = SMI-CT × SMD [31] Mourtzakis et al. [3]; FFM (kg) = 0.30 × L3-SMA + 6.06 Shen et al. MM [2,32,33]; MM (kg) = [(0.166 × L3-SMA + 2.142)] × 1.06; SMI-Shen (kg/m^2) = MT-mass/H^2	NA

Table 1. *Cont.*

Technique	Muscle Biomarker	European Cut-Off Points
BIA	Janssen et al. [34]; MM (kg) = 5.102 + [0.401 × (H^2/R)] + (3.825 × S) − (0.071 × A); SMI-Janssen (kg/m^2) = SMM-Janssen/H^2 MM-Talluri (kg) [c]	Masanés et al. [35] (Spanish): <8.31 Kg/m^2 ♂, <6.68 Kg/m^2 ♀ European [4,5]: <7.00 Kg/m^2 ♂, <5.50 Kg/m^2 ♀
	Kanellakis et al. [36]; FFM (kg) [a] = 12.299 + 0.164 × W + 7.287 × S − 0.116 × (R_z/H) + 0.365 × (X_c/H^2) + 21.570 x H Kotler et al. [37]; FFM (kg) [b] = 0.88 × [($H^{2.24}$/$Z^{0.63}$) × (1.0/37.63)] + 0.16 × W − 3.96 FFM-Talluri (kg) [c]	NA
US	RF-MT (mm)	DRECO study, de Luis et al. [28]: <9.66 mm ♂, <10.4 mm ♀
	RF-CSA (cm^2)	DRECO study, de Luis et al. [28]: <3.48 cm^2 ♂, <2.4 cm^2 ♀
	Quad-MT (mm)	NA
	Fischer et al. (USVALID) [38]; L3-SMA (cm^2) [d] = −54.0 + (21.0 × S) + (0.4 × W) + (0.6 × H) + (15.0 × Quad-MT)	NA

♀: female; ♂male; A: age in years; AU: arbitrary units; BIA: bioelectrical impedance; BMI: Body Mass Index; cm: centimeters; FFM: fat-free mass, H: height; HU: Hounsfield units; kg: kilograms; mm: millimeters; L3-SMA: skeletal muscle area at L3, L3-SMD: skeletal muscle density at L3, NA: not available; MM: muscle mass; RF-CSA: rectus femoris cross-sectional area in mm; RF-MT rectus femoris muscle thickness in mm; R_z: resistance at 50 kHz in ohm (Ω); S: sex (female = 0, male = 1); SMI: Skeletal Muscle Index; US: nutritional ultrasound®; W: weight in kg; X_c: reactance at 50 kHz (Ω); Z: impedance at 50 kHz in ohm (Ω). [a] H expressed in m; [b] H expressed in cm; [c] Proprietary equations are based to a significant degree on computed algorithms developed by Sun S. et al. [39]; [d] H expressed in cm and Quad-MT expressed in cm.

Dynapenia was defined as a maximal handgrip strength below the age-adjusted 10th percentile of normative values developed by Dodds et al. [40], and sarcopenia was defined as the conjunction of muscle atrophy and dynapenia using the EWGSOP-II criteria [5]. Malnutrition was defined using GLIM criteria [41]. Participants were considered to meet the etiological criterion for inflammation. Only involuntary weight loss was taken into consideration, as some participants were under a lifestyle modification to voluntarily reduce weight. Involuntary weight loss was defined as either moderate (>5% within the last 6 months or >10% beyond 6 months) or severe (>10% within the last 6 months or >20% beyond 6 months). Body Mass Index (BMI)-based malnutrition was considered as follows: "moderate" in participants with BMI < 20.0 kg/m^2 if <70 years old or BMI < 22.0 kg/m^2 if >70 years old, and "severe" in participants with BMI < 18.5 kg/m^2 if <70 years old or BMI < 20.0 kg/m^2 if >70 years old. Obesity was defined as BMI $\geq$ 20.0 kg/m^2.

2.3. Data Quality

All techniques (CT segmentation, BIA, US, HGS, and anthropometry) were performed and analyzed by a single researcher with previous experience in body composition analysis (A.J.S.). All participants received both the gold standard (CT) and index techniques (BIA, US, HGS, and anthropometry) in the same day, and in the same order (as previously described). Image analysis was supervised by a certified radiologist (ME.S.-R.) with extensive experience in abdomen imaging. Cancer stagings, treatments, and performance scores were registered in the database as recorded by oncologists (M.V.-A.) in health records. No artificial intelligence-assisted technology was used in data analysis or manuscript preparation.

2.4. Statistical Analysis

The packages *tidyverse* [42], *cowplot* [43], *DescTools* [44], *ggpubr* [45], and *metan* [46] were used in RStudio software (version 2023.06.1+524) [47]. Normality was analyzed with the Shapiro–Wilk test. Normally distributed variables were depicted as mean (standard deviation), and non-normally distributed variables were described as median (interquartile range). A *t*-test (in the presence of normality and homoscedasticity) or a Wilcoxon signed-rank test were used to compare measurements of central tendency in several muscle biomarkers in each technique (CT, BIA, US, and HGS) stratifying by sex (female/male), age (less or more than 65 years), obesity, and malnutrition. These tests were also used to compare measurements of central tendency between techniques (CT vs. BIA, and CT vs. US). Simple correlation between variables was calculated with the Pearson correlation coefficient (*r*). Quantitative agreement between variables was analyzed using the Bland–Altman analysis [48], depicting for each analysis its systematic bias, standard deviation of differences, a linear regression model to analyze dose-dependent bias, and Limits of Agreement (LoA). Quantitative agreement was analyzed using Lin's Concordance Correlation Coefficient (ρ), considering values > 0.99 as "near perfect", 0.95 to 0.99 as "substantial", 0.90 to 0.95 as "moderate", and < 0.90 as "poor" [49]. Associated 95% Confidence Intervals (95%CI) were also calculated for each ρ. Categorical agreements between different muscle atrophy and malnutrition definitions were analyzed with Cohen's kappa [50]. Outliers were not censored, and all measurements were included for statistical analysis. Statistical significance was determined in all two-tailed tests as $p < 0.05$.

3. Results

3.1. Description of the Study Sample

A total of n = 156 participants were measured with all techniques (CT, US, BIA, HGS, and anthropometry) and included for analysis. A flowchart summarizing patient recruitment, exclusions, and final sample size is available as Figure 1. The median time between CT and bedside techniques was 60.0 (20.0) minutes. Possible BIA artifacts (central catheter, ostomy, metallic prothesis, and diuretic) were systematically registered (Table S1), and n = 93 (59.6%) participants were completely artifact-free. No participants had fever or oedema when measurements took place.

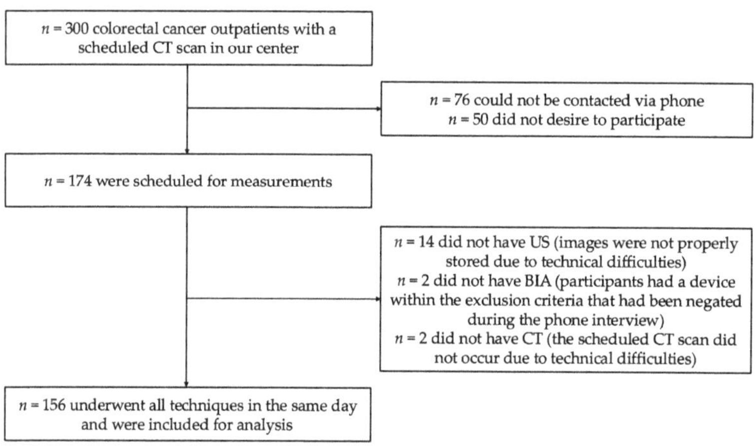

Figure 1. Patient recruitment, exclusions, and final sample size. BIA: bioelectrical impedance analysis; CT: computed tomography; *n* = absolute frequency; US: nutritional ultrasound®.

Demographic and anthropometric data were as follows: (Table 2): *n* = 75 (48.1%) participants were female. The median age was 65.2 (13.6) years. *n* = 54 (34.6%) participants had 70 or more years. Age was 61.5 (9.8) vs. 74.6 (3.7) years ($p < 2.2 \times 10^{-16}$) in young vs. old participants. The median BMI was 27.3 (5.7) kg/m^2, and the modal BMI category was overweight (36.5%). *n* = 41 (26.3%) participants had obesity. Weight was 69.2 (17.0) vs. 90.5 (17.5) kg ($p = 1.457 \times 10^{-14}$) in non-obese vs. obese participants. *n* = 11 (7.0%) participants had malnutrition. All malnutrition cases were "moderate" and due to low BMI, with no significant weight loss in the study sample. Density plots for body mass index (BMI) stratified by age and sex were graphed (Figure S1).

Table 2. Clinical and demographic characteristics of the study sample.

Parameter	Results
Female	n = 75 (48.1%)
Age (years)	M = 65.2 (13.6)
70 years or older	n = 54 (34.6%)
Height (m)	$\bar{x}$ = 1.64 (0.09)
Weight (kg)	M = 73.3 (19.9)
BMI (kg/m^2)	M = 27.3 (5.7)
Obesity	Yes, n = 41 (26.3%) No, n = 115 (73.7%)
BMI as factor	Underweight, n = 8 (5.1%) Normal weight, n = 50 (32.0%) Overweight, n = 57 (36.5%) Grade 1 obesity, n = 27 (17.3%) Grade 2 obesity, n = 10 (6.4%) Grade 3 obesity, n = 4 (2.6%)
GLIM malnutrition	Yes, n = 11 (7.0%) No, n = 145 (93.0%)

n_i: absolute frequency; %: percentage; kg: kilograms; $\bar{x}$ (): mean (standard deviation); M (): median (interquartile range); m: meters.

Tumor-related characteristics were as follows (Table S1): modal ECOG was 0 (64.7%). The most frequent neoplasm was colon (41.6%), and IIIB (20.8%) was the modal TNM stage. Most (91.7%) of the participants had undergone surgery, with right hemi-colectomy (25.9%) being the most frequent surgical procedure. 93.0% of the sample received chemotherapy, mostly with adjuvant intention (62.8%). Monotherapy with capecitabine was the most frequent drug (33.8%). A total of 24.4% of the sample received chemotherapy in the 90 days before the measurements took place. Most of the participants had not received radiotherapy (69.9%).

3.2. Muscle Biomarkers

3.2.1. General Description

All analyzed muscle biomarkers in each technique (CT, BIA, US, and HGS) were stratified by sex, age, BMI, and GLIM criteria. These results and their inter-group comparisons of measures of central tendency are available in Table 3 (CT), Table 4 (BIA), and Table 5 (US and HGS). The most representative biomarkers in each technique have been graphed in Figure 2 (CT), Figure 3 (US), and Figure 4 (BIA) for further clarification and easier visualization.

Table 3. CT-based muscle biomarkers.

		L3 SMA (cm^2)	L3 SMD (HU)	L3 SMI (cm^2/m^2)	SMG (AU)	Shen MM (kg) [2]	Mourtzakis FFM (kg) [3]
Whole sample		$\bar{x}$: 125.8 (29.4)M: 121.2 (45.5) [69.2, 198.6]	$\bar{x}$: 40.7 (8.2) M: 40.8 (10.6) [21.8, 62.8]	$\bar{x}$: 46.3 (8.6) M: 44.9 (12.7) [28.5, 71.3]	$\bar{x}$: 1889.5 (520.6) M: 1873.6 (744.9) [768.3, 3374.8]	$\bar{x}$: 24.4 (5.2) M: 23.6 (8.0) [14.4, 37.2]	$\bar{x}$: 43.8 (8.8) M: 42.4 (13.7) [26.8, 65.6]
Sex							
	Male	145.2	40.3	51.4	2052.4	27.8	49.6
	Female	103.4	41.1	41.0	1713.6	20.50	37.1
	p	$<2.2 \times 10^{-16}$	0.576	1.129×10^{-11}	2.886×10^{-5}	$<2.2 \times 10^{-16}$	$<2.2 \times 10^{-16}$
Age							
	Young	121.2	42.7	44.7	1988.2	23.6	42.1
	Elder	120.2	36.9	45.2	1703.2	23.4	42.4
	p	0.317	2.034×10^{-5}	0.969	7.482×10^{-4}	0.317	0.317
Obesity							
	No	117.8	120.5	43.5	1862.5	23.0	41.4
	Yes	146.0	140.7	51.7	1965.4	28.0	49.9
	p	0.001	8.243×10^{-3}	3.833×10^{-7}	0.288	0.001	0.001
GLIM							
	Negative	122.9	40.2	45.0	1892.3	23.9	42.9
	Positive	108.4	47.0	39.3	1853.8	21.3	38.6
	p	0.041	0.059	0.005	0.804	0.041	0.041

The p-value (p) for the associated central tendency tests in each case is displayed on the right of each category (t-test if assumptions were met, Wilcoxon signed-rank test if not). AU: arbitrary units; cm: centimeters; FFM: fat-free mass; GLIM: Global Leadership Initiative in Malnutrition; HU: Hounsfield units; MM: muscle mass; p: p-value. Range is represented as [minimum, maximum].

Table 4. BIA muscle biomarkers.

	Janssen MM (kg) [34]	Talluri MM (kg)	Kanellakis FFM (kg) [36]	Kotler FFM (kg) [37]	Talluri FFM (kg)	θ (°)
Whole sample	x̄: 22.9 (6.1) M: 23.3 (9.2) [13.6, 37.1]	x̄: 30.8 (7.0) M: 29.9 (9.4) [15.2, 50.5]	x̄: 31.3 (12.0) M: 32.6 (19.1) [6.4, 58.2]	x̄: 48.1 (9.2) M: 47.7 (13.1) [30.6, 74.5]	x̄: 50.7 (9.7) M: 49.9 (14.2) [33.4, 80.1]	x̄: 5.0 (0.7) M: 5.1 (0.9) [2.6, 6.7]
Sex						
Male	26.7	34.9	40.3	52.8	56.8	5.3
Female	17.5	26.0	21.1	40.7	42.6	4.9
p	$<2.2 \times 10^{-16}$	$<2.2 \times 10^{-16}$	$<2.2 \times 10^{-16}$	$<2.2 \times 10^{-16}$	$<2.2 \times 10^{-16}$	0.002
Age						
Young	23.5	29.9	33.5	47.7	50.4	5.3
Elder	22.3	29.0	32.0	47.9	49.1	4.7
p	0.287	0.103	0.865	0.719	0.807	2.44×10^{-6}
Obesity						
No	22.5	29.4	30.5	45.7	48.5	5.2
Yes	26.1	33.5	38.2	53.0	55.2	4.8
p	0.041	8.258×10^{-3}	1.596×10^{-3}	7.969×10^{-4}	5.229×10^{-4}	0.277
GLIM						
Negative	23.5	30.6	33.5	48.7	50.5	
Positive	18.5	23.5	18.8	41.5	41.4	5.1
p	0.050	5.171×10^{-4}	0.003	0.006	9.361×10^{-4}	4.90.327

°: degrees; FFM: fat-free mass; θ: raw phase angle.

Table 5. US-based muscle biomarkers.

	RF-MT (mm)	Quad-MT (mm)	RF-CSA (cm^2)	HGS (kg)
Whole sample	x̄: 14.3(3.3) M: 13.9(3.9) [7.1, 25.9]	x̄: 27.3(7.0) M: 26.6(9.1) [11.7, 48.9]	x̄: 4.2(1.2) M: 4.1(1.4) [1.7, 8.3]	x̄: 34.8 (10.0) M: 33.9 (12.9) [13.3, 64.0]
Sex				
Male	15.4	29.9	4.64	40.0
Female	12.5	23.8	3.60	29.0
p	5.154×10^{-9}	6.309×10^{-9}	8.208×10^{-9}	1.7×10^{-13}
Age				
Young	14.4	26.7	4.19	36.4
Elder	13.5	25.1	3.79	31.6
p	0.082	0.214	0.121	0.006
Obesity				
No	13.3	25.1	3.9	34.6
Yes	14.6	30.0	4.5	35.5
p	3.164×10^{-3}	8.568×10^{-3}	1.794×10^{-3}	0.655
GLIM				
Negative	14.4	27.1	4.18	35.0
Positive	11.7	22.1	3.26	32.1
p	7.204×10^{-3}	2.502×10^{-4}	0.002	0.407

HGS: maximal handgrip strength; RF-CSA: rectus femoris Cross-Sectional Area; RF-MT: rectus femoris muscle thickness; Quad-MT: quadricipital (rectus femoris plus vastus intermedius) muscle thickness.

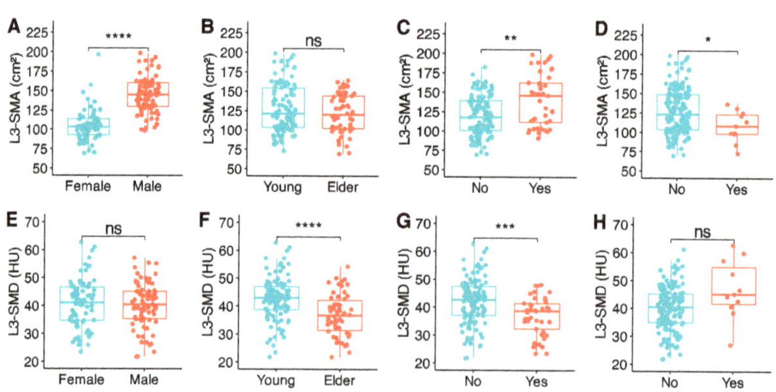

Figure 2. *Cont.*

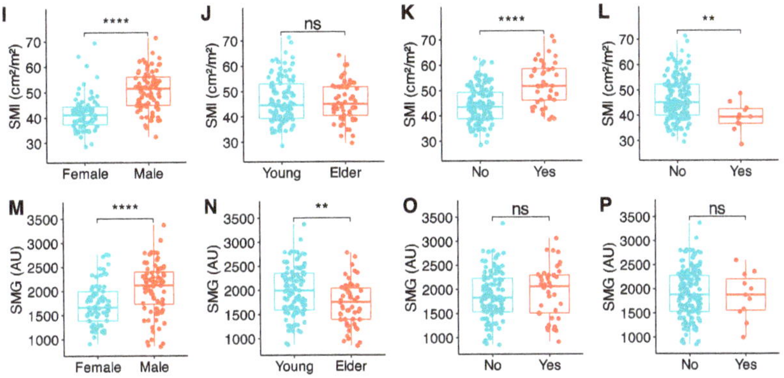

Figure 2. CT-based muscle biomarkers, by rows (from top to down): skeletal muscle area (**A**–**D**), skeletal muscle density (**E**–**H**), skeletal muscle index (**I**–**L**), and skeletal muscle gauge (**D**–**P**). Data are stratified in columns (from left to right) by sex (**A**,**E**,**I**), age (**B**,**F**,**J**), obesity (**C**,**G**,**K**), and malnutrition (**D**,**H**,**L**). Statistical significance for comparisons of central tendency measures is depicted as follows: $p > 0.05$ = ns; $p \leq 0.05$ = *; $p \leq 0.01$ = **; $p \leq 0.001$ = ***; $p \leq 0.0001$ = ****. AU: arbitrary uits; BMI: Body Mass Index; Cm: centimeters; GLIM: Global Leadership Initiative in Malnutrition; HU: Hounsfield units; L3-SMA: skeletal muscle area at L3; L3-SMD: skeletal muscle density at L3; m: meters; SMG: skeletal muscle gauge at L3; SMI: skeletal muscle index at L3M.

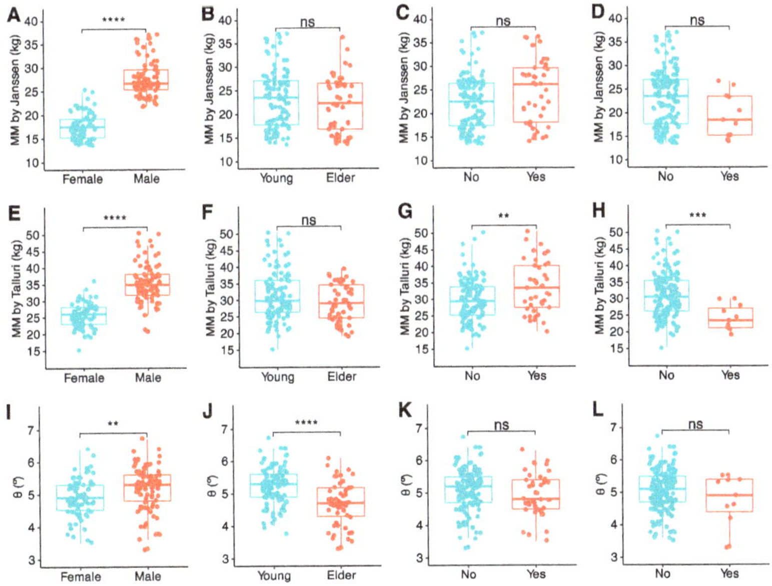

Figure 3. BIA-based muscle biomarkers, by rows (from top to down): Janssen et al. [34] MM (**A**–**D**), Talluri MM (**E**–**H**), and θ (**I**–**L**). Data are stratified in columns (from left to right) by sex (**A**,**E**,**I**), age (**B**,**F**,**J**), obesity (**C**,**G**,**K**), and malnutrition (**D**,**H**,**L**). °: degrees; θ: raw phase angle; MM: muscle mass. Statistical significance for comparisons of central tendency measures is depicted as follows: $p > 0.05$ = ns; $p \leq 0.01$ = **; $p \leq 0.001$ = ***; $p \leq 0.0001$ = ****.

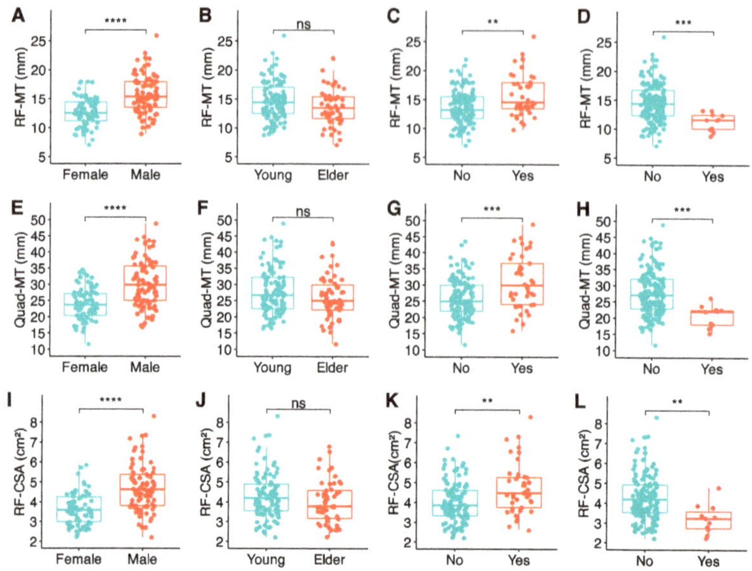

Figure 4. US-based muscle biomarkers, by rows (from top to down): rectus femoris muscle thickness (**A**–**D**), quadricipital muscle thickness (**E**–**H**), and quadricipital muscle area (**I**–**L**). Data are stratified in columns (from left to right) by sex (**A**,**E**,**I**), age (**B**,**F**,**J**), obesity (**C**,**G**,**K**), and malnutrition (**D**,**H**,**L**). Mm: millimeters. RF-MT: rectus femoris muscle thickness in mm; Quad-MT: quadricipital muscle thickness (rectus femoris plus vastus intermedius) in mm; RF-CSA: rectus femoris cross-sectional area in cm^2. Statistical significance for comparisons of central tendency measures is depicted as follows: $p > 0.05$ = ns; $p \leq 0.01$ = **; $p \leq 0.001$ = ***; $p \leq 0.0001$ = ****.

3.2.2. CT Muscle Biomarkers

All variables followed a non-normal distribution, except for L3-SMD and SMG. Female participants had lower muscle surface and mass biomarkers, but had no differences regarding L3-SMD. On the contrary, older participants had worse L3-SMD, but no differences regarding muscle surface and mass biomarkers. Patients with obesity had higher muscle surface and mass biomarkers (even adjusted by height), but also worse L3-SMD. Malnourished patients had worse muscle surface and mass biomarkers, and tended to have worse L3-SMD (Table 3, Figure 2).

3.2.3. BIA Biomarkers

All variables followed a non-normal distribution, except for Talluri MM. Female participants had lower MM, FFM, and θ. On the contrary, older participants had worse θ, but no differences regarding MM or FFM. Patients with obesity had higher MM and FFM. They had worse θ, but without statistical significance. Malnourished patients had worse MM and FFM. They also had worse θ, but again without statistical significance (Table 4, Figure 3).

3.2.4. US Biomarkers and Handgrip Strength

All variables followed a non-normal distribution. Female participants had lower US biomarkers and HGS. Older participants displayed worse HGS, but lacked differences in US biomarkers. Patients with obesity had higher US biomarkers. They had higher HGS, but without statistical significance. Malnourished patients had US biomarkers. They also had lower HGS, in this case without statistical significance (Table 5, Figure 4).

3.3. Muscle Biomarkers: Intra and Inter-Technique Correlation Matrices

For an easier interpretation, muscle biomarkers were separated into two different correlation matrices. The first one includes measured and estimated parameters from BIA, measured and estimated biomarkers from CT, anthropometry, and handgrip strength (Figure 5A). The second one includes US measurements, measured and estimated biomarkers from CT, anthropometry, and handgrip strength (Figure 5B).

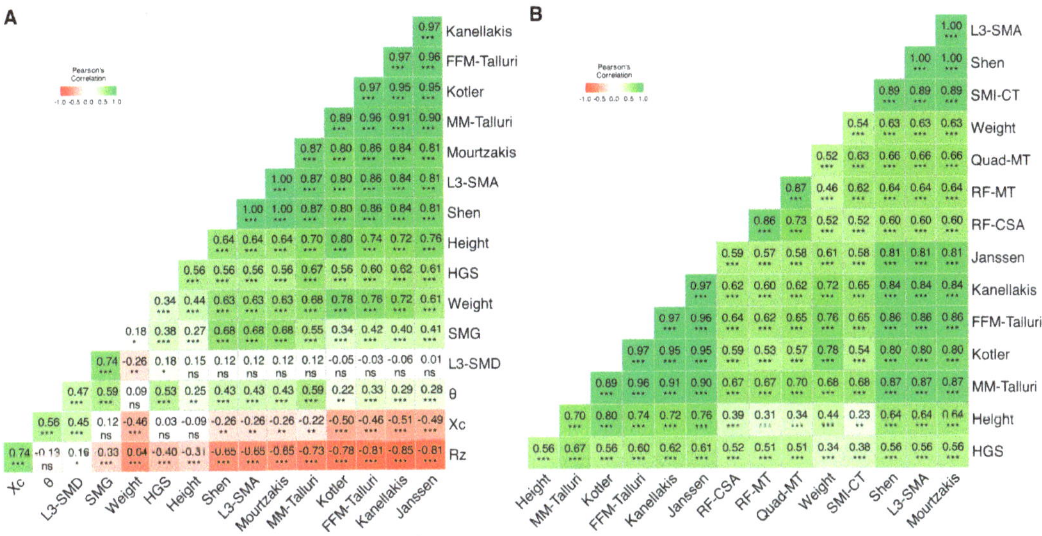

Figure 5. Correlation matrices, based on Spearman's correlation coefficients (r). Direct correlations are shown in shades of green, and inverse correlations are shown in shades of red. Correlation strength is proportional to color intensity. (**A**) BIA-measured (R_z, X_c, and θ) parameters, BIA-estimated FFM (Kanellakis, Kotler, FFM-Talluri) [36,37] and BIA-estimated MM (Janssen, MM-Talluri) [34], CT-measured parameters (SMA, SMD), CT-estimated whole-body MM (Shen) [2] and FFM (Mourtzakis) [3], anthropometry (Height, Weight), and handgrip strength (HGS). (**B**) US-measured (Quad-MT, RF-MT, RF-CSA), BIA-estimated FFM and FM, CT-measured parameters, anthropometry, and handgrip strength. Statistical significance for comparisons of central tendency measures is depicted as follows: $p > 0.05$ = ns; $p \leq 0.05$ = *; $p \leq 0.01$ = **; $p \leq 0.001$ = ***.

3.3.1. Matrix 1: CT, BIA, and HGS

Regarding raw or unbiased BIA measurements:

- R_z had moderate inverse correlations with L3-SMA ($r = -0.65$), weight ($r = -0.65$), and HGS ($r = -0.40$), as well as a moderate direct correlation with X_c ($r = 0.74$).
- Conversely, X_c had moderate direct correlations with θ ($r = 0.56$), and L3-SMD ($r = 0.45$).
- θ had moderate direct correlations with SMG ($r = 0.59$), HGS ($r = 0.53$), L3-SMD ($r = 0.47$), and L3-SMA ($r = 0.43$).

BIA-estimated and CT-estimated whole-body muscle biomarkers were correlated as following:

- L3-SMA (in cm^2) and all the MM equations ($r = 0.87$ Talluri; $r = 0.81$ Janssen) [34] or FFM equations ($r = 0.86$ Talluri, $r = 0.84$ Kanellakis, $r = 0.80$ Kotler) [36,37] displayed high correlation coefficients.
- Whole-body estimated MM by the Shen equation [2] and BIA-based whole-body MM equations ($r = 0.87$ Talluri; $r = 0.81$ Janssen) [34] were also strongly correlated.

- Whole-body estimated FFM by the Mourtzakis equation [3] and BIA-based whole-body FFM equations (r = 0.87 Talluri, r = 0.84 Kanellakis; r = 0.80 Kotler) [36,37] also showed a strong correlation.
- Maximum handgrip strength showed a moderate correlation with these parameters, being the highest for MM Talluri (r = 0.67).

3.3.2. Matrix 2: CT, US, and HGS

All US-based muscle biomarkers had moderate direct correlations with L3-SMA, that ranged from r = 0.56 to r = 0.66, the strongest being with RF-MT (rectus femoris plus vastus intermedius). All three US-based muscle biomarkers also had a moderate or strong correlation with the other two US-based parameters, with the strongest being at RF-MT with Quad-MT (whole-quadriceps muscle thickness, r = 0.87) and RF-MT with RF-CSA (r = 0.86). The correlation with HGS was homogenous amongst all US-based biomarkers (r = 0.51 to r = 0.52).

3.4. *Muscle Biomarkers: Agreement*

3.4.1. Agreement Between CT and BIA

SMI-Janssen and SMI-CT had a moderate linear relation (r = 0.665). The agreement of different equations for whole-body MM estimation using BIA (Janssen, Talluri) [34] with the estimated whole-body MM in CT using the Shen equation [2] was analyzed:

- Janssen-estimated MM [34] had a strong linear relation with Shen [2] (r = 0.809, $p < 2.2 \times 10^{-16}$) (Figure 6A). Quantitative agreement was poor (ρ = 0.772, 95%CI: 0.705, 0.825). Janssen underestimated MM with a 1.5 (3.6) kg systematic bias, a minimal dose-dependent bias, (−5.6, 8.6) kg LoA, and 9/156 (5.7%) measurements outside the LoA (Figure 6B). Grouped measurements were significantly different (23.3 vs. 23.6 kg, $p = 3.609 \times 10^{-8}$) (Figure 6C).
- Talluri-estimated MM had a strong linear relation with Shen [2] (r = 0.865, $p < 2.2 \times 10^{-16}$) (Figure 6D). Quantitative agreement was poor (ρ = 0.538, 95%CI: 0.467, 0.603). Talluri overestimated MM with a −6.4 (3.6) kg systematic bias, a dose-dependent bias, (−13–41, 0.688) kg LoA, and 9/156 (5.7%) measurements outside the LoA (Figure 6E). Grouped measurements were significantly different (29.9 vs. 23.6 kg, $p < 2.2 \times 10^{-16}$) (Figure 6F).

As Janssen-estimated whole-body MM [34] showed the smallest bias in relation to Shen-estimated whole-body MM [2], we studied the influence of possible BIA artifacts using this equation. The Bland–Altman sub-analysis of cases that were completely artifact-free was as follows: 1.6 (3.5) kg with (−5.2, 8,4) kg LoA. Then, we visually inspected the data, looking for bias due to possible artifacts such as central catheters side (Figure S2A), and type (Figure S2B), presence of an ostomy (ileostomy, colostomy, nephrostomy) (Figure S2C), or chronic treatment with a diuretic drug (Figure S2D) in Bland–Altman plots. No systematic bias was found.

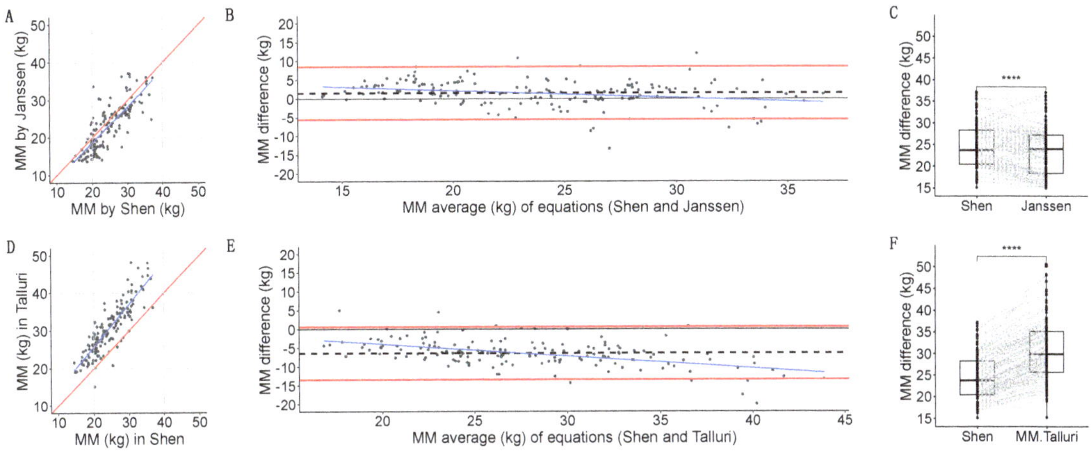

Figure 6. Scatterplot for CT-based MM in kg using Shen [2] equation on the *X*-axis, and different BIA-based equations for muscle mass (MM) in kilograms (kg): Janssen [34] (**A**), and Talluri (**D**) on the Y-axis. Linear regression models are represented as a blue line, and a perfect regression is represented as a red line. Bland–Altman plots for CT-based MM in kg using Shen equation, in comparison with different BIA-based MM equations: Janssen (**B**), and Talluri (**E**). In all cases, averages of MM for both equations are presented on the *X*-axis; differences in MM for both equations are presented on the Y axis. A linear regression model to detect dose-dependent bias is represented as a blue line. Please note how the *Y*-axis has the same scale and range for easier comparisons. Individual measurements are shown as black dots; biases are represented as horizontal dashed black lines; upper and lower limits of agreement are shown as horizontal solid red lines. The absence of differences (Y intercept = 0) between equations is represented as a horizontal solid black line. Boxplots with overlaid point geometry for CT-based MM in kg using Shen equation on the *Y*-axis, and different BIA-based equations for MM in kg: Janssen (**C**), and Talluri (**F**) on the *X*-axis. Please note how the *Y*-axis has the same scale and range for easier comparisons. Each participant is joint by dashed grey lines. Statistical significances for comparisons of central tendency measures is depicted as follows: $p \leq 0.0001$ = ****.

Then, we compared the agreement of different equations for whole-body FFM estimation using BIA (Kanellakis, Kotler, and Talluri) [36,37] with the estimated whole-body FFM in CT using the Mourtzakis equation [3]:

- Kanellakis-estimated FFM [36] had a strong linear relation with Mourtzakis [3] ($r = 0.836$, $p < 2.2 \times 10^{-16}$) (Figure 7A). Quantitative agreement was poor ($\rho = 0.468$, 95%CI: 0.396, 0.534). Kanellakis underestimated FFM with a 12.5 (6.7) kg systematic bias, a linear regression model compatible with a dose-dependent bias, (−0.6, 2.6) kg LoA, and 9/156 (5.7%) measurements outside the LoA (Figure 7B). Grouped measurements were significantly different (32.6 vs. 42.4 kg, $p < 2.2 \times 10^{-16}$) (Figure 7C).
- Kotler-estimated FFM [37] had a strong linear relation with Mourtzakis [3] ($r = 0.802$, $p < 2.2 \times 10^{-16}$) (Figure 7D). Quantitative agreement was poor ($\rho = 0.718$, 95%CI: 0.643, 0.780). Kotler overestimated FFM with a −4.3 (5.7) kg systematic bias, no dose-dependent bias, (−15.4, 6.8) kg LoA, and 9/156 (5.7%) measurements outside the LoA (Figure 7E). Grouped measurements were significantly different (47.7 vs. 42.4 kg, $p = 3.464 \times 10^{-16}$) (Figure 7F).
- Talluri-estimated FFM had a strong linear relation with Mourtzakis [3] ($r = 0.857$, $p < 2.2 \times 10^{-16}$) (Figure 7G). Quantitative agreement was poor ($\rho = 0.666$, 95CI%: 0.595, 0.728). Talluri overestimated FFM with a −6.9 (5.0) kg systematic bias, no dose-dependent bias, (−16.7, 2.9) kg LoA, and 11/156 (7.0%) measurements

outside the LoA (Figure 7H). Grouped measurements were significantly different (49.9 vs. 42.4 kg, $p < 2.2 \times 10^{-16}$) (Figure 7I).

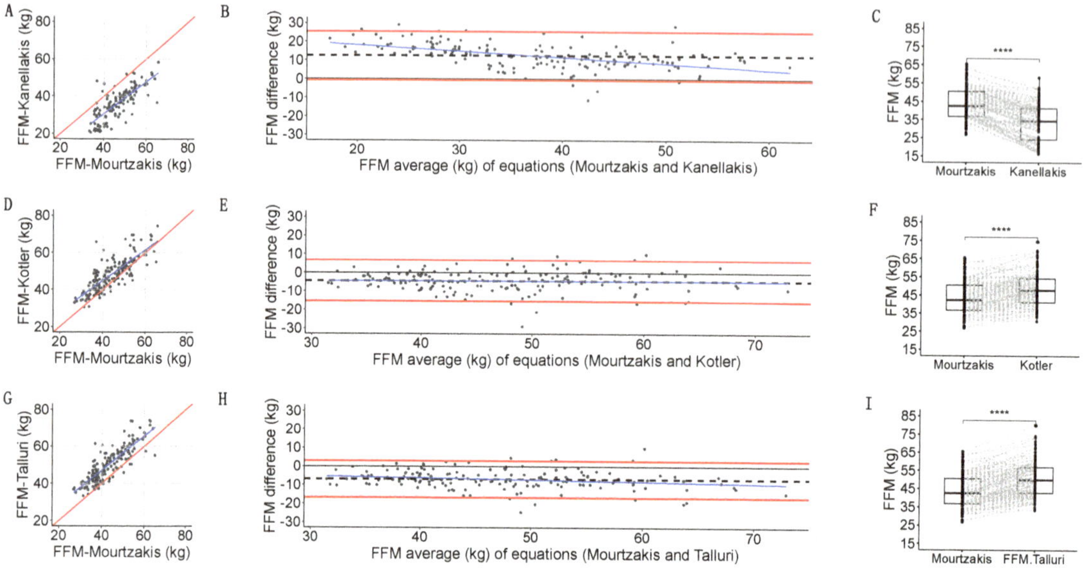

Figure 7. Scatterplot for CT-based FFM in kg using Mourtzakis [3] equation on the *X*-axis, and different BIA-based equations for fat-free mass (FFM) in kilograms (kg): Kanellakis [36] (**A**), Kotler [37] (**D**), and Talluri (**G**) on the *Y*-axis. Bland–Altman plots for CT-based FFM in kg using Mourtzakis equation, in comparison with different BIA-based FFM equations: Kanellakis (**B**), Kotler (**E**), and Talluri (**H**). Boxplots with overlaid point geometry for CT-based FFM in kg using Mourtzakis equation on the *Y* axis, and different BIA-based equations for FFM in kg: Kanellakis (**C**), Kotler (**F**), and Talluri (**I**) on the *X*-axis. Statistical significances for comparisons of central tendency measures is depicted as follows: $p \leq 0.0001$ = ****.

3.4.2. Agreement Between CT and US

We also tested if our dataset could replicate the USVALID (Fischer et al.) [38] equation using the same dependent and independent variables. In our dataset, the following equation with an adjusted R^2 = 0.723 was developed (Table S3): $\text{L3-SMA}(\text{cm}^2) = -74.04 + 12.03 \times Q + 0.56 \times W + 0.70 \times H + 18.86 \times S$, where Q is quadricipital muscle thickness using US (in cm), W is Weight (in kg), H is Height (in cm), and S is Sex (female = 0, male = 1).

Then, we compared the agreement of different equations for L3-SMA estimation using BIA (Fischer, and a new US-based regression model) with the measured L3-SMA in CT:

- Fischer-estimated L3-SMA [38] had a strong linear relation with L3-SMA ($r = 0.849$, $p < 2.2 \times 10^{-16}$) (Figure 8A). Quantitative agreement was poor ($\rho = 0.642$, 95%CI: 0.568, 0.705). Fischer overestimated L3-SMA with a −21.5 (15.2) cm^2 bias, a dose-dependent bias in linear regression, and (−51.9, 8.9) kg LoA (Figure 8B). Grouped measurements were significantly different: 144.6 (40.7) vs. 121.2 (45.5) cm^2 ($p < 2.2 \times 10^{-16}$) (Figure 8C).
- Our new equation had a strong linear relation with L3-SMA ($r = 0.854$, $p < 2.2 \times 10^{-16}$) (Figure 8D). Quantitative agreement was poor ($\rho = 0.696$, 95%CI: 0.626, 0.755). Our equation overestimated L3-SMA with a −17.6 (15.3) cm^2 bias, a dose-dependent bias in linear regression, and (−47.6, 12.3) kg LoA (Figure 8E). Grouped measurements were significantly different: 141.7 (39.6) vs. 121.2 (45.5) cm^2 ($p < 2.2 \times 10^{-16}$) (Figure 8F).

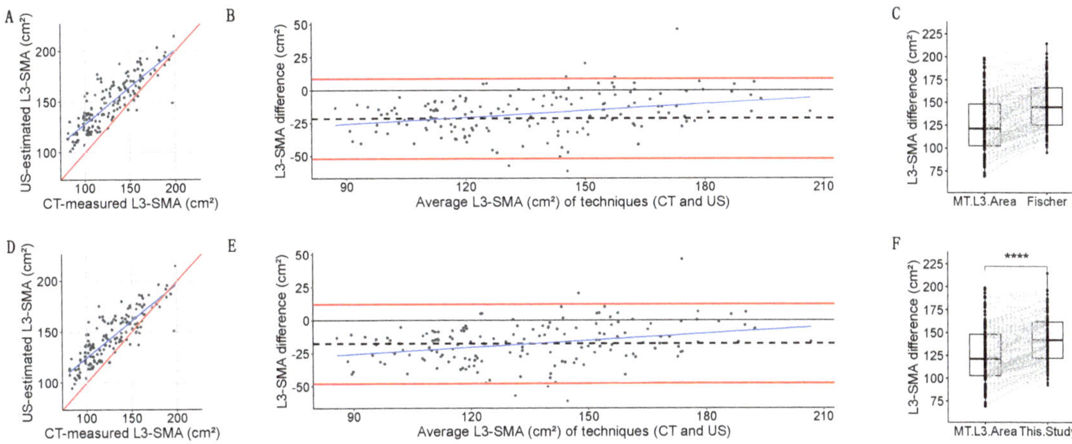

Figure 8. Scatterplot for CT-measured muscle CSA at L3 on the *X*-axis, and US-estimated muscle CSA at L3 on the *Y*-axis using the Fischer et al. equation [38] (**A**) and a similar regression equation with different ß coefficients (**D**). Bland–Altman plots for CT-measured muscle CSA at L3 on the X-axis, and US-estimated muscle CSA at L3 on the *Y*-axis using the Fischer et al. equation (**B**) and a similar regression equation with different ß coefficients (**E**). Boxplots with overlaid point geometry for CT-measured muscle CSA at L3 on the *X*-axis, and US-estimated muscle CSA at L3 on the *Y*-axis using the Fischer et al. equation (**C**) and a similar regression equation with different ß coefficients (**F**). Statistical significance for comparisons of central tendency measures is depicted as follows: $p \leq 0.0001$ = ****.

3.5. Impact of Techniques and Definitions on the Clinical Diagnosis of Muscle Atrophy

3.5.1. Intra-Technique (Between Definitions) Agreement

In CT scans, muscle atrophy based on L3-SMA occurred in 10/156 (6.41%) cases and 76/156 (48.72%) cases applying the Van Vugt et al. [29] and Dolan et al. cut-off points [30], respectively. Qualitative agreement for muscle atrophy was slight, with $k = 0.134$ ($p = 0.797 \times 10^{-3}$). Using CT scans, it could be seen that there were 1/156 (0.64%) and 4/156 (2.56%) cases of sarcopenia applying the Van Vugt et al. [29] and Dolan et al. [30] cut-off points, respectively. Qualitative agreement for sarcopenia was fair, with $k = 0.394$ ($p = 6.240 \times 10^{-10}$). Myosteatosis based on L3-SMD occurred in 2/156 (1.28%) cases and 26/156 (16.66%) cases applying the Van Vugt et al. [29] and Dolan et al. [30] cut-off points, respectively. Qualitative agreement was slight, with $k = 0.122$ ($p = 0.001$). Although SMD was significantly lower in obese participants (120.8 vs. 140.3 HU, p = 0.001), there were no cases of myosteatosis using the Van Vugt et al. [29] definition in this group, with 2/116 cases of myosteatosis in the normal weight group. Using Dolan et al. [30] cut-off points, there were 10/40 (25.00%) cases of myosteatosis amongst obese participants, and 16/116 (13.79%) cases in the normal weight group.

Using Spanish (Masanés) [35] muscle atrophy cut-off points for BIA, muscle atrophy occurred in 38/156 cases (24.4%) and 3/156 cases (1.9%) using Janssen [34] or Talluri equations, respectively. Qualitative agreement between equations was non-existent, with $k = -0.037$ (n.s.) using Spanish (Masanés) [35] cut-off points. There were no cases of atrophy with neither equation using European [4,5] cut-off points. There was a total lack of qualitative agreement between muscle atrophy definitions, and therefore no qualitative agreement regarding sarcopenia.

In US, muscle atrophy based on RF-MT occurred in 16/156 cases (10.26%), while muscle atrophy based on RF-CSA took place in 13/156 cases (8.33%), with both cases using DRECO [28] cut-off points. Qualitative agreement was slight, with $k = 0.127$ (n.s.). Regarding sarcopenia, there were no cases with a RF-MT-based definition of muscle atrophy, and

2/156 (1.28%) cases with a RF-CSA-based based definition of muscle atrophy. Qualitative agreement for sarcopenia was non-existent in US.

3.5.2. Inter-Technique Agreement

Muscle atrophy was defined in all CT cases using Van Vugt et al. [29] cut-off points. No agreement was found between CT and BIA in any case. When using Spanish (Masanés) [35] cut-off points, $k = 0.07$ (n.s.) for CT vs Janssen [34] equation, and $k = -0.03$ (n.s.) for CT vs Talluri equation. With European [4,5] cut-off points, agreement was non-existent with both BIA equations.

In general, CT and US displayed a slight agreement. When comparing CT muscle atrophy using Van Vugt et al. [29] cut-off points versus US muscle atrophy using DRECO cut-off points in RF-MT, a slight agreement was found, with $k = 0.165$ ($p = 0.033$). RF-CSA area also displayed a slight agreement with Van Vugt et al. [29] cut-off points ($k = 0.109$, n.s.). Results were slightly worse when comparing atrophy by Dolan et al. [30] according to L3-SMA measured on CT with the DRECO cut-off points: a slight agreement with RF-MT was found ($k = 0.136$, $p = 0.005$), yet there was no agreement with RF-CSA ($k = 0.069$, n.s.).

4. Discussion

Muscle atrophy and myosteatosis prevalence were generally low in a sample mainly composed of colorectal cancer survivors. The exception was the combinations of Janssen et al. [34] equation (BIA) with Masanés et al. [35] cut-off points, and L3-SMA and L3-SMD (CT) with Dolan et al. [30] cut-off points. Our inter-technique correlations were analogous to similar studies [28,51,52]. In our case, muscle atrophy and myosteatosis prevalence varied widely between techniques and definitions, as previously found [32,33,52]. This may be partly due to the intrinsic and different properties of each body composition technique. But more importantly, the current cut-off points for muscle atrophy and myosteatosis that have been used in the present study are intrinsically heterogeneous, since research groups and expert consensus have calculated them from different samples to act as: (1) a predictor of mortality, (2) a surrogate diagnosis for sarcopenia, or (3) a statistical deviation from a normal population. Therefore, we think that both the type of technique and its selected cut-off points should be taken into consideration when interpreting any body composition analysis study.

GLIM criteria [4,41] associated less muscle surface or mass in all techniques, thus proving a valid definition of malnutrition in our sample. Obesity did not associate worse muscle biomarkers per se. In fact, participants with this definition of obesity had significantly better muscle area or mass biomarkers in both CT and US. These results are in line with previous data that support the use of CT scans instead of a BMI-based approach to detect sarcopenic obesity in this study population [53]. Although some studies show the superiority of SMG as a muscle biomarker [54], we found no differences in SMG regarding the nutritional status of the participants in our sample. It is somehow striking that no statistically significant differences in mass or surface area between young and old participants were found, which may be explained by a modest age difference between groups (74.6 vs. 61.5 years) and sample size.

BIA and CT were not directly interchangeable in our study due to a BIA MM or FFM overestimation, as has happened in previous studies [32,33,52,55–57]. The Janssen et al. [34] equation presented the best diagnostic ability among the MM-estimating BIA equations in regards to whole-body MM estimation using the Shen [2] equation on L3-SMA, a finding also in line with previous evidence [32]. Nevertheless, the associated LoA were still excessively wide and Lin's ρ was poor. The best FFM-estimating BIA equation in our sample was the Kotler et al. [37] equation, in comparison to a whole-body FFM estimation using the Mourtzakis et al. [3] equation on CT scans. With these exceptions, there was a generalized low agreement for muscle atrophy between CT and other valid and widespread BIA equations, both in quantitative and qualitative terms. This supports the recommendation that—if possible—population-specific BIA equations should be used [11,12], and their adequate functioning checked. Due to its intrinsic characteristics, foot-to-hand BIA overestimates the muscularity of the limbs and underestimates that of the torso [58]. This fact could partly explain the discrepancies between CT and BIA. In addition, some patients may be asymmetrically affected by "local sarcopenia" due to their underlying pathology and functionality [16]. In these subjects, body composition analysis techniques that compare skeletal muscle of the trunk (CT) versus that of the extremities (BIA and US) may not coincide, without this really being an error. Nevertheless, participants in this study had no comorbidities that may have caused "local sarcopenia". We found no apparent bias due to the use of central catheters or ostomies, which may be frequent in the population of interest. Our correlation between SMD and raw phase angle was moderate and in the line of previous evidence in colorectal cancer [59].

US biomarkers levels were akin to those of another Spanish colorectal cancer study [51]. Analogous to the USVALID study [38], both CT and US adequately recognized a musculoskeletal sexual dimorphism in our work. As previously reported, GLIM malnutrition was associated with a lower RF-MT [60]. Despite its excellent methodological quality, the USVALID [38] equation displayed a suboptimal performance in our sample, even when muscle biomarkers were strikingly similar in both studies. These studies present differences in operators and measuring devices, and—more importantly—probe locations [61] that may not be interchangeable for skeletal muscle assessment [62]. Nevertheless, our US-based regression equation was equally suboptimal and unable to estimate L3-SMA using the same independent variables with adjusted ß coefficients for our study sample. Therefore, this lack of agreement between CT and US seems due to other reasons, such as patient morphotype. Taking all these findings this into consideration, CT and US were not directly interchangeable in our study, and further research on the validity and usefulness of US as a bedside body composition technique is warranted.

Our study has several strengths. To our knowledge, this is the first study that performed CT, BIA, US, and anthropometry simultaneously in colorectal cancer outpatients, as previous studies in this clinical population have worked with time spans up to one [33] or three months [51], or were conducted in a similarly very close period of time but in a different population [32,52,57]. On the other hand, all measurements were taken by a single trained operator (A.J.S.). This eliminates inter-observer bias, and also makes this a feasibility study, demonstrating that a well-trained endocrinologist could adequately perform all techniques. To our knowledge, this is also the first study that successfully uses the Butterfly iQ+^{TM} device (a handheld POCUS) to assess body composition in this clinical population. These devices may open new possibilities for quick, innocuous, and portable muscle assessment that may be of special interest when patients are unable to attend office appointments, such as hospitalized patients, or those in home care.

This study also has several limitations. Since this is a single-center study, the clinical and morphological characteristics of patients from other centers—and particularly from other countries—may not be superimposable on those of this study. Despite its careful methodology, this study was not pre-registered. Regarding malnutrition definition, our focus was quantitative and qualitative agreement between body composition analysis techniques (CT scans, BIA, and US) and not a traditional nutritional diagnosis, thus why a GLIM—instead of a Subjective Global Assessment (SGA)—approach was selected. Although it has some similarities with previous studies, this research is based on a slightly different population: instead of selecting referred patients to a Nutrition Unit before programed colorectal surgery [33,51], this study actively recruited colorectal cancer outpatients without taking into consideration neither their nutritional risk nor the natural history of the disease when they were invited to participate. Albeit we do not know whether the clinical and morphofunctional characteristics of the patients who did not wish to participate are different from those included, this blind inclusion of participants may have increased sample heterogeneity, potentially decreasing agreement but also increasing external validity. In this regard, patients with possible BIA artifacts (such as a central catheter, ostomy, and diuretic) were included in all analysis and regression equations. Therefore, we believe that these cases could not have favored one equation over the other. Although the inclusion of these participants may have increased our LoA in the Bland–Altman analysis, the artifact-free results were nearly superimposable on the whole sample in that regard, so it was not the case. Regarding US measurements, we do not know to what extent the use of a high-resolution device could have improved our results. Nevertheless, the DRECO study also used a handheld POC US (UProbe L6C) [28]. Besides, differences of vastus lateralis muscle thickness using a POC US vs. a gold-standard device were very small, with substantial or near-perfect intra-rater agreement in previous research [63].

In our study, the diagnosis of muscular atrophy using current definitions was not sufficiently congruent within and between techniques to justify the interchangeable use of these definitions in a similar population. More importantly, quantitative agreement between reference and bedside techniques was not sufficiently intense, accurate, and unbiased to justify the interchangeable use of these techniques in these patients in clinical practice. If a reference technique (CT) is not available, we therefore suggest using a single bedside technique, with a single raw parameter or equation, and a single set of cut-off points, for a more homogeneous follow-up of the muscular status of these patients. We consider that this technique should be chosen based on availability, operator experience, and possible artifacts or contraindications in the individual patient: for example, US could lose definition in patients with an abnormally large subcutaneous adipose panniculus, or BIA could be unreliable in patients with volume overload. As a future line of research, we believe that these limitations could be overcome or mitigated with prospective multicenter studies where both reference and bedside techniques are simultaneously performed, stratifying data by race, gender, and disease status, amongst others. This approach would allow for adjusted prognostic cut-off points on the pure measurements obtained with each technique; as well as regression equations that could transform the results of one technique into another with the highest possible precision, although the use of prediction equations will always introduce a new layer of uncertainty. If the latter were not significantly better than the currently available equations, then a second-best approach could be the stratification of data to find groups of patients where equation performance was sufficiently accurate and unbiased for a direct clinical application.

5. Conclusions

In general, intra-technique agreement with usual operationalized definitions of muscular atrophy was low. Inter-technique agreement regarding the diagnosis of muscular atrophy was equally low. Neither CT and BIA, nor CT and US, were interchangeable. Nevertheless, all techniques adequately recognized the same body composition patterns in the study sample, thus demonstrating biologic plausibility. It seems necessary to continue developing new equations and homogenizing cut-off points with multicenter, prognostic, and prospective studies that may improve agreement between body composition analysis techniques in colorectal cancer outpatients.

Supplementary Materials: The following supporting information can be downloaded at: https://www.mdpi.com/article/10.3390/nu16244312/s1, Figure S1: Density plots for body mass index (BMI); Figure S2: Bland–Altman plots stratified by possible BIA artifacts. Table S1: Possible BIA artifacts; Table S2. Tumor-related characteristics; Table S3. US-based regression model for L3-SMA.

Author Contributions: Conceptualization, A.J.-S.; Data curation, A.J.-S., Formal analysis, A.J.-S.; Funding acquisition, P.P.G.-L. and A.J.-S.; Investigation, A.J.-S.; Methodology, A.J.-S.; Project administration, A.J.-S., M.E.S.-R. and P.P.G.-L.; Resources, A.J.-S., M.E.S.-R., M.V.-A. and P.P.G.-L.; Supervision, P.P.G.-L. and J.L.P.-C.; Visualization, A.J.-S.; Writing—original draft, A.J.-S.; Writing—review and editing, A.J.-S., M.d.C.R.-C. and S.G.-R. All authors have read and agreed to the published version of the manuscript.

Funding: The BIA device (Nutrilab) used in this study was provided by the "Beca FSEEN proyecto de investigación de composición corporal mediante impedanciometría" grant. This study was also supported by the "Beca SANCYD-Fresenius 2021 de investigación al proyecto sobre nuevas técnicas en composición corporal en la valoración nutricional" grant.

Institutional Review Board Statement: The study was conducted in accordance with the Declaration of Helsinki and approved by the Ethics Committee "CEI de los Hospitales Universitarios Virgen Macarena y Virgen del Rocío" (protocol code: 1006-N-22; date of approval: 23 May 2022).

Informed Consent Statement: Informed consent was obtained from all subjects involved in the study.

Data Availability Statement: The data presented in this study are available on request from the corresponding author as per European legislation on data protection.

Conflicts of Interest: The authors declare no conflicts of interest.

Appendix A

Table A1. Van Vugt et al. cutoff points [29] for muscle atrophy and myosteatosis in a European population.

	Men				Women			
	BMI (kg/m^2)				BMI (kg/m^2)			
	Skeletal muscle index (cm^2/m^2)							
Age (years)	17–20	20–25	25–30	30–35	17–20	20–25	25–30	30–35
30–39	36.8	41.3	47.0	52.6	31.0	33.9	37.4	40.9
40–49	35.4	39.9	45.6	51.2	31.0	33.5	36.5	39.5
50–59	34.0	38.6	44.2	49.8	31.0	33.0	35.5	38.0
60–69	32.6	37.2	42.8	48.4	30.9	32.5	34.5	36.4
70–79	31.2	35.8	41.4	47.0	30.7	32.0	33.5	34.8
80–87	29.8	34.4	40.0	45.6	30.6	31.5	32.5	33.2
	Skeletal muscle density (HU)							
30–39	42.5	39.8	36.3	32.8	41.0	37.7	33.6	29.4
40–49	39.6	36.8	33.4	29.9	37.2	34.0	29.8	25.6
50–59	36.6	33.9	30.5	27.0	33.4	30.1	26.0	21.8
60–69	33.7	31.0	27.5	24.0	29.6	26.3	22.2	18.0
70–79	30.7	28.0	24.5	21.1	25.8	22.5	18.3	14.1
80–87	27.7	25.0	21.6	18.1	21.9	18.6	14.4	10.3

Modified from Van Vugt et al. [29]. BMI: Body Mass Index; cm: centimeters; HU: Hounsfield units; kg: kilograms; m: meters.

References

1. Shachar, S.S.; Williams, G.R.; Muss, H.B.; Nishijima, T.F. Prognostic Value of Sarcopenia in Adults with Solid Tumours: A Meta-Analysis and Systematic Review. *Eur. J. Cancer* **2016**, *57*, 58–67. [CrossRef] [PubMed]
2. Shen, W.; Punyanitya, M.; Wang, Z.; Gallagher, D.; St.-Onge, M.-P.; Albu, J.; Heymsfield, S.B.; Heshka, S. Total Body Skeletal Muscle and Adipose Tissue Volumes: Estimation from a Single Abdominal Cross-Sectional Image. *J. Appl. Physiol.* **2004**, *97*, 2333–2338. [CrossRef]
3. Mourtzakis, M.; Prado, C.M.M.; Lieffers, J.R.; Reiman, T.; McCargar, L.J.; Baracos, V.E. A Practical and Precise Approach to Quantification of Body Composition in Cancer Patients Using Computed Tomography Images Acquired during Routine Care. *Appl. Physiol. Nutr. Metab.* **2008**, *33*, 997–1006. [CrossRef] [PubMed]
4. Barazzoni, R.; Jensen, G.L.; Correia, M.I.T.D.; Gonzalez, M.C.; Higashiguchi, T.; Shi, H.P.; Bischoff, S.C.; Boirie, Y.; Carrasco, F.; Cruz-Jentoft, A.; et al. Guidance for Assessment of the Muscle Mass Phenotypic Criterion for the Global Leadership Initiative on Malnutrition (GLIM) Diagnosis of Malnutrition. *Clin. Nutr.* **2022**, *41*, 1425–1433. [CrossRef]
5. Cruz-Jentoft, A.J.; Bahat, G.; Bauer, J.; Boirie, Y.; Bruyère, O.; Cederholm, T.; Cooper, C.; Landi, F.; Rolland, Y.; Sayer, A.A.; et al. Sarcopenia: Revised European Consensus on Definition and Diagnosis. *Age Ageing* **2019**, *48*, 16–31. [CrossRef]
6. Xie, H.; Wei, L.; Liu, M.; Yuan, G.; Tang, S.; Gan, J. Preoperative Computed Tomography-Assessed Sarcopenia as a Predictor of Complications and Long-Term Prognosis in Patients with Colorectal Cancer: A Systematic Review and Meta-Analysis. *Langenbecks Arch. Surg.* **2021**, *406*, 1775–1788. [CrossRef] [PubMed]
7. Derksen, J.W.G.; Kurk, S.A.; Peeters, P.H.M.; Dorresteijn, B.; Jourdan, M.; van der Velden, A.M.T.; Nieboer, P.; de Jong, R.S.; Honkoop, A.H.; Punt, C.J.A.; et al. The Association between Changes in Muscle Mass and Quality of Life in Patients with Metastatic Colorectal Cancer. *J. Cachexia Sarcopenia Muscle* **2020**, *11*, 919–928. [CrossRef] [PubMed]

8. Barbalho, E.R.; Gonzalez, M.C.; Bielemann, R.M.; da Rocha, I.M.G.; de Sousa, I.M.; Bezerra, R.A.; de Medeiros, G.O.C.; Fayh, A.P.T. Is Skeletal Muscle Radiodensity Able to Indicate Physical Function Impairment in Older Adults with Gastrointestinal Cancer? *Exp. Gerontol.* **2019**, *125*, 110688. [CrossRef]
9. Hanna, L.; Nguo, K.; Furness, K.; Porter, J.; Huggins, C.E. Association between Skeletal Muscle Mass and Quality of Life in Adults with Cancer: A Systematic Review and Meta-Analysis. *J. Cachexia Sarcopenia Muscle* **2022**, *13*, 839–857. [CrossRef] [PubMed]
10. Lee, C.M.; Kang, J. Prognostic Impact of Myosteatosis in Patients with Colorectal Cancer: A Systematic Review and Meta-Analysis. *J. Cachexia Sarcopenia Muscle* **2020**, *11*, 1270–1282. [CrossRef]
11. Campa, F.; Coratella, G.; Cerullo, G.; Stagi, S.; Paoli, S.; Marini, S.; Grigoletto, A.; Moroni, A.; Petri, C.; Andreoli, A.; et al. New Bioelectrical Impedance Vector References and Phase Angle Centile Curves in 4367 Adults: The Need for an Urgent Update after 30 Years. *Clin. Nutr.* **2023**, *42*, 1749–1758. [CrossRef] [PubMed]
12. Beaudart, C.; Bruyère, O.; Geerinck, A.; Hajaoui, M.; Scafoglieri, A.; Perkisas, S.; Bautmans, I.; Gielen, E.; Reginster, J.-Y.; Buckinx, F. Equation Models Developed with Bioelectric Impedance Analysis Tools to Assess Muscle Mass: A Systematic Review. *Clin. Nutr. ESPEN* **2020**, *35*, 47–62. [CrossRef] [PubMed]
13. García-Almeida, J.M.; García-García, C.; Vegas-Aguilar, I.M.; Ballesteros Pomar, M.D.; Cornejo-Pareja, I.M.; Fernández Medina, B.; de Luis Román, D.A.; Bellido Guerrero, D.; Bretón Lesmes, I.; Tinahones Madueño, F.J. Nutritional Ultrasound®: Conceptualisation, Technical Considerations and Standardisation. *Endocrinol. Diabetes Nutr.* **2023**, *70* (Suppl. 1), 74–84. [CrossRef]
14. Nakanishi, N.; Tsutsumi, R.; Okayama, Y.; Takashima, T.; Ueno, Y.; Itagaki, T.; Tsutsumi, Y.; Sakaue, H.; Oto, J. Monitoring of Muscle Mass in Critically Ill Patients: Comparison of Ultrasound and Two Bioelectrical Impedance Analysis Devices. *J. Intensive Care* **2019**, *7*, 61. [CrossRef] [PubMed]
15. Sabatino, A.; Regolisti, G.; Bozzoli, L.; Fani, F.; Antoniotti, R.; Maggiore, U.; Fiaccadori, E. Reliability of Bedside Ultrasound for Measurement of Quadriceps Muscle Thickness in Critically Ill Patients with Acute Kidney Injury. *Clin. Nutr.* **2017**, *36*, 1710–1715. [CrossRef]
16. Sanz-Paris, A.; González-Fernandez, M.; Hueso-Del Río, L.E.; Ferrer-Lahuerta, E.; Monge-Vazquez, A.; Losfablos-Callau, F.; Sanclemente-Hernández, T.; Sanz-Arque, A.; Arbones-Mainar, J.M. Muscle Thickness and Echogenicity Measured by Ultrasound Could Detect Local Sarcopenia and Malnutrition in Older Patients Hospitalized for Hip Fracture. *Nutrients* **2021**, *13*, 2401. [CrossRef] [PubMed]
17. Nijholt, W.; Jager-Wittenaar, H.; Raj, I.S.; van der Schans, C.P.; Hobbelen, H. Reliability and Validity of Ultrasound to Estimate Muscles: A Comparison between Different Transducers and Parameters. *Clin. Nutr. ESPEN* **2020**, *35*, 146–152. [CrossRef] [PubMed]
18. Earthman, C.P. Body Composition Tools for Assessment of Adult Malnutrition at the Bedside: A Tutorial on Research Considerations and Clinical Applications. *J. Parenter. Enter. Nutr.* **2015**, *39*, 787–822. [CrossRef]
19. von Elm, E.; Altman, D.G.; Egger, M.; Pocock, S.J.; Gøtzsche, P.C.; Vandenbroucke, J.P. STROBE Initiative Strengthening the Reporting of Observational Studies in Epidemiology (STROBE) Statement: Guidelines for Reporting Observational Studies. *BMJ* **2007**, *335*, 806–808. [CrossRef]
20. Whiting, P.F.; Rutjes, A.W.S.; Westwood, M.E.; Mallett, S.; Deeks, J.J.; Reitsma, J.B.; Leeflang, M.M.G.; Sterne, J.A.C.; Bossuyt, P.M.M. QUADAS-2 Group QUADAS-2: A Revised Tool for the Quality Assessment of Diagnostic Accuracy Studies. *Ann. Intern. Med.* **2011**, *155*, 529–536. [CrossRef] [PubMed]
21. Jiménez-Sánchez, A.; Soriano-Redondo, M.E.; Pereira-Cunill, J.L.; Martínez-Ortega, A.J.; Rodríguez-Mowbray, J.R.; Ramallo-Solís, I.M.; García-Luna, P.P. A Cross-Sectional Validation of Horos and CoreSlicer Software Programs for Body Composition Analysis in Abdominal Computed Tomography Scans in Colorectal Cancer Patients. *Diagnostics* **2024**, *14*, 1696. [CrossRef]
22. Kyle, U.G.; Bosaeus, I.; De Lorenzo, A.D.; Deurenberg, P.; Elia, M.; Manuel Gómez, J.; Lilienthal Heitmann, B.; Kent-Smith, L.; Melchior, J.-C.; Pirlich, M.; et al. Bioelectrical Impedance Analysis—Part II: Utilization in Clinical Practice. *Clin. Nutr.* **2004**, *23*, 1430–1453. [CrossRef] [PubMed]
23. Roberts, H.C.; Denison, H.J.; Martin, H.J.; Patel, H.P.; Syddall, H.; Cooper, C.; Sayer, A.A. A Review of the Measurement of Grip Strength in Clinical and Epidemiological Studies: Towards a Standardised Approach. *Age Ageing* **2011**, *40*, 423–429. [CrossRef]
24. Jiménez-Sánchez, A.; Pereira-Cunill, J.L.; Limón-Mirón, M.L.; López-Ladrón, A.; Salvador-Bofill, F.J.; García-Luna, P.P. A Cross-Sectional Validation Study of Camry EH101 versus JAMAR Plus Handheld Dynamometers in Colorectal Cancer Patients and Their Correlations with Bioelectrical Impedance and Nutritional Status. *Nutrients* **2024**, *16*, 1824. [CrossRef] [PubMed]
25. Oken, M.M.; Creech, R.H.; Tormey, D.C.; Horton, J.; Davis, T.E.; McFadden, E.T.; Carbone, P.P. Toxicity and Response Criteria of the Eastern Cooperative Oncology Group. *Am. J. Clin. Oncol.* **1982**, *5*, 649–655. [CrossRef]
26. Amin, M.B.; Greene, F.L.; Edge, S.B.; Compton, C.C.; Gershenwald, J.E.; Brookland, R.K.; Meyer, L.; Gress, D.M.; Byrd, D.R.; Winchester, D.P. The Eighth Edition AJCC Cancer Staging Manual: Continuing to Build a Bridge from a Population-Based to a More "Personalized" Approach to Cancer Staging. *CA Cancer J. Clin.* **2017**, *67*, 93–99. [CrossRef] [PubMed]
27. Cervantes, A.; Adam, R.; Roselló, S.; Arnold, D.; Normanno, N.; Taïeb, J.; Seligmann, J.; Baere, T.D.; Osterlund, P.; Yoshino, T.; et al. Metastatic Colorectal Cancer: ESMO Clinical Practice Guideline for Diagnosis, Treatment and Follow-Up. *Ann. Oncol.* **2023**, *34*, 10–32. [CrossRef] [PubMed]
28. De Luis Roman, D.; García Almeida, J.M.; Bellido Guerrero, D.; Guzmán Rolo, G.; Martín, A.; Primo Martín, D.; García-Delgado, Y.; Guirado-Peláez, P.; Palmas, F.; Tejera Pérez, C.; et al. Ultrasound Cut-Off Values for Rectus Femoris for Detecting Sarcopenia in Patients with Nutritional Risk. *Nutrients* **2024**, *16*, 1552. [CrossRef] [PubMed]

29. Van Vugt, J.L.A.; Van Putten, Y.; Van Der Kall, I.M.; Buettner, S.; D'Ancona, F.C.H.; Dekker, H.M.; Kimenai, H.J.A.N.; De Bruin, R.W.F.; Warlé, M.C.; IJzermans, J.N.M. Estimated Skeletal Muscle Mass and Density Values Measured on Computed Tomography Examinations in over 1000 Living Kidney Donors. *Eur. J. Clin. Nutr.* **2019**, *73*, 879–886. [CrossRef]
30. Dolan, R.D.; Almasaudi, A.S.; Dieu, L.B.; Horgan, P.G.; McSorley, S.T.; McMillan, D.C. The Relationship between Computed Tomography-derived Body Composition, Systemic Inflammatory Response, and Survival in Patients Undergoing Surgery for Colorectal Cancer. *J. Cachexia Sarcopenia Muscle* **2019**, *10*, 111–122. [CrossRef] [PubMed]
31. Weinberg, M.S.; Shachar, S.S.; Muss, H.B.; Deal, A.M.; Popuri, K.; Yu, H.; Nyrop, K.A.; Alston, S.M.; Williams, G.R. Beyond Sarcopenia: Characterization and Integration of Skeletal Muscle Quantity and Radiodensity in a Curable Breast Cancer Population. *Breast J.* **2018**, *24*, 278–284. [CrossRef]
32. Looijaard, W.G.P.M.; Stapel, S.N.; Dekker, I.M.; Rusticus, H.; Remmelzwaal, S.; Girbes, A.R.J.; Weijs, P.J.M.; Oudemans-van Straaten, H.M. Identifying Critically Ill Patients with Low Muscle Mass: Agreement between Bioelectrical Impedance Analysis and Computed Tomography. *Clin. Nutr.* **2020**, *39*, 1809–1817. [CrossRef]
33. De Luis Roman, D.; López Gómez, J.J.; Muñoz, M.; Primo, D.; Izaola, O.; Sánchez, I. Evaluation of Muscle Mass and Malnutrition in Patients with Colorectal Cancer Using the Global Leadership Initiative on Malnutrition Criteria and Comparing Bioelectrical Impedance Analysis and Computed Tomography Measurements. *Nutrients* **2024**, *16*, 3035. [CrossRef] [PubMed]
34. Janssen, I.; Heymsfield, S.B.; Baumgartner, R.N.; Ross, R. Estimation of Skeletal Muscle Mass by Bioelectrical Impedance Analysis. *J. Appl. Physiol.* **2000**, *89*, 465–471. [CrossRef]
35. Masanes Toran, F.; Culla, A.; Navarro-Gonzalez, M.; Navarro-Lopez, M.; Sacanella, E.; Torres, B.; Lopez-Soto, A. Prevalence of Sarcopenia in Healthy Community-Dwelling Elderly in an Urban Area of Barcelona (Spain). *J. Nutr. Health Aging* **2012**, *16*, 184–187. [CrossRef]
36. Kanellakis, S.; Skoufas, E.; Karaglani, E.; Ziogos, G.; Koutroulaki, A.; Loukianou, F.; Michalopoulou, M.; Gkeka, A.; Marikou, F.; Manios, Y. Development and Validation of a Bioelectrical Impedance Prediction Equation Estimating Fat Free Mass in Greek—Caucasian Adult Population. *Clin. Nutr. ESPEN* **2020**, *36*, 166–170. [CrossRef]
37. Kotler, D.P.; Burastero, S.; Wang, J.; Pierson, R.N. Prediction of Body Cell Mass, Fat-Free Mass, and Total Body Water with Bioelectrical Impedance Analysis: Effects of Race, Sex, and Disease. *Am. J. Clin. Nutr.* **1996**, *64*, 489S–497S. [CrossRef] [PubMed]
38. Fischer, A.; Hertwig, A.; Hahn, R.; Anwar, M.; Siebenrock, T.; Pesta, M.; Liebau, K.; Timmermann, I.; Brugger, J.; Posch, M.; et al. Validation of Bedside Ultrasound to Predict Lumbar Muscle Area in the Computed Tomography in 200 Non-Critically Ill Patients: The USVALID Prospective Study. *Clin. Nutr.* **2022**, *41*, 829–837. [CrossRef] [PubMed]
39. Sun, S.S.; Chumlea, W.C.; Heymsfield, S.B.; Lukaski, H.C.; Schoeller, D.; Friedl, K.; Kuczmarski, R.J.; Flegal, K.M.; Johnson, C.L.; Hubbard, V.S. Development of Bioelectrical Impedance Analysis Prediction Equations for Body Composition with the Use of a Multicomponent Model for Use in Epidemiologic Surveys. *Am. J. Clin. Nutr.* **2003**, *77*, 331–340. [CrossRef] [PubMed]
40. Dodds, R.M.; Syddall, H.E.; Cooper, R.; Benzeval, M.; Deary, I.J.; Dennison, E.M.; Der, G.; Gale, C.R.; Inskip, H.M.; Jagger, C.; et al. Grip Strength across the Life Course: Normative Data from Twelve British Studies. *PLoS ONE* **2014**, *9*, e113637. [CrossRef] [PubMed]
41. Correia, M.I.T.D.; Tappenden, K.A.; Malone, A.; Prado, C.M.; Evans, D.C.; Sauer, A.C.; Hegazi, R.; Gramlich, L. Utilization and Validation of the Global Leadership Initiative on Malnutrition (GLIM): A Scoping Review. *Clin. Nutr.* **2022**, *41*, 687–697. [CrossRef] [PubMed]
42. Wickham, H.; Averick, M.; Bryan, J.; Chang, W.; McGowan, L.D.; François, R.; Grolemund, G.; Hayes, A.; Henry, L.; Hester, J.; et al. Welcome to the Tidyverse. *J. Open Source Softw.* **2019**, *4*, 1686. [CrossRef]
43. Wilke, C. cowplot: Streamlined Plot Theme and Plot Annotations for 'ggplot2'. R Package Version 1.1.3. Available online: https://cran.r-project.org/web/packages/cowplot/index.html (accessed on 17 November 2024).
44. Signorell, A.; Aho, K.; Alfons, A.; Anderegg, N.; Aragon, T.; Arachchige, C.; Arppe, A.; Baddeley, A.; Barton, K.; Bolker, B.; et al. DescTools: Tools for Descriptive Statistics. R Package Version 0.99.58. Available online: https://cran.r-project.org/web/packages/DescTools/index.html (accessed on 17 November 2024).
45. Kassambara, A. Ggpubr: "ggplot2" Based Publication Ready Plots. R Package Version 0.6.0. Available online: https://cran.r-project.org/web/packages/ggpubr/index.html (accessed on 17 November 2024).
46. Olivoto, T. Metan: Multi Environment Trials Analysis. R Package Version 1.18.0. Available online: https://cran.r-project.org/web/packages/metan/index.html (accessed on 17 November 2024).
47. RStudio Team RStudio: Integrated Development for R. Available online: https://www.posit.co/ (accessed on 17 November 2024).
48. Bland, J.M.; Altman, D.G. Statistical Methods for Assessing Agreement between Two Methods of Clinical Measurement. *Lancet* **1986**, *1*, 307–310. [CrossRef] [PubMed]
49. Akoglu, H. User's Guide to Correlation Coefficients. *Turk. J. Emerg. Med.* **2018**, *18*, 91–93. [CrossRef]
50. Cohen, J. A Coefficient of Agreement for Nominal Scales. *Educ. Psychol. Meas.* **1960**, *20*, 37–46. [CrossRef]
51. Guirado-Peláez, P.; Fernández-Jiménez, R.; Sánchez-Torralvo, F.J.; Mucarzel Suárez-Arana, F.; Palmas-Candia, F.X.; Vegas-Aguilar, I.; Amaya-Campos, M.D.M.; Martínez Tamés, G.; Soria-Utrilla, V.; Tinahones-Madueño, F.; et al. Multiparametric Approach to the Colorectal Cancer Phenotypes Integrating Morphofunctional Assessment and Computer Tomography. *Cancers* **2024**, *16*, 3493. [CrossRef]

52. Zuo, J.; Zhou, D.; Zhang, L.; Zhou, X.; Gao, X.; Hou, W.; Wang, C.; Jiang, P.; Wang, X. Comparison of Bioelectrical Impedance Analysis and Computed Tomography for the Assessment of Muscle Mass in Patients with Gastric Cancer. *Nutrition* **2024**, *121*, 112363. [CrossRef] [PubMed]
53. Prado, C.M.M.; Lieffers, J.R.; McCargar, L.J.; Reiman, T.; Sawyer, M.B.; Martin, L.; Baracos, V.E. Prevalence and Clinical Implications of Sarcopenic Obesity in Patients with Solid Tumours of the Respiratory and Gastrointestinal Tracts: A Population-Based Study. *Lancet Oncol.* **2008**, *9*, 629–635. [CrossRef]
54. Zhang, Y.; Zhang, T.; Yin, W.; Zhang, L.; Xiang, J. Diagnostic Value of Sarcopenia Computed Tomography Metrics for Older Patients with or without Cancers with Gastrointestinal Disorders. *J. Am. Med. Dir. Assoc.* **2023**, *24*, 220–227.e4. [CrossRef]
55. Hansen, C.; Tobberup, R.; Rasmussen, H.H.; Delekta, A.M.; Holst, M. Measurement of Body Composition: Agreement between Methods of Measurement by Bioimpedance and Computed Tomography in Patients with Non-Small Cell Lung Cancer. *Clin. Nutr. ESPEN* **2021**, *44*, 429–436. [CrossRef]
56. Souza, N.C.; Gonzalez, M.C.; Martucci, R.B.; Rodrigues, V.D.; De Pinho, N.B.; Qureshi, A.R.; Avesani, C.M. Comparative Analysis Between Computed Tomography and Surrogate Methods to Detect Low Muscle Mass Among Colorectal Cancer Patients. *J. Parenter. Enter. Nutr.* **2020**, *44*, 1328–1337. [CrossRef]
57. Kim, D.; Sun, J.S.; Lee, Y.H.; Lee, J.H.; Hong, J.; Lee, J.-M. Comparative Assessment of Skeletal Muscle Mass Using Computerized Tomography and Bioelectrical Impedance Analysis in Critically Ill Patients. *Clin. Nutr.* **2019**, *38*, 2747–2755. [CrossRef] [PubMed]
58. Di Iorio, B.R.; Terracciano, V.; Bellizzi, V. Bioelectrical Impedance Measurement: Errors and Artifacts. *J. Ren. Nutr. Off. J. Counc. Ren. Nutr. Natl. Kidney Found.* **1999**, *9*, 192–197. [CrossRef]
59. Souza, N.C.; Avesani, C.M.; Prado, C.M.; Martucci, R.B.; Rodrigues, V.D.; De Pinho, N.B.; Heymsfield, S.B.; Gonzalez, M.C. Phase Angle as a Marker for Muscle Abnormalities and Function in Patients with Colorectal Cancer. *Clin. Nutr.* **2021**, *40*, 4799–4806. [CrossRef] [PubMed]
60. López-Gómez, J.J.; García-Benitez, D.; Jiménez-Sahagún, R.; Izaola-Jauregui, O.; Primo-Martín, D.; Ramos-Bachiller, B.; Gómez-Hoyos, E.; Delgado-García, E.; Pérez-López, P.; De Luis-Román, D.A. Nutritional Ultrasonography, a Method to Evaluate Muscle Mass and Quality in Morphofunctional Assessment of Disease Related Malnutrition. *Nutrients* **2023**, *15*, 3923. [CrossRef] [PubMed]
61. Fischer, A.; Anwar, M.; Hertwig, A.; Hahn, R.; Pesta, M.; Timmermann, I.; Siebenrock, T.; Liebau, K.; Hiesmayr, M. Ultrasound Method of the USVALID Study to Measure Subcutaneous Adipose Tissue and Muscle Thickness on the Thigh and Upper Arm: An Illustrated Step-by-Step Guide. *Clin. Nutr. Exp.* **2020**, *32*, 38–73. [CrossRef]
62. e Lima, K.M.M.; da Matta, T.T.; de Oliveira, L.F. Reliability of the Rectus Femoris Muscle Cross-Sectional Area Measurements by Ultrasonography. *Clin. Physiol. Funct. Imaging* **2012**, *32*, 221–226. [CrossRef] [PubMed]
63. Phillip, J.G.; Minet, L.R.; Smedemark, S.A.; Ryg, J.; Andersen-Ranberg, K.; Brockhattingen, K.K. Comparative Analysis of Hand-Held and Stationary Ultrasound for Detection of Sarcopenia in Acutely Hospitalised Older Adults—A Validity and Reliability Study. *Eur. Geriatr. Med.* **2024**, *15*, 1017–1022. [CrossRef]

nutrients

MDPI

Article

Phase Angle and Ultrasound Assessment of the Rectus Femoris for Predicting Malnutrition and Sarcopenia in Patients with Esophagogastric Cancer: A Cross-Sectional Pilot Study

Erika Vieira Maroun [1,2,3], María Argente Pla [1,4,*], María José Pedraza Serrano [5], Bianca Tabita Muresan [3], Agustín Ramos Prol [4], Eva Gascó Santana [4], Silvia Martín Sanchis [4], Ángela Durá De Miguel [4], Andrea Micó García [4], Anna Cebrián Vázquez [4], Alba Durbá Lacruz [4] and Juan Francisco Merino-Torres [1,2,4]

1 Joint Research Unit on Endocrinology, Nutrition and Clinical Dietetics, Health Research Institute La Fe, 46026 Valencia, Spain; erika.vieira@universidadeuropea.es (E.V.M.); merino_jfr@gva.es (J.F.M.-T.)
2 Department of Medicine, Faculty of Medicine, University of Valencia, 46010 Valencia, Spain
3 Facultad Ciencias de la Salud, Universidad Europea de Valencia, 46010 Valencia, Spain; biancatabita.muresan@universidadeuropea.es
4 Endocrinology and Nutrition Department, La Fe University and Polytechnic Hospital in Valencia, 46026 Valencia, Spain; ramos_agu@gva.es (A.R.P.); gasco_evasan@gva.es (E.G.S.); martin_silsan@gva.es (S.M.S.); dura_angdem@gva.es (Á.D.D.M.); mico_and@gva.es (A.M.G.); cebrian_anavaz@gva.es (A.C.V.); durba_alb@gva.es (A.D.L.)
5 Independent Researcher, 46100 Valencia, Spain; majopese@alumni.uv.es
* Correspondence: argente_marpla@gva.es

Abstract: Background: Disease-related malnutrition (DRM) and sarcopenia are prevalent conditions in gastrointestinal cancer patients, whose early diagnosis is essential to establish a nutritional treatment that contributes to optimizing adverse outcomes and improving prognosis. Phase angle (PhA) and rectus femoris ultrasound measurements are considered effort-independent markers of muscle wasting, which remains unrecognized in oncology patients. Objective: This study aimed to evaluate the potential utility of PhA, rectus femoris cross-sectional area (RFCSA), and rectus femoris thickness (RF-Y-axis) in predicting malnutrition and sarcopenia in patients with esophagogastric cancer (EGC). Methods: This was a cross-sectional study of patients diagnosed with EGC. PhA was obtained using bioelectrical impedance vector analysis (BIVA) along with ASMMI. The RFCSA and RF-Y-axis were measured using nutritional ultrasound (NU®). Muscle capacity was assessed using handgrip strength (HGS), and functionality by applying the Short Physical Performance Battery (SPPB). Malnutrition and sarcopenia were determined according to the GLIM and EWGSOP2 criteria, respectively. Results: Out of the 35 patients evaluated, 82.8% had malnutrition and 51.4% had sarcopenia. The RFCSA ($r = 0.582$) and RF-Y-axis ($r = 0.602$) showed significant, moderate correlations with ASMMI, unlike PhA ($r = 0.439$), which displayed a weak correlation with this parameter. However, PhA (OR = 0.167, CI 95%: 0.047–0.591, $p = 0.006$), RFCSA (OR = 0.212, CI 95%: 0.074–0.605, $p = 0.004$), and RF-Y-axis (OR = 0.002, CI 95%: 0.000–0.143, $p = 0.004$) all showed good predicting ability for sarcopenia in the crude models, but only the RF-Y-axis was able to explain malnutrition in the regression model (OR = 0.002, CI 95%: 0.000–0.418, $p = 0.023$). Conclusions: The RF-Y-axis emerged as the only independent predictor of both malnutrition and sarcopenia in this study, likely due to its stronger correlation with ASMMI compared to PhA and RFCSA.

Keywords: esophagogastric cancer; malnutrition; sarcopenia; ultrasound of rectus femoris muscle; phase angle; morphofunctional assessment

1. Introduction

According to the latest data from the Global Cancer Observatory (GLOBOCAN) of 2022, gastrointestinal (GI) cancers are a major public health concern, as they pose the highest lifetime risk of death due to the invasive nature of the disease [1]. In Europe, esophageal and gastric cancers, two of the most lethal malignant GI tumors [2,3], accounted for 189,031 new cases and 142,508 deaths in 2020 [4], resulting in a sixth and third place in terms of mortality, respectively [1].

These patients commonly experience a high rate of nutritional impairment due to symptoms arising from systemic inflammation and local tumor effects, such as dysphagia, nausea, malabsorption, vomiting, diarrhea, or fatigue [5–7]. This leads to inadequate nutritional intake [8,9], which causes involuntary weight loss and reduced muscle mass [10–13]. Therefore, disease-related malnutrition (DRM) and sarcopenia are the most common cancer-related conditions, affecting between 15% and 40% of patients at the time of diagnosis. Moreover, in advanced stages of esophagogastric cancer (EGC), DRM, and sarcopenia may affect up to 75% of patients [14–17].

Currently, in cancer patients, DRM and sarcopenia are associated with adverse outcomes, including a higher likelihood of postoperative complications and reduced response and tolerance to treatment [18]. This results in an increased length of hospital stay, disease burden, and healthcare costs, further worsening patient prognosis and overall survival [19–21]. Hypercatabolic states and, consequently, muscle wasting are often exacerbated by most chemotherapeutic agents and surgery itself, underscoring the importance of evaluating muscle mass as a key component in morphofunctional assessment to identify malnutrition and sarcopenia [22], which can also occur in individuals with normal weight, overweight, or obesity.

The Global Leadership Initiative on Malnutrition (GLIM) has highlighted the role of reduced muscle mass as a phenotypic criterion for diagnosing malnutrition in clinical settings [23]. Similarly, in 2019, the European Working Group on Sarcopenia in Older People 2 (EWGSOP2) updated the definition of this condition, establishing that sarcopenia is probable when low muscle strength is detected; its diagnosis is confirmed by the presence of low muscle quantity or quality and is considered severe when low physical performance is identified [24]. Several techniques are available to assess changes in body composition, such as bioelectrical impedance analysis (BIA) and ultrasound (US), which have the advantages of low cost, high portability, and bedside use [25,26], unlike magnetic resonance imaging (MRI), dual-energy X-ray absorptiometry (DEXA), and computerized tomography scan (CT), currently considered as gold standards for assessing the nutritional status of patients [27].

On the one hand, BIA is a non-invasive method based on the human body's ability to transmit an electrical current, providing bioelectrical impedance vector analysis (BIVA) and phase angle (PhA), both of which elucidate insights into cell membrane integrity and vitality, and body hydration [28–30]. The BIVA approach and PhA are derived from raw measurements, specifically resistance (R) and reactance (Xc), rendering them independent of body weight and free from calculation-inherent errors, which makes them suitable for use in cancer patients [31].

On the other hand, although there is evidence that ultrasound muscle measurements are affected by fluid hydration status [32,33], US has recently proven to be a valuable tool for estimating muscle quantity and quality [34,35]. Although various muscular structures can be evaluated, the rectus femoris (RF) is one of the most referenced ones, since anterior thigh muscles are affected early in catabolic processes [36]. Like PhA, ultrasound-derived rectus femoris cross-sectional area (RFCSA) and muscle thickness or rectus femoris Y-axis (RF-Y-axis) have been proposed as attractive, effort-independent surrogate markers of malnutrition and sarcopenia. Recent studies have demonstrated that lower values of these parameters are linked to reduced muscle mass, strength and/or functionality [37–40].

However, contradictory findings have also been reported [41–43]. In addition, most studies yielding positive results have focused on contexts outside of oncology, including cardiovascular diseases, chronic obstructive pulmonary disease, SARS-CoV-2 disease, or even healthy patients [39,40,44]. Furthermore, research evaluating the effectiveness of PhA has predominantly examined its association with postoperative complication rates, length of hospital stay, quality of life, and survival, rather than with malnutrition and sarcopenia [45,46]. The same has occurred when considering US measurements, as studies have concentrated on establishing correlations between RFCSA, RF-Y-axis, and mortality [38].

Consequently, to date, there is a gap in the literature regarding the ability of certain bioelectrical and ultrasound parameters to reflect nutritional status, including muscle quantity and quality, in EGC patients. Therefore, under the hypothesis that PhA, RFCSA, and RF-Y-axis could play an important role in nutritional screening and subsequent diagnosis by detecting muscle loss, this study was aimed at evaluating the potential utility of PhA, RF-CSA, and RF-Y-axis in identifying malnutrition and sarcopenia according to the GLIM and EWGSOP2 criteria, respectively, in adult patients with EGC.

2. Materials and Methods

2.1. Study Design

This is a cross-sectional pilot study conducted as part of a prospective, single-center research project involving 35 patients diagnosed with esophagogastric cancer. Patients were recruited from the Endocrinology and Nutrition Service at the Hospital Universitario y Politécnico La Fe in Valencia between January and September 2024, after being referred from the departments of esophagogastric surgery or medical oncology.

The inclusion criteria were patients between 18 and 80 years old with histologically confirmed diagnoses, regardless of tumor stage or route of feeding. The exclusion criteria were patients with concomitant non-esophagogastric malignant tumors and those undergoing palliative treatment and patients with ECOG (Eastern Cooperative Oncology Group) >2. Patients diagnosed with severe liver cirrhosis, stage 4 or 5 chronic kidney disease (glomerular filtration rate less than 30 mL/min/1.73 m^2, measured by the equation proposed by the Chronic Kidney Disease Epidemiology Collaboration (CKD-EPI)), heart failure, mental illness, or stroke were excluded. Additionally, patients without all clinical data, such as weight or height and contraindications to BIA, were also excluded. This ensured that, in total, 4 patients were excluded from the present study.

The study was approved by the Clinical Research Ethics Committee of the La Fe Health Research Institute (approval number 2023-1188-1, date of approval: 20 December 2023). Informed consent was obtained from all participants for the anonymous use of their data.

2.2. Clinical and Sociodemographic Data

We collected data related to sex, age, comorbidities such as diabetes, hypertension, dyslipemia, tumor location, tumor–node–metastasis (TNM) cancer staging system, oncology treatment, and ECOG. Information was recruited by interview or medical record. The level of physical activity was assessed using the International Physical Activity Questionnaire (IPAQ) [47]. Based on the results, the participants were classified into three groups: inactive or low physical activity, moderate activity, and high activity.

2.3. Anthropometric Measurements

Height was measured using a stadiometer, and weight was assessed with a calibrated weighing scale (SECA®, Hamburg, Germany), equipped with certified test weights (±0.1 kg). As part of anthropometry, the patients were measured with the patient standing, dressed in light clothing, barefoot, and with the head oriented in the Frankfurt horizontal plane, using a mechanical column scale. The body mass index (BMI) was calculated for each patient and classified according to the World Health Organization (WHO) guidelines. For older patients, the BMI was classified according to the recommendations of the Spanish Society of Gerontology and Geriatrics (SEGG) and the Spanish Society of Clinical Nutrition and Metabolism (SENPE) [48].

Calf (CC) and mid-arm circumferences (MAC) were measured according to recommendations using a flexible, non-elastic measuring tape (SECA® 201, Hamburg, Germany) calibrated in centimeters, with millimeter precision. The CC cut-off was set at <34 cm for men and <33 cm for women (BMI = 18.5–24.9 kg/m^2), with adjustment factors applied for other BMI categories) [49].

2.4. Nutritional Screening and Diagnosis of Malnutrition

Nutritional risk was evaluated using subjective global assessment (SGA) [50]. SGA is the most studied, validated, and widely recognized method for accurately assessing the nutritional status of oncology patients [51,52]. It produces the following global ratings: well nourished (A), moderately malnourished (B), or severely malnourished (C).

The GLIM criteria were used to diagnose malnutrition [23], which requires the presence of at least one etiological and one phenotypic criterion simultaneously. The phenotypic criteria included: (a) unintentional weight loss > 5% over the past six months or >10% over a longer period, (b) a body mass index (BMI) < 18.5 kg/m^2 for individuals under 70 years of age, or <20 kg/m^2 for those aged 70 and older, and (c) reduced muscle mass based on appendicular skeletal muscle mass index (ASMMI) (<7 kg/m^2 in males and <5.5 kg/m^2 in females) or fat-free mass index (FFMI) (<17 kg/m^2 in males and <15 kg/m^2 in females).

We determined that all patients fulfilled the GLIM etiological criteria for chronic disease-related cancer. Dietary intake was estimated using a 24-h dietary recall of 3 days conducted by a trained registered dietician.

2.5. Morphofunctional Assessment

2.5.1. Bioelectrical Impedance Vector Analysis (BIVA)

Impedance measurements were performed using a single-frequency, phase-sensitive impedance analyzer (NUTRILAB®, AKERN®, Pontassieve, Italy), which applies an alternating sinusoidal current of 400 μA at 50 kHz. The measurements were carried out following a standardized and validated technique [53] based on electrode placement (BIATRODES™, Pontassieve, Italy) on the back of the right hand (center of the third proximal phalanx) and on the corresponding foot (proximal to the second and third metatarsophalangeal joints). The position of the patients was supine, with the legs opened at a 45° angle relative to the body's midline, while the upper limbs were positioned 30° away from the trunk. To avoid disturbances, all patients waited five minutes in a supine position to balance the fluid distribution, and they were instructed to abstain from food and drink for a 2 h period before the test [54]. Bioelectrical parameters were analyzed to estimate body composition, including PhA, total body water (TBW), extracellular body water (ECW), intracellular body water (ICW), fat-free mass (FFM), fat mass (FM), body cell mass (BMC), and appendicular skeletal muscle mass (ASMM). To assess the hydration status, the ECW/TBW ratio and TBW/FFM % were used.

2.5.2. Nutritional Ultrasound (NU)®

The U PROBE-L6C® (manufacturer Léleman®, Valencia, Spain) (linear 7.5–10 KHz) ultrasound scanner was used, as implemented by De Luis Román et al. in their disease-related caloric-protein malnutrition echography (DRECO) study [55]. The patient was in a relaxed supine position, with the knee fully extended. Ultrasound scans of the rectus femoris muscle were performed at a point two-thirds of the way between the superior pole of the patella and the anterior superior iliac spine, according to a standardized technique [56]. The probe was covered with a suitable water-soluble transmission gel to ensure proper acoustic contact without compressing the dermal surface. It was aligned perpendicularly to both the longitudinal and transverse axes of the rectus femoris muscle to acquire the transverse image (Figure 1A). We measured, in the transversal axis, the cross-sectional area (RFCSA) in cm^2, muscle thickness (or RF-Y-axis), the RF-X-axis, and leg subcutaneous fat (RF-AT) in cm.

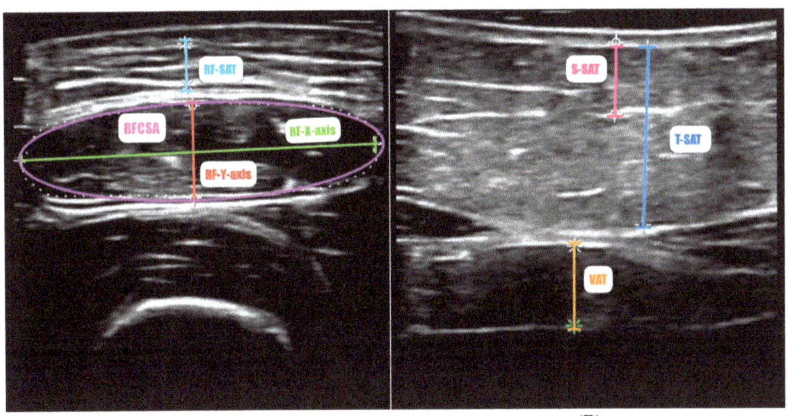

(A) (B)

Figure 1. Measurement of rectus femoris (**A**) and abdominal adipose tissue (**B**) by ultrasound of a patient in our sample. Abbreviations—RFCSA: rectus femoris cross-sectional area; RF-Y-axis: rectus femoris Y-axis or muscle thickness; RF-X-axis: rectus femoris X-axis; RF-SAT: rectus femoris superficial adipose tissue; VAT: visceral adipose tissue; T-SAT: total subcutaneous adipose tissue; S-SAT: superficial subcutaneous adipose tissue.

Adipose tissue assessment at the level of the abdominal wall was performed at the midpoint between the xiphoid process and the umbilicus. Cross-sectional imaging revealed the epidermis, superficial and deep adipose tissue layers, rectus abdominis muscles, and the preperitoneal fat layer between the *linea alba* and the parietal peritoneum. Measurements of total subcutaneous abdominal adipose tissue (T-SAT), superficial subcutaneous abdominal adipose tissue (S-SAT), and preperitoneal or visceral fat (VAT) were taken in centimeters during unforced expiration, perpendicularly to the skin. The procedure was carried out by a single experienced professional to minimize interobserver variability.

2.5.3. Functional and Muscle Strength Assessment

Hand grip strength (HGS) in the dominant hand was measured using a Jamar dynamometer (J A Preston Corporation, New York, NY, USA). The patients were instructed to sit in a chair with a backrest, with both feet on the floor, with the shoulders close to the body in a neutral position and the forearm flexed at 90° without rotation [57,58]. The correct grip was then explained to them and initiated when they were in a comfortable position. They were asked to squeeze as hard as they could after receiving a verbal command; they were then verbally encouraged to achieve better results. Three measurements were recorded with the dominant hand, with 1 min of rest between each measurement, and then averaged.

Physical performance was assessed using the Short Physical Performance Battery (SPPB), which comprises three tests: balance (feet together, semi-tandem, and tandem), walking speed (over a 4-m distance), and the chair rise test. Based on the results, the patients were categorized as dependent/disabled (0–3 points), frail (4–6 points), pre-frail (7–9 points), or autonomous/robust (10–12 points) [59].

2.6. Assessment and Diagnosis of Sarcopenia

Sarcopenia risk was assessed using the validated Spanish version of the SARC-F [60], a five-item self-report questionnaire evaluating patients' perceptions of their limitations in strength, assistance with walking, rising from a chair, climbing stairs, and experiences with falls. The final score was used to classify the patients as having a low probability of sarcopenia (<4 points) or a high probability of sarcopenia (≥4 points) [61].

Sarcopenia was diagnosed using the European Working Group on Sarcopenia in Older People (EWGSOP2) criteria [24]. Patients were classified according to the EWGSOP2 algorithm: (1) probable sarcopenia, defined by low muscle strength as measured by dynamometry (<27 kg in men and <16 kg in women); (2) confirmed sarcopenia, when low muscle strength coexists with low muscle quantity or quality, as determined by ASMMI (<7 kg/m^2 in males and <5.5 kg/m^2 in females); and (3) severe sarcopenia, when low strength and low muscle quantity/quality are accompanied by low physical performance (SPPB test $\leq$ 8 points).

2.7. Statistical Analysis

Continuous variables are presented as mean ± standard deviation (SD) or median with interquartile range (IQR), as appropriate. Categorical variables are expressed as proportions (%). Previously, the Shapiro–Wilk test was performed to check the normality of the data. Comparisons between groups were made with different tests, depending on the nature of the variables, including the Mann–Whitney U test, Fisher's exact test, one-way ANOVA, and the Kruskal–Wallis test, followed by the Bonferroni post hoc test, as appropriate. Inferential statistics were performed with bivariate correlations using the Pearson and Spearman correlation tests, according to normal distribution. To determine whether different variables could predict malnutrition and sarcopenia, binary logistic regression analysis was conducted using a crude model, with the presence or absence of malnutrition and sarcopenia as the dependent variables. Statistical significance was set at $p < 0.05$. All statistical analyses were performed using SPSS version 30.0 (SPSS Inc., Chicago, IL, USA).

3. Results

The study included 35 patients, 26 of whom were male (74.3%), with a mean age of 62.8 ± 8.8 years. A total of 25 (71.4%) patients had esophageal cancer and 14 (40%) were in stage III. The combination of surgery and chemotherapy (CTx) was the most commonly applied therapy (54.3%). Most patients were inactive or considered to have low physical activity (74.3%). The characteristics of the population study, including demographic and clinical variables, screening methods, and anthropometric measurements, are summarized in Table 1.

Table 1. Baseline demographic and disease characteristics of the participants.

Variable	All Patients (n = 35)	Male (n = 26)	Female (n = 9)
Age (years)	62.8 ± 8.8	62.2 ± 9.5	64.8 ± 6.4
Primary site tumor			
Esophageal	25 (71.4%)	21 (80.8%)	4 (44.4%)
Gastric	10 (28.6%)	5 (19.2%)	5 (55.6%)
Tumor stage			
I	3 (8.6%)	0 (0%)	3 (33.3%)
II	10 (28.6)	8 (30.8%)	2 (22.2%)
III	14 (40%)	11 (42.3%)	3 (33.3%)
IV	8 (22.9%)	7 (26.9%)	1 (11.1%)
Comorbidities			
0	7 (20%)	6 (23.1%)	1 (11.1%)
1	8 (22.9%)	6 (23.1%)	2 (22.2%)
≥2	20 (57.1%)	14 (53.8%)	6 (66.7%)
Physical activity			
Low or inactive	26 (74.3%)	19 (73.1%)	7 (77.8%)
Medium	5 (14.3%)	3 (11.5%)	2 (22.2%)
High	4 (11.4%)	4 (15.4%)	0 (0%)
Treatment			
Only CTx	8 (22.9%)	8 (30.8%)	0 (0%)
CTx and RTx	4 (11.4%)	2 (7.7%)	2 (22.2%)
Surgery and CTx	10 (54.3%)	13 (50%)	6 (66.7%)
Surgery, CTx and RTx	4 (11.4%)	3 (11.5%)	1 (11.1%)

Table 1. *Cont.*

Data are expressed as mean ± standard deviations or percentage. The groups were divided by sex variable. Abbreviations—CTx: chemotherapy; RTx: radiotherapy.

Classical and advanced parameters of nutritional status assessment in the study sample, stratified by sex, are shown in Table 2.

Table 2. Morphofunctional assessment parameters stratified by sex.

Variable	All Patients (n = 35)	Male (n = 26)	Female (n = 9)
BMI (kg/m^2)	23.3 ± 5.7	23.5 ± 5.3	22.6 ± 6.9
Underweight	13 (37.1%)	9 (34.6%)	4 (44.4%)
Normal	12 (34.3%)	10 (38.5%)	2 (22.2%)
Overweight	4 (11.4%)	3 (11.5%)	1 (11.1%)
Obesity	6 (17.1%)	4 (15.4%)	2 (22.2%)
Weight loss within past 6 months (%)	14.3 ± 7.9	14.9 ± 8.3	12.3 ± 6.5
<5%	4 (11.4%)	3 (11.5%)	1 (11.1%)
5–10%	5 (14.3%)	2 (7.7%)	3 (33.3%)
>10%	26 (74.3%)	21 (80.8%)	5 (55.6%)
MAC (cm)	26.1 ± 5.3	23.5 ± 5.3	25.2 ± 6.9
CC (cm)	32.9 ± 4.4	33.3 ± 4.5	31.9 ± 4.1
Normal	8 (22.9%)	6 (23.1%)	2 (22.2%)
Low	27 (77.1%)	20 (66.9%)	7 (77.8%)
BIVA-derived parameters			
PhA (°)	4.7 ± 0.9	4.9 ± 0.9	4.3 ± 0.8
ECW/TBW ratio	0.5 ± 0.07	0.48 ± 0.06	0.51 ± 0.08
TBW/FFM (%)	69.7 ± 17.6	71.1 ± 14.7	66.0 ± 24.6
FM (%)	19.6 ± 12	18.7 ± 10.2	22.2 ± 16.6
ASMMI (kg/m^2)	6.8 ± 1.2	7.2 ± 1.06	5.6 ± 0.86
BCM (kg)	24.9 ± 6.1	27.1 ± 5.2	18.8 ± 3.9
Nutritional ultrasound®: rectus femoris muscle			
RFCSA (cm^2)	2.8 ± 1.0	2.9 ± 1.02	2.2 ± 0.8
RF-Y-axis (cm)	0.8 ± 0.3	0.87 ± 0.27	0.77 ± 0.22
RF-X-axis	3.65 ± 0.50	3.76 ± 0.44	3.31 ± 0.55
RF-AT (cm)	0.41 (0.23–0.74)	0.35 (0.24–0.55)	0.78 (0.22–1.42)
Nutritional ultrasound®: abdominal adipose tissue			
T-SAT (cm)	1.4 (0.5–1.9)	1.35 (0.47–1.85)	1.41 (0.82–2.43)
S-SAT (cm)	0.52 (0.28–0.87)	0.47 (0.26–0.79)	0.68 (0.35–1.06)
VAT (cm)	0.55 (0.31–0.73)	0.52 (0.30–0.65)	0.58 (0.33–0.95)
Hand grip strength			
HGS (kg)	27.5 ± 8.4	31.1 ± 6.5	17.3 ± 2.5
Functional test			
SPPB	10 (7–11)	10 (7.7–11.2)	10 (6.5–10.5)

Data are expressed as mean ± standard deviation or median (interquartile range). Abbreviations—BMI: body mass index; MAC: mid-arm circumference; CC: calf circumference;; BIVA: bioelectrical impedance vector analysis; PhA: phase angle; ECW: extracellular water; TBW: total body water; FFM: fat-free mass; FM: fat mass; ASMMI: appendicular skeletal muscle mass index; BCM: body cellular mass; RFCSA: rectus femoris cross-sectional area; RF-Y-axis: rectus femoris Y-axis; RF-X-axis: rectus femoris X-axis; RF-AT: rectus femoris adipose tissue; T-SAT: total subcutaneous adipose tissue; S-SAT: superficial subcutaneous adipose tissue; VAT: visceral adipose tissue; HGS: hand grip strength; SPPB: Short Physical Performance Battery.

According to SGA, 3 (8.6%) patients were classified as well nourished, 14 (40.0%) as mild to moderately malnourished, and 18 (51.4%) as severely malnourished. Similarly, 11 (31.4%) participants exhibited moderate malnutrition, and 18 (51.4%) presented severe malnutrition when applying the GLIM criteria, resulting in an overall malnutrition prevalence of 82.8%. Following the EWGSOP2 criteria, sarcopenia was observed in 18 patients (51.4%), with 8 (22.8%) classified as having confirmed sarcopenia and 10 (28.6%) as having severe sarcopenia, despite only 8 (22.8%) participants being identified as at risk for this condition based on SARC-F findings.

As shown in Table 3, weight loss was the only variable that showed a statistically significant difference between non-malnutrition and stages 1 ($p = 0.010$) and 2 ($p < 0.001$) of this condition. When analyzing BIVA-derived parameters by group pair, the PhA values associated with severe malnutrition (4.3 ± 0.7) were significantly lower than those corresponding to non-malnourished individuals (5.3 ± 0.7; $p = 0.001$). The data for BMI ($p < 0.001$), ASMMI ($p = 0.003$), and BCM ($p = 0.017$) exhibited the same trend.

Table 3. Differences in demographic, clinical, BIVA-derived, and ultrasound data according to the GLIM criteria.

Variable	No Malnutrition (*n* = 6)	Moderate Malnutrition (*n* = 11)	Severe Malnutrition (*n* = 18)	*p*-Value
Sex				0.773
Male	4 (66.7%)	9 (81.8%)	13 (72.2%)	
Female	2 (33.3%)	2 (18.2%)	5 (27.8%)	
Age (years)	60.5 ± 4.8	63.3 ± 10.9	63.3 ± 8.7	0.786
BMI (kg/m^2)	29.3 ± 5.6	25.9 ± 4.8	19.6 ± 3.0	<0.001 ***
Weight loss within past 6 months (%)	4.2 ± 4.3	14.9 ± 5.5	17.3 ± 7.4	<0.001 ***

Table 3. *Cont.*

Variable	No Malnutrition (n = 6)	Moderate Malnutrition (n = 11)	Severe Malnutrition (n = 18)	p-Value
MAC (cm)	31.0 ± 4.6	29.4 ± 4.3	22.4 ± 3.0	<0.001 ***
CC (cm)	36.8 ± 5.3	34.9 ± 3.5	30.3 ± 2.8	<0.001 ***
SGA				
Well nourished (A)	3 (50%)	0 (0%)	0 (0%)	<0.001 ***
Mild to moderately malnourished (B)	2 (33.3%	8 (72.7%)	4 (22.2%)	
Severely malnourished (C)	1 (16.7%)	3 (27.3%)	14 (77.8%)	
BIVA-derived parameters				
PhA (°)	5.3 ± 0.7	5.1 ± 1.02	4.3 ± 0.7	0.016 *
ECW/TBW ratio	0.46 ± 0.04	0.47 ± 0.07	0.50 ± 0.07	0.405
TBW/FFM (%)	62.3 ± 30.3	74.3 ± 2.1	69.7 ± 17.2	0.430
FM (%)	25.7 ± 13.9	21.0 ± 13.6	16.7 ± 9.8	0.255
ASMMI (kg/m^2)	7.7 ± 1.5	7.6 ± 0.8	6.0 ± 0.8	<0.001 ***
BCM (kg)	29.9 ± 4.7	27.6 ± 5.6	21.7 ± 4.9	<0.001 ***
Nutritional ultrasound®: rectus femoris muscle				
RFCSA (cm^2)	3.5 ± 0.9	3.5 ± 0.9	2.1 ± 0.6	<0.001 ***
RF-Y-axis (cm)	1.1 ± 0.3	0.97 ± 0.19	0.68 ± 0.18	<0.001 ***
RF-X-axis (cm)	3.64 ± 0.22	3.96 ± 0.12	3.46 ± 0.11	0.030 *
RF-AT (cm)	0.82 (0.4–1.16)	0.44 (0.34–1.01)	0.30 (0.18–0.50)	0.037 *
Nutritional ultrasound®: abdominal adipose tissue				
T-SAT (cm)	2.08 (1.72–2.59)	1.30 (0.55–2.62)	1.0 (0.36–1.56)	0.012 *
S-SAT (cm)	1.07 (0.73–1.26)	0.62 (0.34–0.95)	0.44 (0.19–0.65)	0.011 *
VAT (cm)	0.63 (0.56–0.97)	0.62 (0.55–0.93)	0.34 (0.24–0.48)	0.004 **

Data are expressed as mean ± standard deviation or median (interquartile range) or percentage. Asterisk indicates significant difference between groups, according to the Mann–Whitney test or Fisher's exact test (*** $p < 0.001$, ** $p < 0.01$, * $p < 0.05$). Abbreviations—BMI: body mass index; MAC: mid-arm circumference; CC: calf circumference; SGA: subjective global assessment; BIVA: bioelectrical impedance vector analysis; PhA: phase angle; ECW: extracellular water; TBW: total body water; FFM: fat-free mass; FM: fat mass; ASMMI: appendicular skeletal muscle mass index; BCM: body cellular mass; RFCSA: rectus femoris cross-sectional area; RF-Y-axis: rectus femoris Y-axis; RF-X-axis: rectus femoris X-axis; RF-AT: rectus femoris adipose tissue; T-SAT: total subcutaneous adipose tissue; S-SAT: superficial subcutaneous adipose tissue; VAT: visceral adipose tissue.

Regarding US measurements, both RF-CSA ($p < 0.001$) and RF-Y-axis ($p < 0.001$) showed significant differences between the non-malnutrition and severe malnutrition groups. Although the %FM measured by BIVA did not reveal noteworthy variations among any of the groups, significant differences were observed between the RF adipose tissue values of the two groups ($p = 0.020$). Differences between malnutrition groups and sociodemographic and clinical variables such as physical activity, primary site tumor, comorbidities, tumor stage, and treatment were not found.

In relation to sarcopenia diagnosis, significant differences were observed in sex ($p = 0.003$) and age ($p = 0.021$) across the four groups, as well as in the SARC-F score. All patients without sarcopenia were men. Table 4 shows that the PhA values for individuals with confirmed (4.5 ± 0.8; $p = 0.009$) and severe sarcopenia (4.1 ± 0.5, $p < 0.001$) were significantly lower than those for patients without this condition (5.6 ± 0.7). This finding was also evident in the values obtained for BCM ($p = 0.011$, $p < 0.001$) and ASMMI ($p < 0.001$, $p < 0.001$). Like BCM and ASMMI, both RF-CSA and RF-y-axis showed significant differences between the non-sarcopenia group and the confirmed ($p < 0.001$) and severe sarcopenia groups ($p = 0.027$, $p = 0.039$).

Table 4. Differences in demographic, clinical, BIVA-derived, and ultrasound data according to the EWGSOP2 criteria.

Variable	No Sarcopenia (n = 12)	Probable Sarcopenia (n = 5)	Confirmed Sarcopenia (n = 8)	Severe Sarcopenia (n = 10)	p-Value
Sex					0.003 **
Male	12 (100%)	1 (20%)	5 (62.5%)	8 (80%)	
Female	0 (0%)	4 (80%)	3 (37.5%)	2 (20%)	
Age (years)	57.7 ± 9.4	68.8 ± 6.5	61.2 ± 6.9	67.2 ± 7.1	0.021 *
BMI (kg/m^2)	27.3 ± 5.2	26.9 ± 5.5	18.5 ± 3.2	20.3 ± 2.6	<0.001 ***
MAC (cm)	30.4 ± 3.8	29.2 ± 5.5	20.4 ± 2.3	23.9 ± 2.4	<0.001 ***
CC (cm)	36.7 ± 4.2	33.3 ± 3.4	30.3 ± 3.1	30.3 ± 2.5	<0.001 ***
SARC-F					<0.001 ***
No risk	12 (100%)	2 (40%)	8 (100%)	5 (50%)	
Sarcopenia risk	0 (0%)	3 (60%)	0 (0%)	5 (50%)	
BIA-derived parameters					
PhA (°)	5.6 ± 0.7	4.5 ± 0.9	4.5 ± 0.8	4.1 ± 0.5	<0.001 ***
ECW/TBW ratio	0.47 ± 0.04	0.48 ± 0.09	0.48 ± 0.07	0.51 ± 0.07	0.550
TBW/FFM (%)	74.15 ± 1.97	60.13 ± 33.3	73.4 ± 0.29	66.0 ± 24.5	0.407
FM (%)	19.4 ± 12.7	25.2 ± 19.1	14.2 ± 8.9	21.4 ± 8.4	0.408
ASMMI (kg/m^2)	7.98 ± 0.95	6.73 ± 0.57	5.92 ± 0.96	6.08 ± 0.69	<0.001 ***
BCM (kg)	30.2 ± 3.6	23.5 ± 6.3	22.7 ± 6.3	21.1 ± 3.9	<0.001 ***
Nutritional ultrasound®: rectus femoris muscle					
RFCSA (cm^2)	3.56 ± 0.76	2.80 ± 0.60	1.82 ± 0.49	2.53 ± 1.05	<0.001 ***
RF-Y-axis (cm)	1.05 ± 0.22	0.86 ± 0.13	0.58 ± 0.18	0.80 ± 0.21	<0.001 ***
RF-X-axis (cm)	3.79 ± 0.11	3.75 ± 0.20	3.49 ± 0.99	3.55 ± 0.23	0.520
RF-AT (cm)	0.48 (0.36–0.85)	1.10 (0.28–1.84)	0.26 (0.15–0.48)	0.30 (0.18–0.49)	0.072
Hand grip strength					
HGS (kg)	35.9 ± 4.9	19.5 ± 7.1	25.4 ± 5.2	23.3 ± 6.2	<0.001 ***
Functional test					
SPPB	11.5 (10–12)	10 (7.5–10.5)	10 (9–10.75)	6 (5–7.25)	<0.001 ***

Data are expressed as mean ± standard deviation or median (interquartile range) or percentage. Asterisk indicates significant difference between groups, according to the Mann–Whitney test or Fisher's exact test (*** $p < 0.001$, ** $p < 0.01$, * $p < 0.05$) Abbreviations—BMI: body mass index; MAC: mid-arm circumference; CC: calf circumference; BIVA: bioelectrical impedance vector analysis; PhA: phase angle; ECW: extracellular water; TBW: total body water; FFM: fat-free mass; FM: fat mass; ASMMI: appendicular skeletal muscle mass index; BCM: body cellular mass; RFCSA: rectus femoris cross-sectional area; RF-Y-axis: rectus femoris Y-axis; RF-X-axis: rectus femoris X-axis; RF-AT: rectus femoris adipose tissue; HGS: hand grip strength; SPPB: Short Physical Performance Battery.

Significant differences were also observed between the non-sarcopenia and sarcopenia probable groups when comparing the data for PhA (p = 0.044). The same pattern was noted for the other two diagnostic components of sarcopenia, showing significantly higher HGS values in patients without sarcopenia compared to those with probable (p = 0.037), confirmed (p = 0.002), and severe sarcopenia (p < 0.001). SPPB values in patients with severe sarcopenia were also significantly lower than those in the other groups (p < 0.001).

As with malnutrition, we did not find differences between sarcopenia groups and other sociodemographic and clinical variables.

All the primary variables examined—PhA, RFCSA, and RF-Y-axis—were significantly correlated with ASMMI, the key parameter used to diagnose malnutrition and sarcopenia (Figure 2).

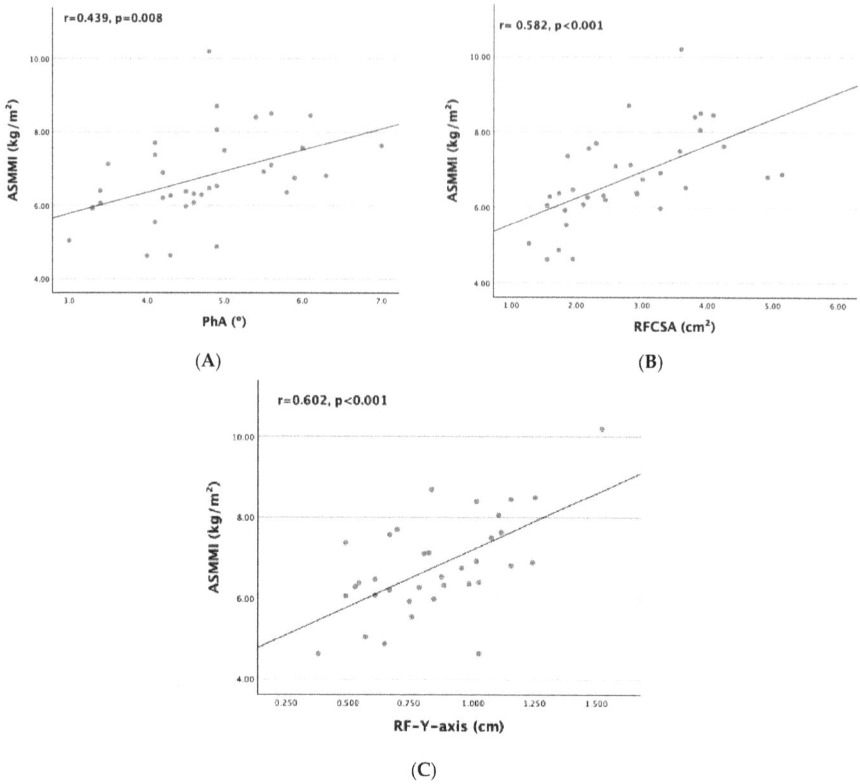

Figure 2. Scatter plot graphs of correlation between ASMMI and (**A**) PhA, (**B**) RFCSA, and (**C**) RF-Y-axis.

As shown in Table 5, the RF-Y-axis was the only muscle mass-related measure significantly correlated with all three diagnostic components of malnutrition, namely weight loss (r = −0.386, p = 0.022), BMI (r = 0.599, p < 0.001), and ASMMI (r = 0.602, p < 0.001). PhA was not correlated with either BMI or weight loss. In contrast, adipose tissue markers such as RF-AT (r = 0.742, p < 0.001), T-SAT (r = 0.826, p < 0.001), and S-SAT (r = 0.799, p < 0.001) showed high correlations with BMI, as well as FM (r = 0.543, p < 0.001), but low correlations with weight loss. These findings suggest that the RF-Y-axis may perform better than the other parameters as a predictor of malnutrition.

Table 5. Correlations between BIVA-derived parameters, ultrasound measurements, and components of malnutrition diagnosis according to GLIM criteria (%weight loss, BMI, and ASMMI).

Variable	% Weight Loss		BMI (kg/m^2)		ASMMI (kg/m^2)	
	r	*p*-Value	r	*p*-Value	r	*p*-Value
BIA-derived parameters						
PhA (°)	−0.093	0.596	0.288	0.094	0.439	0.008 **
ECW/TBW ratio	0.244	0.157	0.244	0.158	−0.246	0.154
TBW/FFM (%)	0.156	0.378	0.261	0.136	0.169	0.338
FM (%)	−0.232	0.181	0.543	<0.001 ***	0.204	0.240
BCM (kg)	−0.313	0.067	0.397	0.018 *	0.837	<0.001 ***
Nutritional ultrasound®: rectus femoris muscle						
RFCSA (cm^2)	−0.311	0.069	0.531	0.001 ***	0.582	<0.001 ***
RF-Y-axis (cm)	−0.386	0.022 *	0.599	<0.001 ***	0.602	<0.001 ***
RF-AT (cm)	−0.420	0.012 *	0.742	<0.001 ***	0.245	0.156
Nutritional ultrasound®: abdominal adipose tissue						
T-SAT (cm)	−0.491	0.005 **	0.826	<0.001 ***	0.399	0.026 *
S-SAT (cm)	−0.459	0.009 **	0.799	<0.001 ***	0.416	0.020 *
VAT (cm)	−0.092	0.112	0.607	<0.001 ***	0.278	0.130

Asterisk indicates significant correlation (*** $p < 0.001$, ** $p < 0.01$, * $p < 0.05$). Abbreviations—BMI: body mass index; ASMMI: appendicular skeletal muscle mass index; PhA: phase angle; ECW: extracellular water; TBW: total body water; FFM: fat-free mass; FM: fat mass; BCM: body cellular mass; RFCSA: rectus femoris cross-sectional area; RF-Y-axis: rectus femoris Y-axis; RF-AT: rectus femoris adipose tissue; T-SAT: total subcutaneous adipose tissue; S-SAT: superficial subcutaneous adipose tissue; VAT: visceral adipose tissue.

As detailed in Table 6, regarding the diagnostic components of sarcopenia, PhA exhibited statistically significant direct correlations with HGS (r = 0.556, $p < 0.001$), ASMMI (r = 0.439, $p = 0.008$), and SPPB (r = 0.475, $p = 0.004$), similar to BCM; however, the correlations with PhA were weaker. The RF-Y-axis showed the strongest association with ASMMI (r = 0.602, $p < 0.001$), but did not correlate with HGS, unlike RFCSA (r = 0.447, $p = 0.007$). Neither ultrasound measure was correlated with SPPB. These results suggest that PhA may provide a better prediction of sarcopenia than either the RFCSA or RF-Y-axis.

Table 6. Correlations between BIVA-derived parameters, ultrasound measurements, and components of sarcopenia diagnosis according to the EWGSOP2 (HGS, ASMMI, SPPB).

Variable	HGS (kg)		ASMMI (kg/m^2)		SPPB	
	r	*p*-Value	r	*p*-Value	r	*p*-Value
BIA-derived parameters						
PhA (°)	0.556	<0.001 ***	0.439	0.008 **	0.475	0.004 **
ECW/TBW ratio	−0.257	0.135	−0.246	0.154	−0.376	0.026 *
TBW/FFM (%)	0.223	0.204	0.169	0.338	0.124	0.483
BCM (kg)	0.751	<0.001 ***	0.837	<0.001 ***	0.461	0.005 **
Nutritional ultrasound®: rectus femoris muscle						
RFCSA (cm^2)	0.447	0.007 **	0.582	<0.001 ***	0.233	0.178
RF-Y-axis (cm)	0.315	0.065	0.602	<0.001 ***	0.151	0.388

Asterisk indicates significant correlation (*** $p < 0.001$, ** $p < 0.01$, * $p < 0.05$). Abbreviations—HGS: hand grip strength; ASMMI: appendicular skeletal muscle mass index; SPPB: Short Physical Performance Battery; PhA: phase angle; ECW: extracellular water; TBW: total body water; FFM: fat-free mass; BCM: body cellular mass; RFCSA: rectus femoris cross-sectional area; RF-Y-axis: rectus femoris Y-axis.

As shown in Figure 3, a positive correlation was found between RF ultrasound measurements and BIVA-derived parameters. RFCSA showed a moderate positive correlation with PhA (r = 0.564, $p < 0.001$) and BCM (r = 0.533, $p < 0.001$). The RF-Y-axis revealed a weak positive correlation with PhA (r = 0.457, $p = 0.006$) and BCM (r = 0.445, $p = 0.007$).

The unadjusted binary logistic regression models aimed at predicting the presence of malnutrition demonstrated that higher values of the RF-Y-axis (OR = 0.002, IC 95%: 0.000–0.418, $p = 0.023$) are protective factors against this condition. As shown in Table 7, for each one-cm increase in the RF-Y-axis, the likelihood of not having malnutrition is 500 times higher. PhA, RFCSA, and RF-AT failed to predict malnutrition in this case.

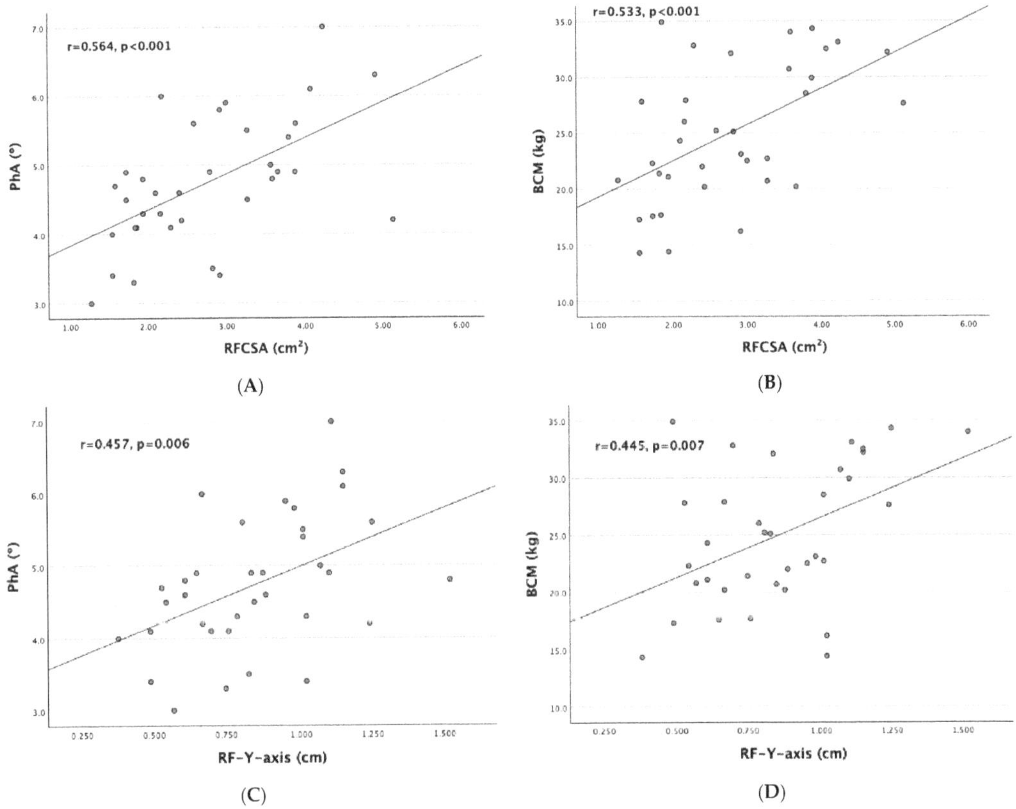

Figure 3. Scatter plot graphs of correlation between RF ultrasound measurements and BIVA-derived parameters: (**A**) RFCSA with PhA, (**B**) RFCSA with BCM, (**C**) RF-Y-axis with PhA, and (**D**) RF-Y-axis with BCM.

Table 7. Crude logistic regression analysis evaluating PhA, RFCSA, RFT, T-SAT, and S-SAT with GLIM malnutrition and EWGSOP2 sarcopenia.

	Malnutrition		Sarcopenia	
Variables	**OR**	***p*-Value**	**OR**	***p*-Value**
PhA (°)	0.430 (0.152–1.217)	0.112	0.167 (0.047–0.591)	0.006 **
BCM (kg)	0.817 (0.673–0.993)	0.042 *	0.797 (0.682–0.932)	0.005 **
Nutritional ultrasound®: rectus femoris muscle				
RFCSA (cm^2)	0.401 (0.155–1.037)	0.060	0.212 (0.074–0.605)	0.004 **
RF-Y-axis (cm)	0.002 (0.000–0.418)	0.023 *	0.002 (0.000–0.143)	0.004 **
RF-AT (cm)	0.220 (0.035–1.369)	0.105		
Nutritional ultrasound®: abdominal adipose tissue				
T-SAT (cm)	0.192 (0.043–0.851)	0.030 *		
S-SAT (cm)	0.019 (0.001–0.448)	0.014 *		

Asterisk indicates statical significance (** $p < 0.01$, * $p < 0.05$). Abbreviations—PhA: phase angle; BCM: body cellular mass; RFCSA: rectus femoris cross-sectional area; RF-Y-axis: rectus femoris Y-axis; RF-AT: rectus femoris adipose tissue; T-SAT: total subcutaneous adipose tissue; S-SAT: superficial subcutaneous adipose tissue.

Then, the crude analyses for predicting sarcopenia indicated that higher values of PhA (OR = 0.167, IC 95%: 0.047–0.591, $p = 0.006$) and ultrasound measurements of the rectus femoris, namely RFCSA (OR = 0.212, IC 95%: 0.074–0.605, $p = 0.004$) and RF-Y-axis (OR = 0.002, IC 95%: 0.000–0.143, $p = 0.004$), are protective against this condition. Specifically, the likelihood of being free from sarcopenia increases by 5.99 times with each one-degree increase in PhA. Similarly, for every one-centimeter increase in RFCSA and the RF-Y-axis, the probability of not having sarcopenia rises by 4.72 and 500 times, respectively.

It is worth noting that BCM, like the RF-Y-axis, showed good predictive ability in both crude models for malnutrition and sarcopenia. However, the estimation of this parameter relies on predictive BIA equations, which require data such as weight and height that are not always available. For this reason, attention has been focused on the results corresponding to PhA, RFCSA, and RF-Y-axis. Multivariable logistic regression models were not conducted due to the limited sample size.

4. Discussion

To the best of our knowledge, this is the first study to investigate the potential usefulness of phase angle and nutritional ultrasound in identifying the presence of malnutrition and sarcopenia in European patients with EGC using the most recent diagnostic criteria (GLIM and EWGSOP2). Only two studies have assessed the predictive value of PhA in patients with gastrointestinal cancer, one focusing solely on malnutrition [62] and the other including sarcopenia [63]. In fact, when considering ultrasound, only one study used RF-CSA and RF-Y-axis to predict these two deleterious conditions in head and neck cancer patients [64], while another one used it to anticipate 12-month mortality in a similar sample [38].

Our investigation identified that malnutrition was highly prevalent in esophageal and gastric cancer patients (82.8%), with 31.4% of patients showing moderate malnutrition and 51.4% with severe malnutrition. These values are higher than those found in most studies with the same population and similar methodology [63,65–67]. Moreover, these investigations have emphasized that patients who are candidates for oncological surgery, such as most of those included in our study, are twice as likely to present with malnutrition. A study recorded 72.2% malnutrition in patients after esophagogastric cancer surgery [68].

Moreover, this research showed that sarcopenia was highly prevalent in the patients analyzed with EGC, representing 51.5% of them. As with undernutrition, these results are significantly higher compared to other studies [69,70]. The discrepancies observed can primarily be attributed to differences in methodology, as most studies have used different diagnostic criteria or another technique to assess body composition, such as CT scans. Only one study included the EWGSOP2 diagnostic algorithm for sarcopenia, which found 43.3% sarcopenic patients [71]. However, in studies that included patients who underwent esophagectomy or gastrectomy [72,73], the prevalence of sarcopenia increased considerably (57.4% and 57.7%, respectively), more closely resembling our results.

Clinical characteristics, such as tumor site, tumor stage, and type of treatment, did not show significant differences between the malnutrition and sarcopenia groups, likely due to sample heterogeneity, which resulted in very small frequencies in each subgroup. However, statistically significant differences were observed in some BIVA-derived parameters, such as PhA, ASMMI, and BCM. This trend has also been recorded in multiple studies carried out in oncology patients [29,74,75]. PhA was positively correlated with all the components of sarcopenia diagnosis (ASMMI, HGS, and SPPB). Zuo et al. previously reported a similar correlation in gastric cancer patients [63]. Unlike the results observed in our study, they also found a positive correlation between PhA and all the nutritional indices used to diagnose malnutrition according to the GLIM criteria.

Interestingly, BCM was the parameter most strongly correlated with the diagnostic components of malnutrition and sarcopenia. Also, the crude analyses for predicting these two conditions demonstrated that a higher value of BCM is a protective factor against malnutrition and sarcopenia. These results are consistent with those reported by Herrera-Martínez et al. in a large cohort of patients with head and neck cancer [76]. Their results demonstrated that BCM was more strongly associated with malnutrition (OR = 0.88, 95% CI = 0.84–0.93, $p < 0.001$) and sarcopenia (OR = 0.81, 95% CI = 0.76–0.87, $p < 0.001$) compared to PhA (OR = 0.54, 95% CI = 0.40–0.71, $p < 0.001$) (OR = 0.47, 95% CI = 0.33–0.66, $p < 0.001$).

However, the present study focused on parameters such as PhA given its clinical significance, but in our study, phase angle was not able to predict malnutrition, although it could predict sarcopenia. Conversely, the study by Yang et al., using logistic regression models, confirmed PhA as a valuable indicator of malnutrition in patients with gastrointestinal cancer (OR = 0.548, 95% CI = 0.385–0.780, $p < 0.001$) [62]. A potential explanation for the discrepancies could be the altered hydration status and the small size of our study sample. The mean ECW/TBW index that we found exceeded the reference value established by Ge et al. [77] for the oncologic population with sarcopenia, evidencing a state of overhydration (ECW/TBW ≥ 0.385), which may interfere with correlations involving PhA.

The use of NU®-derived parameters based on muscle area and thickness (RFCSA and RF-Y-axis, respectively) may contribute to the assessment of malnutrition and sarcopenia. We found a moderate positive correlation between RFCSA and R-Y-axis with ASMMI, as previously described by Hida et al. [78]. Like Lopez-Gómez et al. [79], we also detected a weak correlation between RFCSA and HGS, which indicates that RF ultrasound measurements could be related not only to muscle quantity but also to muscle strength. This is supported by previous research on the role of ultrasound in the prediction of sarcopenia in elderly patients. It was revealed that the RFCSA and RF-Y-axis were the best indicators for detecting the loss of muscle mass and strength [80].

The RF-Y-axis was the only marker capable of predicting both sarcopenia and malnutrition. Furthermore, it exhibited the strongest correlation with ASMMI when considering PhA and RFCSA. Ozturk et al. also disclosed that the RF-Y-axis had a slightly greater positive correlation with skeletal muscle mass for the diagnosis of malnutrition using GLIM criteria in hospitalized internal medicine patients [81].

Due to the limited literature using these ultrasound measurements as markers of malnutrition and sarcopenia, making direct comparisons was challenging. In cancer patients, we have only the data reported by two Spanish studies [64,79]. On the one hand, Fernández-Jiménez et al. described that high levels of the RFCSA (OR = 0.81 (0.68–0.98), $p < 0.05$) and RF-Y-axis (OR = 0.31 (0.15–0.61), $p < 0.001$) were associated with a decreased risk of malnutrition, as defined by the GLIM criteria. Sarcopenia showed the same trend (OR = 0.64 (0.49–0.82), $p < 0.001$) for RFCSA and (OR = 0.27 (0.11–0.68), $p < 0.01$) for RF-Y-axis. On the other hand, Lopez-Gómez only found statistical differences in the RFCSA with sarcopenia diagnosis (sarcopenia: 2.47 cm^2 (± 0.54 cm^2); no sarcopenia: 3.65 cm^2 (± 1.34 cm^2); $p = 0.02$), but no differences with malnutrition.

Concerning adipose tissue, assessed using NU®, we found that all abdominal measurements (T-SAT, S-SAT, and VAT) and RF adipose tissue were significantly different between malnutrition groups. Additionally, T-SAT and S-SAT were correlated with all the components of malnutrition diagnosis, and they could predict malnutrition in the crude logistic regression analysis. As expected and described by other studies [64], US adipose tissue measurements did not show any relation with sarcopenia parameters, since they are highly associated with methods of assessing fat deposition and distribution.

Furthermore, we found a significant correlation between RFCSA and R-Y-axis with PhA, BCM, and ASMMI, which is consistent with a previous study in a longitudinal cohort of patients with cancer [38] and with the DRECO study [55]. These findings may support the integration of BIVA and NU® as part of the morphofunctional assessment for monitoring and optimizing the nutritional status of cancer patients, with both techniques being easily accessible in routine clinical practice.

There were several limitations to the current study. First, this was a cross-sectional study with a small sample size and a low proportion of women. Multicenter trials including a larger number of patients with EGC are needed for further validation. Second, multivariate logistic regression models were not conducted, which weakened the results by excluding important confounding factors such as age, type of treatment, and BMI. Third, the lack of consensus regarding cut-off values for PhA, RFCSA, RF-Y-axis, and RF-AT limited the ability to compare the results with previous studies. In addition, the cross-sectional nature of the study prevented participant follow-up. Therefore, prospective studies that include patients with different types of GI cancer are essential in order to establish causal relationships derived from nutritional intervention, thereby obtaining results that can be extrapolated to the oncological population.

5. Conclusions

In conclusion, the RF-Y-axis is the only parameter that appears to be a promising and useful independent predictor of both malnutrition and sarcopenia in this sample of EGC patients. These results reinforce the implementation of RF-Y-axis in routine clinical practice and its use as a potential low muscle quantity or quality criterion in the EWGSOP2 criteria and as a potential phenotypic criterion for muscle mass loss in the GLIM criteria. Nevertheless, PhA and RFCSA demonstrated good performance in predicting sarcopenia, but not malnutrition in the same population. This suggests the need for a larger sample to demonstrate stronger correlations between these two markers and ASMMI in order to effectively determine their usefulness as predictors not only of the presence but also of the severity of malnutrition and sarcopenia.

This study represents the initial exploration of an ongoing prospective nutritional follow-up project aimed at improving the process of identifying patients who require multimodal interventions, as well as assessing the outcomes of these interventions in terms of body composition and function. In this way, the research conducted would allow the results obtained to be translated into a more practical, effective, and objective morphofunctional assessment, thereby supporting the work of health professionals.

Author Contributions: Conceptualization, E.V.M., M.J.P.S., B.T.M. and M.A.P.; methodology, E.V.M.; formal analysis, E.V.M. and M.J.P.S.; investigation, E.V.M., M.J.P.S., M.A.P., A.R.P., E.G.S., S.M.S., Á.D.D.M., A.M.G., A.C.V. and A.D.L.; resources, J.F.M.-T.; data curation, E.V.M. and M.J.P.S.; writing—original draft preparation, E.V.M. and M.J.P.S.; writing—review and editing, E.V.M., M.J.P.S., B.T.M. and M.A.P.; visualization, E.V.M.; supervision, M.A.P., B.T.M. and J.F.M.-T.; project administration, E.V.M., M.A.P. and J.F.M.-T.; funding acquisition, J.F.M.-T. All authors have read and agreed to the published version of the manuscript.

Funding: E.V.M is supported by a predoctoral fellowship ("Formación del Profesorado Universitario" Ref: FPU23/03502), and this research was funded by SENPE Foundation ("Grant for the best research project presented in Clinical Nutrition on morphofunctional assessment in patients with gastrointestinal tract disease").

Institutional Review Board Statement: The study was conducted in accordance with the Declaration of Helsinki and approved by the Clinical Research Ethics Committee of the La Fe Health Research Institute (number 2023-1188-1, approval date 20 December 2023).

Informed Consent Statement: Informed consent was obtained from all subjects involved in the study.

Data Availability Statement: Data are contained within the article.

Conflicts of Interest: The authors declare no conflicts of interest.

References

1. Bray, F.; Laversanne, M.; Sung, H.; Ferlay, J.; Siegel, R.L.; Soerjomataram, I.; Ahmedin, J. Global Cancer Statistics 2022: GLOBOCAN Estimates of Incidence and Mortality Worldwide for 36 Cancers in 185 Countries. *CA Cancer J. Clin.* **2024**, *74*, 229–263. [CrossRef] [PubMed]
2. Xie, Y.; Shi, L.; He, X.; Luo, Y. Gastrointestinal Cancers in China, the USA, and Europe. *Gastroenterol. Rep.* **2021**, *9*, 91–104. [CrossRef] [PubMed]
3. Jardim, S.R.; de Souza, L.M.P.; de Souza, H.S.P. The Rise of Gastrointestinal Cancers as a Global Phenomenon: Unhealthy Behavior or Progress? *Int. J. Environ. Res. Public Health* **2023**, *20*, 3640. [CrossRef]
4. Giusti, F.; Martos, C.; Bettio, M.; Negrão Carvalho, R.; Zorzi, M.; Guzzinati, S.; Rugge, M. Geographical and Temporal Differences in Gastric and Oesophageal Cancer Registration by Subsite and Morphology in Europe. *Front. Oncol.* **2024**, *14*, 1250107. [CrossRef]
5. Movahed, S.; Norouzy, A.; Motlagh, A.G.; Eslami, S.; Khadem-Rezaiyan, M.; Emadzadeh, M.; Nematy, M.; Ghayour-Mobarhan, M.; Tabrizi, F.V.; Bozzetti, F.; et al. Nutritional Status in Patients with Esophageal Cancer Receiving Chemoradiation and Assessing the Efficacy of Usual Care for Nutritional Managements. *Asian Pac. J. Cancer Prev.* **2020**, *21*, 2315. [CrossRef]
6. Ajani, J.A.; D'Amico, T.A.; Bentrem, D.J.; Cooke, D.; Corvera, C.; Das, P.; Enzinger, P.C.; Enzler, T.; Farjah, F.; Gerdes, H.; et al. Esophageal and Esophagogastric Junction Cancers, Version 2.2023, NCCN Clinical Practice Guidelines in Oncology. *J. Natl. Compr. Canc Netw.* **2023**, *21*, 393–422. [CrossRef]
7. Wöll, E.; Amann, A.; Eisterer, W.; Gerger, A.; Grünberger, B.; Rumpold, H.; Weiss, L.; Winder, T.; Greil, R.; Prager, G.W. Treatment Algorithm for Patients With Gastric Adenocarcinoma: Austrian Consensus on Systemic Therapy—An Update. *Anticancer Res.* **2023**, *43*, 2889–2897. [CrossRef]
8. Jordan, T.; Mastnak, D.M.; Palamar, N.; Kozjek, N.R. Nutritional Therapy for Patients with Esophageal Cancer. *Nutr. Cancer* **2018**, *70*, 23–29. [CrossRef]
9. Peterson, S.J.; Mozer, M. Differentiating Sarcopenia and Cachexia Among Patients with Cancer. *Nutr. Clin. Pract.* **2017**, *32*, 30–39. [CrossRef]
10. Ferrara, M.; Samaden, M.; Ruggieri, E.; Vénéreau, E. Cancer Cachexia as a Multiorgan Failure: Reconstruction of the Crime Scene. *Front. Cell Dev. Biol.* **2022**, *10*, 960341. [CrossRef]
11. Ma, L.; Poulin, P.; Feldstain, A.; Chasen, M.R. The Association between Malnutrition and Psychological Distress in Patients with Advanced Head-and-Neck Cancer. *Curr. Oncol.* **2013**, *20*, 554–560. [CrossRef] [PubMed]
12. Arends, J.; Bachmann, P.; Baracos, V.; Barthelemy, N.; Bertz, H.; Bozzetti, F.; Fearon, K.; Hütterer, E.; Isenring, E.; Kaasa, S.; et al. ESPEN Guidelines on Nutrition in Cancer Patients. *Clin. Nutr.* **2017**, *36*, 11–48. [CrossRef] [PubMed]
13. Muscaritoli, M.; Lucia, S.; Farcomeni, A.; Lorusso, V.; Saracino, V.; Barone, C.; Plastino, F.; Gori, S.; Magarotto, R.; Carteni, G.; et al. Prevalence of Malnutrition in Patients at First Medical Oncology Visit: The PreMiO Study. *Oncotarget* **2017**, *8*, 79884–79896. [CrossRef] [PubMed]
14. Brown, L.R.; Laird, B.J.A.; Wigmore, S.J.; Skipworth, R.J.E. Understanding Cancer Cachexia and Its Implications in Upper Gastrointestinal Cancers. *Curr. Treat. Options Oncol.* **2022**, *23*, 1732–1747. [CrossRef]
15. Curtis, A.R.; Livingstone, K.M.; Daly, R.M.; Marchese, L.E.; Kiss, N. Associations between Dietary Patterns and Malnutrition, Low Muscle Mass and Sarcopenia in Adults with Cancer: A Scoping Review. *Int. J. Environ. Res. Public Health* **2022**, *19*, 1769. [CrossRef]
16. Bossi, P.; Delrio, P.; Mascheroni, A.; Zanetti, M. The Spectrum of Malnutrition/Cachexia/Sarcopenia in Oncology According to Different Cancer Types and Settings: A Narrative Review. *Nutrients* **2021**, *13*, 1980. [CrossRef]
17. Arends, J. Malnutrition in Cancer Patients: Causes, Consequences and Treatment Options. *Eur. J. Surg. Oncol.* **2024**, *50*, 107074. [CrossRef]
18. Van Soom, T.; El Bakkali, S.; Gebruers, N.; Verbelen, H.; Tjalma, W.; van Breda, E. The Effects of Chemotherapy on Energy Metabolic Aspects in Cancer Patients: A Systematic Review. *Clin. Nutr.* **2020**, *39*, 1863–1877. [CrossRef]
19. Lee, D.U.; Fan, G.H.; Hastie, D.J.; Addonizio, E.A.; Han, J.; Prakasam, V.N.; Karagozian, R. The Clinical Impact of Malnutrition on the Postoperative Outcomes of Patients Undergoing Gastrectomy for Gastric Cancer: Propensity Score Matched Analysis of 2011–2017 Hospital Database. *Clin. Nutr. ESPEN* **2021**, *46*, 484–490. [CrossRef]
20. Browning, A.F.; Chong, L.; Read, M.; Hii, M.W. Economic Burden of Complications and Readmission Following Oesophageal Cancer Surgery. *ANZ J. Surg.* **2022**, *92*, 2901–2906. [CrossRef]

21. Del Giorno, R.; Quarenghi, M.; Stefanelli, K.; Rigamonti, A.; Stanglini, C.; De Vecchi, V.; Gabutti, L. Phase Angle Is Associated with Length of Hospital Stay, Readmissions, Mortality, and Falls in Patients Hospitalized in Internal-Medicine Wards: A Retrospective Cohort Study. *Nutrition* **2021**, *85*, 111068. [CrossRef] [PubMed]
22. Ballesteros-Pomar, M.D.; Gajete-Martín, L.M.; Pintor-De-la-maza, B.; González-Arnáiz, E.; González-Roza, L.; García-Pérez, M.P.; González-Alonso, V.; García-González, M.A.; de Prado-Espinosa, R.; Cuevas, M.J.; et al. Disease-Related Malnutrition and Sarcopenia Predict Worse Outcome in Medical Inpatients: A Cohort Study. *Nutrients* **2021**, *13*, 2937. [CrossRef] [PubMed]
23. Cederholm, T.; Jensen, G.L.; Correia, M.I.T.D.; Gonzalez, M.C.; Fukushima, R.; Higashiguchi, T.; Baptista, G.; Barazzoni, R.; Blaauw, R.; Coats, A.; et al. GLIM Criteria for the Diagnosis of Malnutrition—A Consensus Report from the Global Clinical Nutrition Community. *Clin. Nutr.* **2019**, *38*, 1–9. [CrossRef] [PubMed]
24. Cruz-Jentoft, A.J.; Bahat, G.; Bauer, J.; Boirie, Y.; Bruyère, O.; Cederholm, T.; Cooper, C.; Landi, F.; Rolland, Y.; Sayer, A.A.; et al. Sarcopenia: Revised European Consensus on Definition and Diagnosis. *Age Ageing* **2019**, *48*, 16–31. [CrossRef]
25. Kokura, Y.; Nishioka, S.; Maeda, K.; Wakabayashi, H. Ultrasound Utilized by Registered Dietitians for Body Composition Measurement, Nutritional Assessment, and Nutritional Management. *Clin. Nutr. ESPEN* **2023**, *57*, 173–180. [CrossRef]
26. Lima, J.; Foletto, E.; Cardoso, R.C.B.; Garbelotto, C.; Frenzel, A.P.; Carneiro, J.U.; Carpes, L.S.; Barbosa-Silva, T.G.; Gonzalez, M.C.; Silva, F.M. Ultrasound for Measurement of Skeletal Muscle Mass Quantity and Muscle Composition/Architecture in Critically Ill Patients: A Scoping Review on Studies' Aims, Methods, and Findings. *Clin. Nutr.* **2024**, *43*, 95–110. [CrossRef]
27. Manfrinato Miola, T.; Santos Da Conceição, E.L.; De Oliveira Souza, J.; Vieira Barbosa, P.N.; José, F.; Coimbra, F.; Galvão, A.; Bitencourt, V. CT Assessment of Nutritional Status and Lean Body Mass in Gastric and Esophageal Cancer. *Appl. Cancer Res.* **2018**, *38*, 12. [CrossRef]
28. da Silva, B.R.; Orsso, C.E.; Gonzalez, M.C.; Sicchieri, J.M.F.; Mialich, M.S.; Jordao, A.A.; Prado, C.M. Phase Angle and Cellular Health: Inflammation and Oxidative Damage. *Rev. Endocr. Metab. Disord.* **2022**, *24*, 543. [CrossRef]
29. Branco, M.G.; Mateus, C.; Capelas, M.L.; Pimenta, N.; Santos, T.; Mäkitie, A.; Ganhão-Arranhado, S.; Trabulo, C.; Ravasco, P. Bioelectrical Impedance Analysis (BIA) for the Assessment of Body Composition in Oncology: A Scoping Review. *Nutrients* **2023**, *15*, 4792. [CrossRef]
30. Bellido, D.; García-García, C.; Talluri, A.; Lukaski, H.C.; García-Almeida, J.M. Future Lines of Research on Phase Angle: Strengths and Limitations. *Rev. Endocr. Metab. Disord.* **2023**, *24*, 563. [CrossRef]
31. Norman, K.; Herpich, C.; Müller-Werdan, U. Role of Phase Angle in Older Adults with Focus on the Geriatric Syndromes Sarcopenia and Frailty. *Rev. Endocr. Metab. Disord.* **2023**, *24*, 429–437. [CrossRef] [PubMed]
32. Stanley, B.; Greig, C.; Jackson, T.; Lewis, D.; Moorey, H.; Majid, Z.; Masud, T.; Pinkney, T.; Welch, C. Investigating the Impact of Fluid Status on the Ultrasound Assessment of Muscle Quantity and Quality in the Diagnosis of Sarcopenia—A Multidimensional Cross-Sectional Study. *BMC Geriatr.* **2023**, *23*, 493. [CrossRef] [PubMed]
33. Cheng, D.; Luo, H.; Ren, S.; Wang, N.; Wu, J. The Effects of Fluid Hydration Status on Ultrasound Muscle Measurement in Hemodialysis Patients. *J. Ren. Nutr.* **2023**, *33*, 214–218. [CrossRef] [PubMed]
34. Nijholt, W.; Jager-Wittenaar, H.; Raj, I.S.; van der Schans, C.P.; Hobbelen, H. Reliability and Validity of Ultrasound to Estimate Muscles: A Comparison between Different Transducers and Parameters. *Clin. Nutr. ESPEN* **2020**, *35*, 146–152. [CrossRef]
35. Chen, Y.L.; Liu, P.T.; Chiang, H.K.; Lee, S.H.; Lo, Y.L.; Yang, Y.C.; Chiou, H.J. Ultrasound Measurement of Rectus Femoris Muscle Parameters for Discriminating Sarcopenia in Community-Dwelling Adults. *J. Ultrasound Med.* **2022**, *41*, 2269–2277. [CrossRef]
36. Nies, I.; Ackermans, L.L.G.C.; Poeze, M.; Blokhuis, T.J.; Ten Bosch, J.A. The Diagnostic Value of Ultrasound of the Rectus Femoris for the Diagnosis of Sarcopenia in Adults: A Systematic Review. *Injury* **2022**, *53*, S23–S29. [CrossRef]
37. Nijholt, W.; Scafoglieri, A.; Jager-Wittenaar, H.; Hobbelen, J.S.M.; van der Schans, C.P. The Reliability and Validity of Ultrasound to Quantify Muscles in Older Adults: A Systematic Review. *J. Cachexia Sarcopenia Muscle* **2017**, *8*, 702. [CrossRef]
38. García-García, C.; Vegas-Aguilar, I.M.; Rioja-Vázquez, R.; Cornejo-Pareja, I.; Tinahones, F.J.; García-Almeida, J.M. Rectus Femoris Muscle and Phase Angle as Prognostic Factor for 12-Month Mortality in a Longitudinal Cohort of Patients with Cancer (AnyVida Trial). *Nutrients* **2023**, *15*, 522. [CrossRef]
39. Simón-Frapolli, V.J.; Vegas-Aguilar, I.M.; Fernández-Jiménez, R.; Cornejo-Pareja, I.M.; Sánchez-García, A.M.; Martínez-López, P.; Nuevo-Ortega, P.; Reina-Artacho, C.; Estecha-Foncea, M.A.; Gómez-González, A.M.; et al. Phase Angle and Rectus Femoris Cross-Sectional Area as Predictors of Severe Malnutrition and Their Relationship with Complications in Outpatients with Post-Critical SARS-CoV2 Disease. *Front. Nutr.* **2023**, *10*, 1218266. [CrossRef]
40. Deng, M.; Yan, L.; Tong, R.; Zhao, J.; Li, Y.; Yin, Y.; Zhang, Q.; Gao, J.; Wang, Q.; Zhou, X.; et al. Ultrasound Assessment of the Rectus Femoris in Patients with Chronic Obstructive Pulmonary Disease Predicts Sarcopenia. *Int. J. Chronic Obstr. Pulm. Dis.* **2022**, *17*, 2801–2810. [CrossRef]
41. Gomes, T.L.N.; Soares, J.D.P.; Borges, T.C.; Pichard, C.; Pimentel, G.D. Phase Angle Is Not Associated with Fatigue in Cancer Patients: The Hydration Impact. *Eur. J. Clin. Nutr.* **2020**, *74*, 1369–1373. [CrossRef] [PubMed]
42. Matias, C.N.; Cavaco-Silva, J.; Reis, M.; Campa, F.; Toselli, S.; Sardinha, L.; Silva, A.M. Phase Angle as a Marker of Muscular Strength in Breast Cancer Survivors. *Int. J. Environ. Res. Public Health* **2020**, *17*, 4452. [CrossRef] [PubMed]

43. Valentino, N.P.; Gomes, T.L.N.; Barreto, C.S.; Borges, T.C.; Soares, J.D.P.; Pichard, C.; Laviano, A.; Pimentel, G.D. Low Phase Angle Is Associated with the Risk for Sarcopenia in Unselected Patients with Cancer: Effects of Hydration. *Nutrition* **2021**, *84*, 111122. [CrossRef] [PubMed]
44. Yokomachi, J.; Fukuda, T.; Mizushima, Y.; Nozawa, N.; Ishizaka, H.; Matsumoto, K.; Kambe, T.; Inoue, S.; Nishikawa, K.; Toyama, Y.; et al. Clinical Usefulness of Phase Angle as an Indicator of Muscle Wasting and Malnutrition in Inpatients with Cardiovascular Diseases. *Asia Pac. J. Clin. Nutr.* **2023**, *32*, 297–307. [CrossRef]
45. Gulin, J.; Ipavic, E.; Mastnak, D.M.; Brecelj, E.; Edhemovic, I.; Kozjek, N.R. Phase Angle as a Prognostic Indicator of Surgical Outcomes in Patients with Gastrointestinal Cancer. *Radiol. Oncol.* **2023**, *57*, 524–529. [CrossRef]
46. Conde Frio, C.; Härter, J.; Santos, L.P.; Orlandi, S.P.; Gonzalez, M.C. Phase Angle, Physical Quality of Life and Functionality in Cancer Patients Undergoing Chemotherapy. *Clin. Nutr. ESPEN* **2023**, *57*, 331–336. [CrossRef]
47. Sember, V.; Meh, K.; Sorić, M.; Jurak, G.; Starc, G.; Rocha, P. Validity and Reliability of International Physical Activity Questionnaires for Adults across EU Countries: Systematic Review and Meta Analysis. *Int. J. Environ. Res. Public Health* **2020**, *17*, 7161. [CrossRef]
48. Wanden-Berghe, C. Valoración antropométrica. In *Valoración Nutricional en el Anciano. Recomendaciones Prácticas de los Expertos en Geriatría y Nutrición (SENPE y SEGG)*; Galénitas-Nigra Trea: Madrid, Spain, 2007; pp. 77–96.
49. Gonzalez, M.C.; Mehrnezhad, A.; Razaviarab, N.; Barbosa-Silva, T.G.; Heymsfield, S.B. Calf Circumference: Cutoff Values from the NHANES 1999–2006. *Am. J. Clin. Nutr.* **2021**, *113*, 1679–1687. [CrossRef]
50. Detsky, A.S.; Mclaughlin, J.; Baker, J.P.; Johnston, N.; Whittaker, S.; Mendelson, R.A.; Jeejeebhoy, K.N. What Is Subjective Global Assessment of Nutritional Status? *JPEN J. Parenter. Enteral Nutr.* **1987**, *11*, 8–13. [CrossRef]
51. De Groot, L.M.; Lee, G.; Ackerie, A.; van der Meij, B.S. Malnutrition Screening and Assessment in the Cancer Care Ambulatory Setting: Mortality Predictability and Validity of the Patient-Generated Subjective Global Assessment Short Form (PG-SGA SF) and the GLIM Criteria. *Nutrients* **2020**, *12*, 2287. [CrossRef]
52. Du, H.; Liu, B.; Xie, Y.; Liu, J.; Wei, Y.; Hu, H.; Luo, B.; Li, Z. Comparison of Different Methods for Nutrition Assessment in Patients with Tumors. *Oncol. Lett.* **2017**, *14*, 165. [CrossRef] [PubMed]
53. Lukaski, H.C.; Bolonchuk, W.W.; Hall, C.B.; Siders, W.A. Validation of Tetrapolar Bioelectrical Impedance Method to Assess Human Body Composition. *J. Appl. Physiol.* **1986**, *60*, 1327–1332. [CrossRef] [PubMed]
54. Artero, A.; Sáez Ramírez, T.; Muresan, B.T.; Ruiz-Berjaga, Y.; Jiménez-Portilla, A.; Sánchez-Juan, C.J. The Effect of Fasting on Body Composition Assessment in Hospitalized Cancer Patients. *Nutr. Cancer* **2023**, *75*, 1610–1618. [CrossRef] [PubMed]
55. de Luis Roman, D.; García Almeida, J.M.; Bellido Guerrero, D.; Guzmán Rolo, G.; Martín, A.; Primo Martín, D.; García-Delgado, Y.; Guirado-Peláez, P.; Palmas, F.; Tejera Pérez, C.; et al. Ultrasound Cut-Off Values for Rectus Femoris for Detecting Sarcopenia in Patients with Nutritional Risk. *Nutrients* **2024**, *16*, 1552. [CrossRef]
56. García-Almeida, J.M.; García-García, C.; Vegas-Aguilar, I.M.; Ballesteros Pomar, M.D.; Cornejo-Pareja, I.M.; Fernández Medina, B.; de Luis Román, D.A.; Bellido Guerrero, D.; Bretón Lesmes, I.; Tinahones Madueño, F.J. Nutritional Ultrasound®: Conceptualisation, Technical Considerations and Standardisation. *Endocrinol. Diabetes Nutr.* **2023**, *70*, 74–84. [CrossRef]
57. Trampisch, U.S.; Franke, J.; Jedamzik, N.; Hinrichs, T.; Platen, P. Optimal Jamar Dynamometer Handle Position to Assess Maximal Isometric Hand Grip Strength in Epidemiological Studies. *J. Hand Surg. Am.* **2012**, *37*, 2368–2373. [CrossRef]
58. Sánchez Torralvo, F.J.; Porras, N.; Abuín Fernández, J.; García Torres, F.; Tapia, M.J.; Lima, F.; Soriguer, F.; Gonzalo, M.; Rojo Martínez, G.; Olveira, G. Normative Reference Values for Hand Grip Dynamometry in Spain. Association with Lean Mass. *Nutr. Hosp.* **2018**, *35*, 98–103. [CrossRef]
59. Santamaría-Peláez, M.; González-Bernal, J.J.; Da Silva-González, Á.; Medina-Pascual, E.; Gentil-Gutiérrez, A.; Fernández-Solana, J.; Mielgo-Ayuso, J.; González-Santos, J. Validity and Reliability of the Short Physical Performance Battery Tool in Institutionalized Spanish Older Adults. *Nurs. Rep.* **2023**, *13*, 1354–1367. [CrossRef]
60. Parra-Rodríguez, L.; Szlejf, C.; García-González, A.I.; Malmstrom, T.K.; Cruz-Arenas, E.; Rosas-Carrasco, O. Cross-Cultural Adaptation and Validation of the Spanish-Language Version of the SARC-F to Assess Sarcopenia in Mexican Community-Dwelling Older Adults. *J. Am. Med. Dir. Assoc.* **2016**, *17*, 1142–1146. [CrossRef]
61. Malmstrom, T.K.; Morley, J.E. SARC-F: A Simple Questionnaire to Rapidly Diagnose Sarcopenia. *J. Am. Med. Dir. Assoc.* **2013**, *14*, 531–532. [CrossRef]
62. Yang, J.; Xie, H.; Wei, L.; Ruan, G.; Zhang, H.; Shi, J.; Shi, H. Phase Angle: A Robust Predictor of Malnutrition and Poor Prognosis in Gastrointestinal Cancer. *Nutrition* **2024**, *125*, 112468. [CrossRef] [PubMed]
63. Zuo, J.; Zhou, D.; Zhang, L.; Zhou, X.; Gao, X.; Zhang, J.X.; Ding, X.; Hou, W.; Wang, C.; Jiang, P.; et al. Phase Angle—A Screening Tool for Malnutrition, Sarcopenia, and Complications in Gastric Cancer. *Clin. Nutr. ESPEN* **2024**, *59*, 334–342. [CrossRef] [PubMed]

64. Fernández-Jiménez, R.; García-Rey, S.; Roque-Cuéllar, M.C.; Fernández-Soto, M.L.; García-Olivares, M.; Novo-Rodríguez, M.; González-Pacheco, M.; Prior-Sánchez, I.; Carmona-Llanos, A.; Muñoz-Jiménez, C.; et al. Ultrasound Muscle Evaluation for Predicting the Prognosis of Patients with Head and Neck Cancer: A Large-Scale and Multicenter Prospective Study. *Nutrients* **2024**, *16*, 387. [CrossRef] [PubMed]
65. Liu, C.; Lu, Z.; Li, Z.; Xu, J.; Cui, H.; Zhu, M. Influence of Malnutrition According to the GLIM Criteria on the Clinical Outcomes of Hospitalized Patients With Cancer. *Front. Nutr.* **2021**, *8*, 774636. [CrossRef]
66. dos Santos, M.L.D.; Leite, L.D.O.; Lages, I.C.F. Prevalence of malnutrition, according to the glim criteria, in patients who are the candidates for gastrointestinal tract surgery. *Arq. Bras. Cir. Dig.* **2022**, *35*, e1663. [CrossRef]
67. Xu, L.B.; Shi, M.M.; Huang, Z.X.; Zhang, W.T.; Zhang, H.H.; Shen, X.; Chen, X.D. Impact of Malnutrition Diagnosed Using Global Leadership Initiative on Malnutrition Criteria on Clinical Outcomes of Patients with Gastric Cancer. *JPEN J. Parenter. Enteral Nutr.* **2022**, *46*, 385–394. [CrossRef]
68. Murnane, L.C.; Forsyth, A.K.; Koukounaras, J.; Shaw, K.; King, S.; Brown, W.A.; Mourtzakis, M.; Tierney, A.C.; Burton, P.R. Malnutrition Defined by GLIM Criteria Identifies a Higher Incidence of Malnutrition and Is Associated with Pulmonary Complications after Oesophagogastric Cancer Surgery, Compared to ICD-10-Defined Malnutrition. *J. Surg. Oncol.* **2023**, *128*, 769–780. [CrossRef]
69. Anconina, R.; Ortega, C.; Metser, U.; Liu, Z.A.; Suzuki, C.; McInnis, M.; Darling, G.E.; Wong, R.; Taylor, K.; Yeung, J.; et al. Influence of Sarcopenia, Clinical Data, and 2-[18F] FDG PET/CT in Outcome Prediction of Patients with Early-Stage Adenocarcinoma Esophageal Cancer. *Eur. J. Nucl. Med. Mol. Imaging* **2022**, *49*, 1012–1020. [CrossRef]
70. Sales-Balaguer, N.; Sorribes-Carreras, P.; Morillo Macias, V. Diagnosis of Sarcopenia and Myosteatosis by Computed Tomography in Patients with Esophagogastric and Pancreatic Cancer. *Cancers* **2024**, *16*, 2738. [CrossRef]
71. Kim, M.; Lee, C.; Kang, B.K.; Ha, T.K.; Choi, Y.Y.; Lee, S.J. Sarcopenia Assessed with DXA and CT Increases the Risk of Perioperative Complications in Patients with Gastrectomy. *Eur. Radiol.* **2023**, *33*, 5150–5158. [CrossRef]
72. Şahin, M.E.H.; Akbaş, F.; Yardimci, A.H.; Şahin, E. The Effect of Sarcopenia and Sarcopenic Obesity on Survival in Gastric Cancer. *BMC Cancer* **2023**, *23*, 911. [CrossRef] [PubMed]
73. Tegels, J.J.W.; Van Vugt, J.L.A.; Reisinger, K.W.; Hulsewé, K.W.E.; Hoofwijk, A.G.M.; Derikx, J.P.M.; Stoot, J.H.M.B. Sarcopenia Is Highly Prevalent in Patients Undergoing Surgery for Gastric Cancer but Not Associated with Worse Outcomes. *J. Surg. Oncol.* **2015**, *112*, 403–407. [CrossRef] [PubMed]
74. Vegas-Aguilar, I.M.; Guirado-Peláez, P.; Fernández-Jiménez, R.; Boughanem, H.; Tinahones, F.J.; Garcia-Almeida, J.M. Exploratory Assessment of Nutritional Evaluation Tools as Predictors of Complications and Sarcopenia in Patients with Colorectal Cancer. *Cancers* **2023**, *15*, 847. [CrossRef] [PubMed]
75. Ji, W.; Liu, X.L.; Liu, P.; He, Y.W.; Zhao, Y.X.; Zheng, K.; Cui, J.W.; Li, W. The Efficacy of Fat-Free Mass Index and Appendicular Skeletal Muscle Mass Index in Cancer Malnutrition: A Propensity Score Match Analysis. *Front. Nutr.* **2023**, *10*, 1172610. [CrossRef]
76. Herrera-Martínez, A.D.; Prior-Sánchez, I.; Fernández-Soto, M.L.; García-Olivares, M.; Novo-Rodríguez, C.; González-Pacheco, M.; Martínez-Ramirez, M.J.; Carmona-Llanos, A.; Jiménez-Sánchez, A.; Muñoz-Jiménez, C.; et al. Improving the Nutritional Evaluation in Head Neck Cancer Patients Using Bioelectrical Impedance Analysis: Not Only the Phase Angle Matters. *J. Cachexia Sarcopenia Muscle* **2024**, *15*, 2426–2436. [CrossRef]
77. Ge, Y.Z.; Ruan, G.T.; Zhang, Q.; Dong, W.J.; Zhang, X.; Song, M.M.; Zhang, X.W.; Li, X.R.; Zhang, K.P.; Tang, M.; et al. Extracellular Water to Total Body Water Ratio Predicts Survival in Cancer Patients with Sarcopenia: A Multi-Center Cohort Study. *Nutr. Metab.* **2022**, *19*, 34. [CrossRef]
78. Hida, T.; Ando, K.; Kobayashi, K.; Ito, K.; Tsushima, M.; Kobayakawa, T.; Morozumi, M.; Tanaka, S.; Machino, M.; Ota, K.; et al. Ultrasound Measurement of Thigh Muscle Thickness for Assessment of Sarcopenia. *Nagoya J. Med. Sci.* **2018**, *80*, 519. [CrossRef]
79. López-Gómez, J.J.; Plaar, K.B.S.; Izaola-Jauregui, O.; Primo-Martín, D.; Gómez-Hoyos, E.; Torres-Torres, B.; De Luis-Román, D.A. Muscular Ultrasonography in Morphofunctional Assessment of Patients with Oncological Pathology at Risk of Malnutrition. *Nutrients* **2022**, *14*, 1573. [CrossRef]
80. Ozturk, Y.; Koca, M.; Burkuk, S.; Unsal, P.; Dikmeer, A.; Oytun, M.G.; Bas, A.O.; Kahyaoglu, Z.; Deniz, O.; Coteli, S.; et al. The Role of Muscle Ultrasound to Predict Sarcopenia. *Nutrition* **2022**, *101*, 111692. [CrossRef]
81. Ozturk, Y.; Deniz, O.; Coteli, S.; Unsal, P.; Dikmeer, A.; Burkuk, S.; Koca, M.; Cavusoglu, C.; Dogu, B.B.; Cankurtaran, M.; et al. Global Leadership Initiative on Malnutrition Criteria with Different Muscle Assessments Including Muscle Ultrasound with Hospitalized Internal Medicine Patients. *JPEN J. Parenter. Enteral Nutr.* **2022**, *46*, 936–945. [CrossRef]

MDPI AG
Grosspeteranlage 5
4052 Basel
Switzerland
Tel.: +41 61 683 77 34

Nutrients Editorial Office
E-mail: nutrients@mdpi.com
www.mdpi.com/journal/nutrients

www.ingramcontent.com/pod-product-compliance
Lightning Source LLC
Chambersburg PA
CBHW040819250926
51850CB00007BA/1208
* 9 7 8 3 7 2 5 8 4 5 9 5 8 *